Copyright © 2020 by Edna Brown -All rights reserved.

No part of this publication may be reproduced, distributed, or transmitted in any form or by any means, including photocopying, recording, or other electronic or mechanical methods, without the prior written permission of the publisher, except in the case of brief quotations embodied in reviews and certain other non-commercial uses permitted by copyright law.

This Book is provided with the sole purpose of providing relevant information on a specific topic for which every reasonable effort has been made to ensure that it is both accurate and reasonable. Nevertheless, by purchasing this Book you consent to the fact that the author, as well as the publisher, are in no way experts on the topics contained herein, regardless of any claims as such that may be made within. It is recommended that you always consult a professional prior to undertaking any of the advice or techniques discussed within.This is a legally binding declaration that is considered both valid and fair by both the Committee of Publishers Association and the American Bar Association and should be considered as legally binding within the United States.

CONTENTS

INTRODUCTION..**12**
BREAKFAST AND BRUNCH RECIPES **14**
1. Sour Cream Chicken................................. 14
2. Delectable Breakfast Meal....................... 14
3. Creamy Oregano Chorizo Mushroom 14
4. Simple Chicken Soup 14
5. Broccoli And Tomatoes Casserole 14
6. Egg Casserole 14
7. Chicken Tikka Masala............................... 14
8. Chicken Green Chile Soup 15
9. Cauliflower Hash Browns Slow Casserole............ 15
10. Breakfast Meat Bowl................................ 15
11. Breakfast Tender Chicken Strips 15
12. Kale With Eggs 15
13. Breakfast Bacon And Eggs 15
14. Smoked Sausages With Grits 16
15. Feta Cheese And Kale Breakfast Casserole......... 16
16. Egg Casserole With Italian Cheeses, Sun-dried Tomatoes And Herbs 16
17. Sweet Pepper Hash................................... 16
18. Homemade Vegetable Stock 16
19. Sausage And Spinach 17
20. Pork Stew... 17
21. Chicken Chorizo Soup.............................. 17
22. The Better Quiche Lorraine 17
23. Chicken Fajitas 17
24. Spicy Pepper Chicken Soup 17
25. Veggie Casserole 18
26. Pork Breakfast Sausages 18
27. Sausages And Peppers Hash 18
28. Cheesy Turmeric Eggs 18
29. Cauliflower Hash Brown 18
30. Ham & Cheese Broccoli Brunch Bowl 18
31. Minced Pork Zucchini Lasagna 18
32. Egg Bars... 19
33. Paprika Shrimp 19
34. Greek Crockpot Breakfast Casserole.................... 19
35. Crockpot Mediterranean Frittata 19
36. Turkey-stuffed Peppers........................... 19
37. Creamy Asparagus Bake........................... 19
38. Simple Ham And Egg Casserole............................ 20
39. Sausage-stuffed Eggplants...................... 20
40. Superb Chicken, Bacon, Garlic Thyme Soup....... 20
41. Paprika And Shallots Omelet................... 20
42. Breakfast Pie 20
43. Mexican Breakfast Casserole................... 20
44. Kale Muffins... 21
45. Smoked Salmon Casserole....................... 21
46. Cheesy Green Omelet............................... 21
47. Salmon And Avocado Breakfast Bake................... 21
48. Coconut Flour "porridge" With Blueberries And Cinnamon 21
49. Full-flavored Pot Roast 22
50. Egg Quiche 22
51. Cod Bites 22
52. Delightful Chicken-chorizo Spicy Soup 22
53. Stuffed Breakfast Peppers(2)................... 22
54. Ricotta Eggs 22
55. Creamy Green Tea 23
56. Green Beans Casserole............................. 23
57. Egg & Mushroom Breakfast 23
58. Coconut Avocado And Chicken Mix 23
59. Avocado And Zucchini Bake..................... 23
60. Mexican Chicken Soup.............................. 23
61. Lovely Lentil Sausage Soup 24
62. Chives And Sprouts Casserole.................. 24
63. Pork Chops With Cumin Butter And Garlic 24
64. Ranch Chicken 24
65. Baked Mushrooms With Pesto & Ricotta 24
66. Walnuts Yogurt 24
67. Chicken With Green Beans 25
68. Sausage And Peppers................................ 25
69. Thai-inspired Chicken Soup...................... 25
70. Delicious Bacon & Cheese Frittata 25
71. Spinach Casserole.................................... 25
72. Ricotta Cheese And Almond Mini Pancakes....... 26
73. Bacon And Spiced Egg Bake...................... 26
74. Rice & Shrimp Frittata.............................. 26
75. Oozing Ground Beef Shawarma................. 26
76. Barbecue Beef Stew.................................. 26
77. Dill And Avocado Frittata......................... 26
78. Chicken Meatballs.................................... 27
79. Tasty Sausage & Eggplant Bake................ 27
80. Breakfast Ground Beef Casserole 27
81. Cilantro Pork Meatballs........................... 27
82. Stuffed Peppers.. 27
83. Creamy Chicken Soup............................... 28
84. Vanilla Pancakes(2).................................. 28
85. Zucchini Quiche.. 28
86. Onion Zucchini Hash................................ 28
87. Cinnamon Eggs... 28
88. Mushroom Spinach Breakfast................... 28
89. Mediterranean Meatloaf 28
90. Mouth-watering Cauliflower & Cheese Bake..... 29
91. Green Chile Chicken Soup 29
92. Berry Pudding... 29
93. Roasted Chicken With Lemon & Parsley Butter 29
94. Breakfast Shredded Pork 29
95. Breakfast Meatloaf................................... 29
96. Basil Sprouts And Eggs 30
97. Cheesy Chicken Pot.................................. 30

98. Chili Tomatoes Bowls......................................30
99. Coconut Chip Rice Pudding.........................30
100. Veggie Pot Pie..30
101. Avocado Boats 30
102. Breakfast Sausage Casserole.....................30
103. Feta Eggs 31
104. Pork Shoulder Roast..................................31
105. Coconut Sausage Mix................................31
106. Beef Meatloaf...31
107. Cream Of Zucchini Soup............................31
108. Crack Chicken(2)......................................32
109. Mushroom And Brie "melters".....................32
110. Lovely Sausage Casserole Breakfast.............32
111. Puff Spinach Salmon..................................32
112. Sesame Ginger Chicken.............................32
113. Eggplant Parmesan....................................32
114. Salmon And Asparagus With Herb Butter 33
115. Ham And Kale Bake 33
116. Salmon Cutlets..33
117. Keto Porridge 33
118. Warm Ricotta, Cream, Berry And Macadamia
Whip...33
119. Breakfast Cream And Egg Soufflé 34
120. Chicken Muffins...34
121. Coconut Sausages 34
122. Egg Hash Browns.......................................34
123. Egg, Kale, And Mozzarella Casserole 34
124. Bacon And Spinach Frittata 34
125. French Onion Meatloaf................................34
126. Onion Broccoli Cream Cheese Quiche.............35
127. Mushroom Casserole..................................35
128. Lemon Thyme Chicken...............................35
129. Bacon Topped Hash Browns........................35
130. Balsamic Pot Roast....................................35
131. Reuben Soup With Thousand Islan Dressing.. 36
132. Brussel Sprouts Eggs..................................36
133. Shallot Parmesan Zucchini Asparagus Frittata
....36
134. Steak And Salsa..36
135. Peppers And Eggs Mix 36
136. Avocado Tuna Balls 37
137. Summery Bell Pepper + Eggplant Salad...........37
138. Tuscan Garlic Chicken 37
139. Chili Frittata...37
140. Almond Avocado Mix 37
141. Mini Mushroom & Sausage Quiche 37
142. Kale Frittata 38
143. Bone Broth 38
144. Herb Chicken & Mushroom Stew....................38
145. Chia Seeds Pudding....................................38
146. Cheese & Cauliflower Bake...........................38
147. Cauliflower Breakfast Cake With Capsicum And
Chorizo...39
148. Healthy Slow Cooker Frittata 39
149. Oriental Lamb..39
150. Warming Bean And Veg Soup.......................39
SIDE DISHES RECIPES......................................40
151. Mushroom Stew 40
152. Zucchini Pasta...40
153. Brussel Sprouts With Parmesan....................40
154. Garlic Artichoke...40
155. Broccoli & Cauliflower & Blue Cheese Casserole
....40
156. Broccoli Stew..40
157. Swiss Chard Mix 40
158. Red Cabbage Sauté.....................................41
159. Oregano Green Beans..................................41
160. Red Cabbage Slices....................................41
161. Garlicky Mashed Cauliflower........................41
162. Party Sausages..41
163. Moroccan Eggplant Mash 41
164. Pumpkin Nut Bread 42
165. Paprika Green Beans...................................42
166. Cauliflower Garlic Bread..............................42
167. Oregano Beans And Cucumber......................42
168. Zucchini And Radish Mix 42
169. Pesto Spaghetti Squash 42
170. Cabbage And Tomatoes...............................42
171. Slow Cooker Spaghetti Squash......................43
172. Cauliflower Croquettes................................43
173. Masala Broccoli..43
174. Flax Meal Coffeecake..................................43
175. Paprika Spaghetti Squash............................43
176. Soft Keto Kale Salad 43
177. Coconut Celery...44
178. Spiced Fennel Slices...................................44
179. Green Bean And Avocado Salad.....................44
180. Garlic Peppers...44
181. Glazed Spiced Carrots.................................44
182. Artichoke And Broccoli Mix..........................44
183. Herbed Mushrooms....................................44
184. Rosemary Bok Choy....................................45
185. Pumpkin Cubes..45
186. Collard Greens And Mushrooms 45
187. Eggplant Hash...45
188. Garlic Eggplant Mix....................................45
189. Garlic Green Beans With Gorgonzola 45
190. Mushroom And Kale 46
191. Zucchini Spaghetti......................................46
192. Lime Cauliflower...46
193. Brussels Sprouts 46
194. Garlic Green Beans.....................................46
195. Keto Leeks 46
196. Swiss Chard Saute 46
197. Zucchini And Cabbage 46
198. Quinoa Brussels Sprout Salad 47
199. Brussels Sprouts Au Gratin..........................47
200. Nutmeg Artichokes 47

201. Cauliflower Puree With Parmesan 47
202. Kale Mash With Blue Cheese 47
203. Rutabaga Wedges 47
204. Saucy Beans 48
205. Okra Stew 48
206. Seasoned Carrots 48
207. Broccoli Cheese Florets 48
208. Green Bean Casserole 48
209. Bacon Wrapped Cauliflower 48
210. Paprika Peppers 49
211. Creamy Eggplant Salad 49
212. Creamy Green Beans 49
213. Spinach Mix 49
214. Layered Mushrooms 49
215. Asparagus And Onion Mix 49
216. Eggplant Gratin 49
217. Lime Zucchini Noodles 50
218. Peanut Butter & Chocolate Cake 50
219. Grated Zucchini With Cheese 50
220. Rosemary Cauliflower 50
221. Cilantro Cauliflower Rice 50
222. Cauliflower Casserole 50
223. Cranberry Brussels Sprouts Mix 50
224. Mozzarella Zucchinis And Leeks 51
225. Glazed Leeks 51
226. Tomato And Radish 51
227. Bok Choy And Radishes 51
228. Chard And Radishes 51
229. Dill Broccoli 51
230. Curry Mushrooms 51
231. Zucchini Gratin 52
232. Tomato Gratin With Bell Pepper 52
233. Vegetable Stew 52
234. Mayo Salad 52
235. Tomato And Eggplant Salad 52
236. Coconut Cauliflower Mash 52
237. Greens Mix 53
238. Chinese Broccoli 53
239. Coconut Radish Mix 53
240. Tofu And Green Beans 53
241. Sesame Snow Peas 53
242. Ginger Peppers 53
243. Zucchini Slices With Mozzarella 53
244. Sautéed Bell Peppers 54
245. Celery Puree 54
246. Spicy Kale 54
247. Tender Green Cabbage 54
248. Bbq Smokies 54
249. Cheesy Spaghetti Squash 54
250. Thyme Mushrooms 54
251. Garlicky Cauliflower Florets 55
252. Hot Green Beans 55
253. Rhubarb And Zucchini Mix 55
254. Curry Cauliflower 55

255. Cowboy Mexican Dip 55
256. Artichoke Spinach 55
257. Marinated Mushrooms 55
258. Radish And Tomato Salad 56
259. Mashed Cauliflower 56
260. Butter Zucchini 56
261. Hot Tomatoes 56
262. Cabbage Steaks 56
263. Broccoli And Cauliflower Bake 56
264. Cherry Tomatoes Sauté 57
265. Tomato And Spaghetti Squash 57
266. Savoury Almond Bread 57
267. Butter Mushrooms 57
268. Garlic Cauliflower Steaks 57
269. Green Beans 57
270. Leeks And Cauliflower Mash 57
271. Parsley And Tomato Green Beans 58
272. Curled Rutabaga 58
273. Cumin Green Beans 58
274. Mint Peppers 58
275. Thai Cabbage 58
MAIN DISHES RECIPES 59
276. Sardine Pate 59
277. Cod Fillet In Coconut Flakes 59
278. Keto Chili 59
279. Duck Rolls 59
280. Pulled Pork Salad 59
281. Chicken Liver Sauté 59
282. Tuscan Chicken 60
283. Chicken In Bacon 60
284. Spicy Bacon Strips 60
285. Pork-jalapeno Bowl 60
286. Cayenne Pepper Drumsticks 60
287. Autumn Pork Stew 60
288. Rosemary Leg Of Lamb 60
289. Marinated Beef Tenderloin 61
290. Peppered Steak 61
291. Handmade Sausage Stew 61
292. Sesame Seed Shrimp 61
293. Keto Beef Ribs 61
294. Lamb Stew 61
295. Keto Pork Tenderloin 62
296. Asian Chopped Beef 62
297. Marinated Greek Style Pork 62
298. Corned Beef 62
299. Ground Pork Bowl 62
300. Paprika Pork Sausages 62
301. Pork Shoulder 63
302. Garlic Pork Belly 63
303. Prawn Stew 63
304. Delicious Turmeric Beef Stew 63
305. Keto Bbq Chicken Wings 63
306. Chicken Marsala 63
307. Chicken Liver Pate 64

308. Keto Adobo Chicken 64
309. Chili Verde 64
310. Keto Lasagna 64
311. Thyme Lamb Chops 64
312. Duck Breast 64
313. Spare Ribs 64
314. Creamy Chicken Thighs 65
315. Bacon Meatloaf 65
316. Garlic Duck Breast 65
MEAT RECIPES...**66**
317. Chicken Liver With Anchovies 66
318. Pork Roast With Cheese 66
319. Pork Butt Carnitas 66
320. Green Chile Chicken 66
321. Pork Filled Avocado 66
322. Pork Tomatillo Salsa 66
323. Chicken And Zucchinis 67
324. Lamb And Spinach 67
325. Cheddar Chicken 67
326. Lamb And Leeks 67
327. Chicken And Hot Sauce 67
328. Pumpkin Beef Chili 67
329. Chicken Fillets And Mustard Sauce 67
330. Chicken And Tomato Sauce 68
331. Chicken And Walnuts 68
332. Chipotle Barbacoa Recipe 68
333. Chili Chicken 68
334. Ground Pork And Veggies 68
335. Chicken Ginger Curry 68
336. Saucy Goose Satay 69
337. Herbed Lamb Loin Chops 69
338. Savoury Lamb Chili 69
339. Thai Chicken Curry 69
340. Duck And Vegetable Stew 69
341. Wine Dipped Pork Ribs 69
342. Mushroom Cream Goose Curry 70
343. Fennel Chicken Mix 70
344. Chicken And Spring Onions 70
345. Ground Beef And Broccoli 70
346. Lamb Curry 70
347. Stuffed Chicken Breasts 70
348. Beef Stuffed Mushrooms 71
349. Southwest Jalapeno Beef 71
350. Lemon Beef 71
351. Chicken With Nuts 71
352. Caraway Ribs 71
353. Dinner Lamb Shanks 71
354. Chicken With Lemon Parsley Butter 72
355. Mint Lamb Roast 72
356. Pork Roast With Cabbage Stir Fry 72
357. Pork Shoulder And Zucchinis 72
358. Chicken And Okra 72
359. Chili Lamb 72
360. Indian Lamb Stew 73
361. Debdoozie's Beef Chili 73
362. Mozzarella Chicken 73
363. Paprika Drumsticks 73
364. Beef And Asparagus 73
365. Butter Turkey And Olives 73
366. Vegetable Beef Stew 74
367. Crockpot Chicken Adobo 74
368. Chicken With Celery Stick 74
369. Parmesan Pork Schnitzel 74
370. Passata Mixed Pulled Pork 74
371. Lamb Chops With Dill Butter 74
372. Rosemary Rainbow Pork Sautee 74
373. Steak And Dill Sauce 75
374. Lamb, Celery And Tomatoes 75
375. Garlic Creamy Beef Steak 75
376. Mustard Rubbed Lamb Chops 75
377. Sweet Passata Dipped Steaks 75
378. Lamb Pepper Stew 75
379. Pork Tenderloin With Swiss Chard 76
380. Cajun Lamb 76
381. Chunky Chicken Salsa 76
382. Lamb Tomato Stew 76
383. Coconut Milk Turkey Breast 76
384. Chicken And Cabbage 76
385. Pork Roast With Cinnamon 77
386. Chicken And Tomatoes 77
387. Beef With Bok Choy 77
388. Butter And Lemon Lamb 77
389. Chicken And Creamy Onions And Peppers 77
390. Basil Chicken 77
391. Green Chile Shredded Beef Cabbage Bowl 77
392. Beef And Cauliflower 78
393. Cumin Chicken 78
394. Chicken Cubes And Pesto 78
395. Coconut Lamb Stew 78
396. Irish Chop Stew 78
397. Chives Chicken Teriyaki 78
398. Lamb Leg With Thyme 79
399. Pork Brisket Bo Kho 79
400. Chicken And Eggplant 79
401. Chili Lamb Skewers 79
402. Lamb Shanks And Olives 79
403. Beef Lasagna 79
404. Ground Duck Chili 80
405. Lemongrass Pork Meatballs 80
406. Blue Cheese Casserole 80
407. Lime Chicken Drumsticks 80
408. Paprika Chicken 80
409. Nutmeg Chicken 81
410. Chicken Stew 81
411. Lamb Mushroom Curry 81
412. Stevia Pork Mix 81
413. Tangy Lamb Meat Balls 81
414. Jalapeno Pork Tenderloin Soup 81

415. Char Siu Glazed Pork..................................82
416. Pork Tenderloin And Kale.........................82
417. Herbed Lamb Stew..................................82
418. Pork Carne Asada 82
419. Pork Roast 82
420. Chicken Dipped In Tomatillo Sauce...................82
421. Dill Turkey...83
422. Meatballs With Saucy Mushrooms....................83
423. Thyme And Coriander Brisket 83
424. Tarragon Lamb Chops 83
425. Lamb Chops Curry....................................83
426. Pomegranate Lamb....................................83
427. Pork Mushroom Stew 84
428. Beef And Broccoli 84
429. Chicken With Romano Cheese 84
430. Pork With Green Onion Sauce.....................84
431. Slow CookerWhole Chicken........................84
432. Creamy Chicken.......................................85
433. Barbecue Beef Short Ribs..........................85
434. Spicy Mexican Luncheon...........................85
435. Mustard Beef...85
436. Full Meal Turmeric Lamb..........................85
437. Slow CookerBeef Shank.............................85
438. Vegetable Lamb Stew................................86
439. Pozole Blanco..86
440. Dijon Chicken...86
441. Garlic Sirloin...86
FISH AND SEAFOOD RECIPES..............................87
442. Thyme Sea Bass.......................................87
443. Butter-dipped Lobsters..............................87
444. Creamy Vanilla Custard.............................87
445. Fish And Salsa Bowl.................................87
446. Butter Glazed Mussels...............................87
447. Calamari Rings And Broccoli......................87
448. Citrus Enriched Salmon.............................87
449. Shrimp Mushroom Alfredo.........................88
450. Cod Soup...88
451. Herbed Shrimp 88
452. Warming Mussels Tomato Soup...................88
453. Shrimp Curry..88
454. Salmon With Leeks And Cream 88
455. Shrimp Tomato Medley..............................89
456. Fish And Tomato Stew...............................89
457. Shrimp And Zucchini................................89
458. Coffee Creams With Toasted Seed Crumble
Topping...89
459. Cod & Peas With Sour Cream.....................89
460. Slow CookerTuna Steaks............................89
461. Tilapia And Radish Bites............................90
462. Shrimp & Pepper Stew..............................90
463. Chili Squid...90
464. Creamy Seafood Chowder..........................90
465. Luscious Herbed Clams.............................90
466. Dinner Mussels..90

467. Salmon Casserole.....................................90
468. Creamy Tuna..91
469. Cinnamon Mackerel..................................91
470. Lime Cod And Shrimps..............................91
471. Cheesy Tuna...91
472. Salty-sweet Almond Butter And Chocolate
Sauce..91
473. Fish And Bacon Soup................................91
474. Nutritious Salmon Dinner..........................91
475. Coconut Squares With Blueberry Glaze...........92
476. Balsamic Mussels.....................................92
477. Maple Glazed Salmon Fillet........................92
478. Cider Soaked Pancetta Clams......................92
479. Cod Platter...92
480. Tuna And Cabbage Mix.............................92
481. Seafood Stew..93
482. Salmon And Garlic Greens..........................93
483. Jalapeno Cheese Oysters.............................93
484. Chocolate And Blackberry Cheesecake Sauce 93
485. Sage Halibut...93
486. Cajun Shrimp...93
487. Salmon And Spinach Bake..........................94
488. Peanut Butter, Chocolate And Pecan Cupcakes
....94
489. Salmon Cake...94
490. Tangy Pepper Oysters................................94
491. Shrimp Bake...94
492. Spiced Shrimp..94
493. Fish Curry Delight....................................95
494. Shrimp And Salmon Skewers......................95
495. Coconut Catfish.......................................95
496. Balsamic Salmon......................................95
497. Ambrosia..95
498. Shrimp Creole...96
499. Balsamic Scallops.....................................96
500. Oregano Crab...96
501. Creamy Lobster.......................................96
502. Prawn And Sausage Crock Pot Casserole.........96
503. Herbed Swordfish Delight...........................96
504. Sea Bass And Celery..................................97
505. Shrimp And Fennel Soup...........................97
506. Slow Cooked Coconut Lime Mussels...............97
507. Seafood Jambalaya....................................97
508. Cod Patties..97
509. Lobster Dinner..97
510. Parsley Salmon..97
511. Curried Shrimp.......................................98
512. Salmon With Juicy Shallots.........................98
513. Oregano Salmon......................................98
514. Lemon-butter Fish....................................98
515. Caraway Cod..98
516. Coconut, Chocolate&Almond Truffle Bake.......98
517. Saffron Tilapia...99
518. Salmon Curry...99

519. Mouth-watering Casserole 99
520. Tilapia And Tomatoes.......................... 99
521. Tomato Shrimps................................ 99
522. Lemon Crab Legs 99
523. Stevia Salmon 100
524. Mozzarella Shrimp Parcels 100
525. Chocolate Covered Bacon Cupcakes 100
526. Salmon And Cauliflower Chowder 100
527. Marinara Shrimp...............................100
528. Slow Cooked Sesame Prawns 100
529. Parmesan Salmon 101
530. Fish Curry 101
531. Mozzarella Fish...............................101
532. Salmon And Asparagus 101
533. Elegant Dinner Mussels 101
534. Macadamia Fudge Truffles 101
535. Salmon And Radish Soup 102
536. Butter Salmon And Avocado 102
537. Lemon Cheesecake..............................102
538. Slow Cooked Whole Fish With Ginger 102
539. Creamy Sea Bass 102
540. Mediterranean Cod Salad 102
541. Ginger Mackerel 103
542. Coconut Fish Curry 103
543. Shrimp Salad..................................103
544. Nutmeg Halibut 103
545. Crab Dip 103
546. Keto Coconut Hot Chocolate 103
547. Lemon Salmon 104
548. Mustard Shrimp 104
549. Vanilla And Strawberry Cheesecake 104
550. Spicy Tuna 104
551. Citrus Rich Octopus Salad 104
552. Creamy Clam Chowder Luncheon 104
553. Rich Salmon Soup 104
554. Shrimp And Green Beans 105
555. Chocolate, Berry& Macadamia Layered Jars .105
556. Dark Chocolate And Peppermint Pots 105
557. Chili Shrimp And Okra.........................105
558. Flounder With Shrimp..........................105
559. Italian Shrimp Tortillas 106
560. Avocado And Shrimp............................106
561. Turmeric Calamari 106
562. Citrus Glazed Salmon 106
563. Salmon With Mushroom..........................106
564. Scallops With Romanesco 106
565. Lemon Cod.....................................107
566. Wine Sauce Glazed Cod 107
SNACKS AND APPETIZERS RECIPES 108
567. Spicy Pecans 108
568. Garlic Pork Slices 108
569. Tomato Chicken Wings 108
570. Cheddar Dip..................................108
571. Garlic Chicken Wings 108

572. Zucchini Bread 108
573. Pizza 108
574. Chili Dip 109
575. Applesauce 109
576. Pork Bites 109
577. Cayenne Shrimps 109
578. Zucchini Bites 109
579. Tofu Bites 109
580. Bacon Wrapped Duck Roll 109
581. Molten Lava Cake 110
582. Keto Bread Sticks 110
583. Turkey Meatballs 110
584. Mini Muffins 110
585. Keto Crackers 110
586. Pecans Bowls 110
587. Paprika Almonds 110
588. Nacho Cheese Dip 111
589. Marvelous Turkey Magic Sandwich 111
590. Ketogenic Chicken Sandwich...................111
591. Cherry Marmalade 111
592. Slow CookerSpecial Cheesy Steak Sandwich 111
593. Chicken Tenders 111
594. Parmesan Cream Green Beans...................112
595. Keto Tortillas With Cheese 112
596. Meatloaf Burger For Keto Diet................112
597. Oregano Dip 112
598. Radish Spinach Medley 112
599. Ginger Tea Drink 112
600. Masala Hazelnuts 113
601. Bacon Pepper Quiche 113
602. Spiced Lemon Drink 113
603. Dairy-free Fudge 113
604. Caprese Meatballs 113
605. Bbq Beef Sandwich............................113
606. Delicious Custard 114
607. Carrots Dessert..............................114
608. Crockpot Milk Tea 114
609. Mini Chicken Meatballs 114
610. Almond Granola 114
611. Eggplant Fries 114
612. Chicken Bites 114
613. Spicy & Salty Keto Nuts 114
614. Flavorful Mexican Cheese Dip 115
615. Bacon And Roasted Garlic Spinach Dip 115
616. Turkey Bites And Sauce 115
617. Chicken And Cauliflower Pizza 115
618. Worcestershire Chicken 115
619. Broccoli Balls...............................115
620. Sweet And Spicy Chicken Wings 116
621. Salsa Beef Dip 116
622. Sandwich With Roasted Pork 116
623. Yummy Pumpkin Custard 116
624. Chili Walnuts 116
625. Fish Bites 116

626. Shrimp Skewers 116
627. Cauliflower Popcorn..116
628. Truffle Hot Chocolate.......................................117
629. Lemon Blueberry Custard Cake.......................117
630. Jalapeno Fritters 117
631. Masala Green Beans Bowl...............................117
632. Bacon Dip...117
633. Herb Mixed Radish...117
634. Cheesecake...118
635. Artichoke Hummus 118
636. Eggplant Bacon Fries 118
637. Mushroom Stuffed Meatballs............................118
638. Creamy Dip...118
639. Herbed Cherry Tomatoes 118
640. Lamb Steak Sandwich For Keto Diet 118
641. Parmesan Green Beans 119
642. Peanut Butter Swirl Cake 119
643. Pulled Pork..119
644. Pork Nuggets...119
645. Pork Belly Bites 119
646. Mocha Pudding Cake..119
647. Savory Pine Nuts Cabbage 120
648. Pizza Dip...120
649. Spinach Rolls 120
650. Cheese Sticks 120
651. Chestnut Cream 120
652. Shrimp Meatballs..121
653. Crab Dip With Mushrooms...................................121
654. Asian Pork With Keto Tortillas 121
655. Glazed Walnuts...121
656. Bacon Chicken Chowder......................................121
657. Crunchy Bacon..121
658. Gingerbread..121
659. Salmon Spread..122
660. Ground Chicken Pepper Meatballs.....................122
661. Spiced Punch..122
662. Beef & Mushroom – Super Combo Sandwich
....122
663. Viennese Coffee 122
664. Carrots And Cauliflower Spread.........................123
665. Ketogenic Sloppy Joes From Crock Pot 123
666. Eggplant Bread 123
667. Seasoned Mini Meatballs 123
668. Mozzarella Broccoli Bites.....................................123
669. Cocktail Shrimp 123
670. Garlic Bread With Cheese....................................123
671. Mushroom Skewers 124
672. Cauliflower Fritters 124
673. Nutmeg Fennel 124
674. Sausage Bites And Sauce 124
675. Sugar-free Fudge..124
676. Chicken Dip 124
677. Cauliflower Bites...125
678. Coconut Mushrooms Caps 125
679. Cauliflower Bread.. 125
680. Smoked Hazelnuts.. 125
681. Zucchini Tots With Cheese................................... 125
682. Citrus Rich Cabbage 125
683. Creamy Mustard Asparagus 126
684. Butter Pork Ribs 126
685. Buffalo Chicken Wings... 126
686. Wrapped Prawns In Bacon 126
687. Sweet Kahlua Coffee 126
688. Onion Rings 126
689. Cinnamon Pecans... 126
690. Hot Spiced Wine 127
691. Cheesy Zucchini Crisps.. 127
DESSERT RECIPES 128
692. Keto Brownies... 128
693. Tapioca Pudding 128
694. Sunflower Seeds Cookies 128
695. Blueberry Pie... 128
696. Pudding Cake 128
697. Lime Vanilla Bites 128
698. Mini Pumpkin Cakes 129
699. Spoon Cake... 129
700. Mocha Brownie.. 129
701. Zucchini And Pumpkin Pie 129
702. Coffee Cream 129
703. Flax Seeds Balls 129
704. Chocolate Walnut Pie 130
705. Tender Lime Cake 130
706. Snowball Cookies.. 130
707. Almond Cocoa Cake 130
708. Chocolate Cheese Cake 130
709. Espresso Cookie 130
710. Walnut Balls 130
711. Cinnamon Almonds... 131
712. Lemon Cake 131
713. Nutmeg Raspberry Crisp 131
714. Berry Brownies 131
715. Chocolate Cheesecake... 131
716. Chia Bites.. 132
717. Cinnamon Swirls 132
718. Chocolate Muffins 132
719. Avocado And Walnuts Balls.................................. 132
720. Avocado Bars 132
721. Pumpkin Pie Bars 132
722. Raspberry Cake 133
723. Cinnamon Cake 133
724. Red Berry Gummies 133
725. Zucchini Muffins... 133
726. Almond Cheese Cake 133
727. Chocolate Cream Custard 133
728. Sesame Cookies 134
729. Red Velvet Cupcakes 134
730. Delicious Breakfast Cake 134
731. Orange Cheese Cake 134

732. Keto Soufflé 134
733. Chocolate Fudge 135
734. Vanilla Cake 135
735. Almond Coffee Cream 135
736. Vanilla Cream 135
737. Lemon Cheese Cake 135
738. Maple Custard 135
739. Keto Cobbler 135
740. Raspberry Custard Trifle 136
741. Lavender Cookies 136
742. Pecan Pie 136
743. Mint Cake 136
744. Carrot Walnut Cake 136
745. Ricotta And Pecan Cupcakes 137
746. Keto Sweet Bread 137
747. Strawberry Jam 137
748. Green Tea Cupcakes 137
749. Cocoa Pudding Cake 137
750. Dessert Pancakes 137
751. Peanut Butter Bars 138
752. Lavender Crème Brule 138
753. Sweet Zucchini Muffins 138
754. Keto Peanut Butter Cookies 138
755. Almond Cookies 138
756. Keto Cheesecake 138
757. Rutabaga Cake 139
758. Super Fudgy Brownies 139
759. Lava Cake 139
760. Rhubarb Crumble 139
761. Avocado Mousse 139
762. Blackberry Pancake 139
763. Almond Spread 140
764. Coconut Bars(1) 140
765. Chewy Seed And Nut Bars 140
766. Pineapple Cheese Cake 140
767. Peanut Pie 140
768. Soft Bacon Cookies 140
769. Cinnamon And Blackberry Pie 141
770. Candied Almonds 141
771. Keto Almond Scones 141
772. Mascarpone Fudge 141
773. Pumpkin Cake 141
774. Walnut Muffins 141
775. Chocolate Crème Brule 142
776. Almond Roll 142
777. Caramel Cheesecake 142
778. Cinnamon Cup Cake 142
779. Strawberries Cake 142
780. Keto Flan 143
781. Avocado Muffins 143
782. Coconut Bars(2) 143
783. Walnut Cake 143
784. Spiced Strawberry Pudding 143
785. Rhubarb Bars 143
786. Walnut Squares 144
787. Keto Chocolate Bars.................................... 144
788. Slow-cooked Cranberry Custard 144
789. Crème Brûlée 144
790. Low Carb Sweet Pecans 144
791. Traditional Egg Custard 144
792. Zucchini Cake 145
793. Blueberry Crisp 145
794. Pound Cake 145
795. Vanilla Avocado Cookies 145
796. Chocolate Mousse 145
797. Sweet Sesame Buns 145
798. Crockpot Lemon Custard 145
799. Lemon Scones 146
800. Chocolate Pudding 146
801. Vanilla Bars 146
802. Granola 146
803. Raspberry & Coconut Cake 146
804. Delightful Crème Brule 146
805. Strawberry Cobbler 147
806. Almond Blondies 147
807. Gingerbread Cookies 147
808. Pumpkin Custard 147
809. Toffee Pudding 147
810. Berry & Coconut Cake 147
811. Biscuits 147
812. Vanilla Rolls 148
813. Cream Cheese Cookies 148
814. Keto Fudge 148
815. Cherry Cheese Cake 148
816. Vanilla Pudding 148
OTHER FAVORITE KETO RECIPES 149
817. Balsamic Beef Pot Roast 149
818. Pork Mexican Wraps 149
819. Crockpot Carnitas Taco 149
820. Herbed Green Beans.................................... 149
821. Spiced Nut "snackers" 149
822. Low Carb Taco Soup 149
823. Shrimp Soup 150
824. Spinach Soup 150
825. Spiced Chicken 150
826. Mashed Broccoli 150
827. Garlicky Shrimp 150
828. Chard Chicken Soup 150
829. Carrots With Mushroom Sauce 151
830. Broccoli Mushroom Hash 151
831. Creamy Smoked Salmon Soup 151
832. Lamb Chops 151
833. Thai Turkey Legs 151
834. Ground Turkey And Mushrooms 151
835. Chicken Soup 151
836. Green Bean Leg Of Lamb 152
837. Mushrooms Squash...................................... 152
838. Zucchini And Shrimp................................... 152

839. Ginger Broccoli Stew 152
840. Beef And Cabbage Roast 152
841. Ham Soup 153
842. Creamy Coconut Fennel 153
843. Cinnamon Beef 153
844. Smoked Fish Dip 153
845. Lamb Barbacoa 153
846. Garlic And Chili Brussel's Sprouts With Spicy Mayo Dip 153
847. Tomato Chili 154
848. Crockpot Pork With Picante Sauce 154
849. Cream & Cheese Broccoli Soup 154
850. Chicken Chili Soup 154
851. Paprika Zucchini 154
852. Veggie Shrimps 154
853. Kale And Chicken Broth Soup 155
854. Red Pepper Dip With Warming Spices And Avocado Oil 155
855. Zucchini Eggplant Spread 155
856. Hot Beef Stew With Mushrooms(1) 155
857. Orange Sauce Pork Chops 155
858. Creamy Lemon Chicken Kale Soup 155
859. Lemon Pork Stew 156
860. Parmesan Tomatoes 156
861. Stockman's Beef Tail 156
862. Crockpot Kalua Pig 156
863. Dill Mixed Fennel Bulbs 156
864. Kale And Shrimp 156
865. Chicken In Salsa Verde 157
866. Lamb And Rosemary Stew 157
867. Apricot Salsa Salmon 157
868. Cauliflower Rice Mix 157
869. Butcher Style Cabbage Rolls – Pork & Beef Version 157
870. Asian Chicken Lettuce Wraps 157
871. Radish Soup 158
872. Garlic Lamb Roast 158
873. Coconut Okra 158
874. Beef Noodles With Broccoli & Tomato(1) 158
875. Capers Eggplant Stew 158
876. Sour Cream Soup 158
877. Chimichurri Pork Roast 159
878. Broccoli Yogurt Dip 159
879. Swiss Vegetable Soup 159
880. Lamb Shanks 159
881. Veggies Dish 160
882. Capers Zucchini Dip...160
883. Mushrooms Balsamic Mix 160
884. Creamy Portobello Mix 160
885. Chilli Con Steak 160
886. Bacon, Paprika, And Cauliflower Soup 160
887. Mexican Chicken Low Carb Soup 160
888. Lamb & Feta Meatballs 161

889. Mini Lamb And Eggplant Skewers With Yogurt Dip 161
890. Creamy Parmesan Green Beans 161
891. Simple Chicken Chilli 161
892. Sausage Stew 161
893. Balsamic Collard Greens 161
894. Slightly Addictive Pork Curry 162
895. Crispy Zucchini Wedges.................................... 162
896. Butter Green Peas 162
897. Greek Style Lamb Shanks 162
898. Brussel Sprouts Saute 162
899. Pork Carnitas 162
900. Beef Noodles With Broccoli & Tomato(2) 163
901. Butternut Pumpkin Soup.................................. 163
902. Slow CookerCreole Seafood 163
903. Mexican Flavor Chicken Soup........................ 163
904. Cabbage Stew 163
905. Lamb Shanks With Tomatoes 163
906. Beef And Mushrooms 164
907. Chicken Cacciatore With Zoodles................... 164
908. Ground Beef Soup 164
909. Shredded Pork Tacos 164
910. Green Beans, Leeks And Artichokes 164
911. Rustic Crockpot Ham... 164
912. Cauliflower Rice And Tomatoes 165
913. Lemongrass Short Ribs 165
914. Spicy Salmon With Spinach 165
915. Eggplant Mushroom Soup................................ 165
916. Broccoli Soup.. 165
917. Bacon And Zucchinis 165
918. Pesto Salmon With Vegetables........................ 166
919. Turkey Squash Stew 166
920. Red Wine Beef Stew 166
921. Chinese Pulled Pork 166
922. Coconut Halibut... 166
923. Rabbit & Mushroom Stew 166
924. Scallops In Lemon Butter 167
925. Salmon Stew.. 167
926. Mushroom Soup 167
927. Hot Sweet Ribs 167
928. Paprika Bok Choy 167
929. Coriander Broccoli 167
930. Spinach Leeks Dip 167
931. Butter Green Beans... 168
932. Pot Roast Beef Brisket 168
933. Cauliflower Bowls 168
934. Beef Stew... 168
935. Coconut Pulled Pork.. 168
936. Zucchini Dip... 168
937. Cauliflower Bolognese On Zucchini Noodles 169
938. Bacon Beef Bolognese... 169
939. Lamb With Mint And Green Beans 169
940. Fish Stock.. 169
941. Nutritious Bean Bowl... 169

942. Chicken And Spinach Stew 170
943. Creamy Coconut Cauliflower 170
944. Dill Leeks..170
945. Rich Creamy Endives 170
946. Cider Dipped Greens With Bacon 170
947. Korean Barbecue Beef 170
948. Spinach Stuffed Portobello 170
949. Cheesy Tuna Casserole...................................171
950. Bacon And Cauliflower Soup 171
951. Ground Lamb Casserole 171
952. Lazy Man's Pork Ribs.....................................171
953. Broccoli Sauté 171
954. Cube Steak 171
955. Vegetable Salad 172
956. Trout & Broccoli Chowder.............................172
957. Chicken And Egg Soup 172
958. French Onion Soup..172
959. Beef Stroganoff..172
960. Kale And Celery Stock...................................172
961. Nutty Green Beans With Avocado 173
962. Zucchini Balls 173
963. Steak And Tomato Salad 173
964. Buttermilk Curry...173
965. Spinach And Tomato Soup.............................173
966. Sugar Snap Peas Soup 173
967. Creamy Eggplant Soup 174
968. Pork And Chive Meatballs.............................174
969. Chipotle Barbacoa 174
970. Beet And Goat Cheese 174
971. Pork Chops 174
972. Coco-loco Shrimp... 174
973. Tuna-zucchini Spaghetti 175
974. Winter Keto Stew... 175
975. Mayo Artichokes Hearts................................. 175
976. Smoky Barbecue Pulled Pork 175
977. Zesty Garlic Pulled Pork................................. 175
978. Lamb And Coconut Stew................................ 175
979. Creamy Broccoli 176
980. Hot Eggplant Mix... 176
981. Swiss Cheese Onion Soup.............................. 176
982. Okra Sauté... 176
983. Slow CookerHungarian Goulash..................... 176
984. Tuna Steaks 176
985. Lamb And Eggplant Stew 177
986. Red Cabbage And Walnuts............................. 177
987. Shrimp And Tomatoes..................................... 177
988. German-style Pork Stew 177
989. Chili-lime Chicken Wings 177
990. Lime Green Beans.. 177
991. Tomato Cheese Soup 178
992. Sausage Soup 178
993. Chicken Cordon Bleu Soup............................. 178
994. Cheddar Artichoke 178
995. Keto Slow Cooker Chili 178
996. Squash And Zucchinis 178
997. Fish With Tomatoes.. 179
998. Saucy Ranch Pork 179
999. Cauliflower With Eggplants............................. 179
1000. Cheese Asparagus 179
1001. Cod And Vegetables 179

INTRODUCTION

How does the keto diet work?

The keto diet aims to force your body into using a different type of fuel. Instead of relying on sugar (glucose) that comes from carbohydrates (such as grains, legumes, vegetables, and fruits), the keto diet relies on ketone bodies, a type of fuel that the liver produces from stored fat. Burning fat seems like an ideal way to lose pounds. But getting the liver to make ketone bodies is tricky:

- It requires that you deprive yourself of carbohydrates, fewer than 20 to 50 grams of carbs per day (keep in mind that a medium-sized banana has about 27 grams of carbs).
- It typically takes a few days to reach a state of ketosis.
- Eating too much protein can interfere with ketosis.

What do you eat?

Because the keto diet has such a high fat requirement, followers must eat fat at each meal. In a daily 2,000-calorie diet, that might look like 165 grams of fat, 40 grams of carbs, and 75 grams of protein. However, the exact ratio depends on your particular needs. Some healthy unsaturated fats are allowed on the keto diet — like nuts (almonds, walnuts), seeds, avocados, tofu, and olive oil. But saturated fats from oils (palm, <u>coconut</u>), lard, butter, and cocoa butter are encouraged in high amounts. Protein is part of the keto diet, but it doesn't typically discriminate between lean protein foods and protein sources high in saturated fat such as beef, pork, and bacon. What about fruits and vegetables? All fruits are rich in carbs, but you can have certain fruits (usually berries) in small portions. Vegetables (also rich in carbs) are restricted to leafy greens (such as kale, Swiss chard, spinach), cauliflower, broccoli, Brussels sprouts, asparagus, bell peppers, onions, garlic, mushrooms, cucumber, celery, and summer squashes. A cup of chopped broccoli has about six carbs.

Keto diet risks

<u>A ketogenic diet has numerous risks</u>. Top of the list: it's high in saturated fat. McManus recommends that you keep saturated fats to no more than 7% of your daily calories because of the link to heart disease. And indeed, the keto diet is associated with an increase in "bad" LDL cholesterol, which is also linked to heart disease.

Other potential keto risks include these:

Nutrient deficiency. "If you're not eating a wide variety of vegetables, fruits, and grains, you may be at risk for deficiencies in micronutrients, including selenium, magnesium, phosphorus, and vitamins B and C," McManus says.

Liver problems. With so much fat to metabolize, the diet could make any existing liver conditions worse.

Kidney problems. The kidneys help metabolize protein, and McManus says the keto diet may overload them. (The current recommended intake for protein averages 46 grams per day for women, and 56 grams for men).

Constipation. The keto diet is low in fibrous foods like grains and legumes.

Fuzzy thinking and mood swings. "The brain needs sugar from healthy carbohydrates to function. Low-carb diets may cause confusion and irritability," McManus says. Those risks add up — so make sure that you talk to a doctor and a registered dietitian before ever attempting a ketogenic diet.

7 Things You Need to Know About Slow Cookers
What is Slow Cooking?

Slow cooking is nothing more than the classic technique of <u>braising</u> in which meats or poultry and vegetables are tightly covered and slowly simmered in liquid until succulent and tender. The only difference is that instead of doing the cooking on top of the stove or in the oven, all the magic happens in an appliance made especially for the job—a covered ceramic or stainless steel crock which sits inside an electrical unit that surrounds the crock with gentle heat. Because slow cooking is much more hands-off for the cook than braising, it's an ideal option for anyone with a busy schedule.

Slow Cooker 101

1.   Although synonymous with cold weather meals like stews and chilis, more and more people are turning to their slow cooker for everyday use; it's just as useful in conquering dinner with a variety of different meals you can plan week after week. Slow cooking is the equalizer for weeknight dinner when it comes to tougher, less expensive cuts of meat like brisket or pork shoulder, where they can simmer until fork-tender. Yum!

2.   Look for a cooker that has a removable ceramic or stainless steel insert for easy cleaning. The insert should have sturdy tabbed handles for moving it from the cooker to the table. And while not absolutely necessary, an insert that can be used on the stove or in the oven to brown meats for an added layer of flavor is a nice feature (note that traditional ceramic-style crocks are not safe for stovetop browning). Read the manufacturer's instructions to determine if your insert is capable of stovetop browning.

3.   Check for a well-fitting lid. This is critical to the success of recipes as well as an indication of the quality of construction. Some slow cookers are designed with clamps on the sides to keep the lid in place during transport—a nice feature when taking a dish to a potluck.

4.   The heating elements of most slow cookers are on the bottom of the unit, but high-quality models have elements wrapped around the body as well and tend to cook foods more evenly. Appliances with this wrap-around feature are usually more expensive than those with bottom-only elements.

5.   Make sure the slow cooker insert is perfectly clean before using and thaw all ingredients before putting them in the slow cooker.

6.   For best results, don't fill the crock more than 2/3 full, and resist the temptation to remove the lid during cooking.

7.   Because hot steam will collect under the lid, raise it carefully and away from you when food is done.

BREAKFAST AND BRUNCH RECIPES

1. Sour Cream Chicken

Servings: 4   Cooking Time: 6 Hours

Ingredients:

½ cup of chicken stock	1 batch of taco seasoning
1 can of diced green chilies and tomatoes	2 pounds of chicken breast

Directions:
Add all the ingredients to the slow cooker.   Cook on low for 6 hours.   Divide onto plates and serve.
Nutrition Info: Calories: 262 Fat: 13 grams Fiber: 2.5 grams Protein: 32 grams Carbohydrates: 23 grams

2. Delectable Breakfast Meal

Servings: 1   Cooking Time: 1.5 Hours

Ingredients:

1/4 cups of brown swerve	1/2 cup of raisins
1 cup of water	1 cup of flaxseed meal
1/2 teaspoon of cinnamon powder	1/2 cup of walnuts, diced

Directions:
Start by throwing all the Ingredients: into the Crockpot.   Cover your crockpot and select the Low settings for 1 1/2 hours.   Remove the crockpot's lid.   Serve fresh.
Nutrition Info: Calories 238 Total Fat 23.2 g Saturated Fat 13 g Cholesterol 61 mg Total Carbs 4.8 g Sugar 0 g Fiber 0.9 g Sodium 115 mg Potassium 303 mg Protein 13.3 g

3. Creamy Oregano Chorizo Mushroom

Servings: 8   Cooking Time: 4 Hours 30 Minutes

Ingredients:

3 tbsp. oregano	1 cup milk
2 large onions	2 eggs
1 lb. fresh mushrooms of any kind	1 lb. chorizo style Mexican sausage
1 lb. cream cheese	

Directions:
Slice the bell peppers into thick slices.   Chop onion into large pieces.   Halve or quarter-chop mushrooms depending on preference.   Turn on slow cooker to high and begin to brown the chorizo, allowing the grease to bubble.   Cook onions, peppers and mushrooms for a few moments in chorizo grease.   Combine the creamed cheese, oregano, milk and eggs until blended smoothly. Pour milk and egg mixture on top of the meat in the crockpot and set to low heat.   Cover and let cook for four hours. Serve hot and enjoy!
Nutrition Info: Calories: 516 Carb: 11g Fat: 42g Protein: 22g

4. Simple Chicken Soup

Servings: 6   Cooking Time: 6 Hours

Ingredients:

4 cups water	3 carrots, diced
1/2 tsp black pepper	3 celery stalks, diced
1 tbsp. herb de Provence	1 onion, chopped
1 tsp apple cider vinegar	1 tsp sea salt

Directions:
Add all ingredients to the slow cooker and stir well. Cover and cook on low for 6 hours.   Remove chicken from slow cooker and shred using a fork. Return shredded chicken to the slow cooker and stir well.   Serve and enjoy.
Nutrition Info: Calories 207 Fat 7.3 g Carbohydrates 5.1 g Sugar 2.4 g Protein 28.7 g Cholesterol 87 mg Fiber 1.3 g Net carbs 3.8 g

5. Broccoli And Tomatoes Casserole

Servings: 6   Cooking Time: 4 Hours

Ingredients:

Butter	2 c. cheddar cheese, shredded
Pepper and salt	8 eggs, beaten
1 ¼ c. cooked bacon, crumbled	½ c. whole milk
1 ½ c. cherry tomatoes, halved	1 bunch scallions, sliced

Directions:
Spray cooking spray on the interior of the Crockpot. Toss the broccoli and butter. Season with pepper and salt.   Press the vegetable mixture at the bottom of the Crockpot. Add the bacon and tomatoes on top. Add the cheddar cheese.   Mix the eggs and milk.   Pour the egg mixture over the vegetable layers. Sprinkle the scallions.   Close the lid and cook on low for 4 hours.
Nutrition Info: Calories: 486. Carbohydrates: 8.1 Protein: 21.3g Fat: 17g Sugar: 2.9g Sodium: 845mg Fiber: 5.4g

6. Egg Casserole

Servings: 4   Cooking Time: 2 Hours

Ingredients:

1 tomato, sliced	1 oz fresh dill, chopped
3 eggs	
5 oz asparagus, chopped	1 teaspoon olive oil
4 oz Parmesan, chopped	¾ teaspoon salt
	1 teaspoon paprika

Directions:
Mix up together olive oil, salt, paprika, chopped asparagus, and fresh dill.   Place the mixture in the slow cooker.   Add a layer of the sliced tomato. Beat the eggs and pour over the tomatoes then close the lid.   Cook the casserole for 2 hours on High or until the eggs are solid.   Enjoy!
Nutrition Info:calories 178, fat 11, fiber 2.1, carbs 7.5, protein 15.7

7. Chicken Tikka Masala

Servings: 2   Cooking Time: 6 Hours

Ingredients:

3 tsp Garam Masala   1/2 cup heavy cream
5 oz. diced tomatoes   1/2 cup coconut milk

Directions:
Put chicken to crockpot and add grated ginger knob on top.   Also add the seasonings: 1 tsp onion powder, 2 minced cloves of garlic, 1 tsp paprika and 2 tsp salt. Mix.   Add tomatoes and coconut oil. Mix.   Cook for 6 hours on low.   When cooked, add heavy cream to thicken the curry.
Nutrition Info: Calories: 493 Fat: 41.2 g Net carbs: 5.8 g Protein: 46 g

8. Chicken Green Chile Soup

Servings: 8   Cooking Time: 7 Hours 30 Minutes
Ingredients:

8 oz. cream cheese, softened	4 oz. can green chilies, diced
1 tsp garlic powder	15 oz. salsa
1 tsp onion powder	32 oz. chicken broth
1 tbsp. chili powder	Pepper
2 tbsp. ground cumin	Salt
3/4 cup water	

Directions:
Add all ingredients except cream cheese into the slow cooker and stir well.   Cover and cook on low for 7 hours.   Remove chicken from slow cooker and shred using a fork.   Return shredded chicken to the slow cooker along with cream cheese and stir well to combine.   Cover and cook on low for 30 minutes more.   Stir well and serve.
Nutrition Info: Calories 307 Fat 17.5 g Carbohydrates 6.8 g Sugar 2.3 g Protein 30.4 g Cholesterol 107 mg Fiber 1.6 g Net carbs 5.2 g

9. Cauliflower Hash Browns Slow Breakfast Casserole

Servings: 10   Cooking Time: 5-7 Hours
Ingredients:

Milk - ½ cup	Cauliflower, shredded - 1 head
Dry mustard - ½ teaspoon	Small onion, diced - 1
Kosher salt - 1 teaspoon	Packaged pre-cooked breakfast sausages, sliced – 5 ounces
Pepper - ½ teaspoon	
Additional salt and pepper to season the layers – as required	Shredded cheddar cheese – 8 ounces

Directions:
First of all, grease a 6-quart slow cooker properly with cooking spray.   Mix well all the item likes the eggs, milk, dry mustard, salt, and pepper.   From the shredded cauliflower, take one-third portion and layer it in the bottom of the slow crock pot. After that place one-third of the sliced onion on top.   Use pepper and salt to season and top it with one-third portion of sausage and cheese.   Repeat the same process by maintaining two layers.   Pour the eggs mixture over slow cooker   Cook on low for 5-7 hours and wait until eggs set properly and the top color is browned.
Nutrition Info: Calories 87.7 Calories from Fat 49 Total Fat 5.4 g Cholesterol 1mg Total Carbohydrates 2.2g Dietary Fiber 1.2g Protein 8g

10. Breakfast Meat Bowl

Servings: 4   Cooking Time: 3 Hours
Ingredients:

4 oz ground chicken	1 garlic clove, chopped
4 oz ground beef	
1 teaspoon tomato puree	1 teaspoon turmeric
	1 teaspoon paprika
1 tablespoon butter	

Directions:
Mix together the ground chicken and ground beef. Sprinkle the meat mixture with the tomato puree and chopped garlic clove.   Add turmeric and paprika.   Stir the mixture well.   Place the butter in the slow cooker and add the ground meat mixture. Close the lid and cook the meal for 3 hours on High. When the meat is cooked, transfer it to serving bowls. Enjoy!
Nutrition Info:calories 145, fat 6.9, fiber 0.4, carbs 3, protein 17

11. Breakfast Tender Chicken Strips

Servings: 5   Cooking Time: 5 Hours
Ingredients:

1-pound chicken fillets	1 teaspoon dried dill
2 tablespoons butter	1 teaspoon dried parsley
1 teaspoon dried oregano	2 tablespoons full-fat cream

Directions:
Cut the chicken fillets into the strips.   Then sprinkle the chicken strips with the dried dill, oregano, and parsley.   Toss the poultry with the full-fat cream.   Place the butter in the slow cooker and add the chicken strips.   Then close the lid and cook the chicken strips for 5 hours on Low.   Stir the cooked chicken strips and transfer onto a serving platter.   Enjoy!
Nutrition Info:calories 222, fat 12.1, fiber 0.2, carbs 0.6, protein 26.6

12. Kale With Eggs

Servings: 4   Cooking Time: 3 Hours
Ingredients:

1 garlic clove, minced	4 bacon strips, diced
4 eggs, room temperature	Salt and black pepper- to taste
	Cooking spray

Directions:
Start by greasing the base of your Crockpot. Whisk kale with all other Ingredients: and spread into the crockpot.   Make four wells into this mixture and crack on egg into each well.   Cover your crockpot and select the Low settings for 3 hours. Remove the crockpot's lid.   Serve.
Nutrition Info: Calories 393 Total Fat 15.8 g Saturated Fat 10.3 g Cholesterol 47 mg Total Carbs 4.1 g Sugar 0.4 g Fiber 0.4 g Sodium 421 mg Protein 12.6 g

13. Breakfast Bacon And Eggs

Servings: 5   Cooking Time: 2 Hours
Ingredients:

5 eggs, beaten

6 oz bacon, chopped

1 onion, chopped

2 tablespoons butter

¼ teaspoon cayenne pepper

¾ teaspoon salt

Directions:
Place the chopped bacon in the slow cooker and sprinkle with salt and cayenne pepper.   Add butter and cook for 1 hour on High.   Then add the chopped onion and stir the mixture.   Add the eggs into the slow cooker and close the lid.   Cook the meal for 1 hour on High.   When the eggs are solid, the meal is cooked.   Enjoy!

Nutrition Info:calories 297, fat 23.2, fiber 0.5, carbs 2.9, protein 18.4

14. Smoked Sausages With Grits

Servings: 4   Cooking Time: 4 Hours

Ingredients:

A pinch of salt and black pepper

1 ½ cups of keto grits

1 ½ teaspoon of thyme, diced

4 ½ cups of water

1/4 teaspoon of garlic powder

16 oz. Cheddar cheese, shredded

1 cup of almond milk

Cooking spray

4 eggs, whisked

Directions:
Boil water in a suitable cooking pot after placing it over medium heat.   Add grits to the water and cover them for 5 minutes, then take them off from the heat.   Stir cheese and mix well until it melts. Stir in almond milk, salt, pepper, garlic powder, eggs, and thyme.   Add the grits mixture and all other Ingredients: to the Crockpot.   Cover your crockpot and select the Low settings for 4 hours. Remove the crockpot's lid.   Serve.

Nutrition Info: Calories 226 Total Fat 17.1 g Saturated Fat 10.6 g Cholesterol 56 mg Total Carbs 6.7 g Sugar 2.9 g Fiber 2.4 g Sodium 88 mg Protein 14.1 g

15. Feta Cheese And Kale Breakfast Casserole

Servings: 6   Cooking Time: 4 Hours

Ingredients:

2 teaspoons olive oil

¾ cup feta cheese, crumbled

12 eggs, beaten

Salt and pepper to taste

Directions:
Mix all ingredients in a large mixing bowl until well combined.   Place in a Ziploc bag and write the date when the recipe is made.   Place inside the freezer.   Once you are ready to cook the meal, allow to thaw on the countertop for at least 2 hours. Pour the ingredients into the crockpot and close the lid.   Cook on high for 3 hours or on low for 4 hours.

Nutrition Info: Calories: 397 Carbohydrates: 4g Protein: 32.2g Fat: 29.4g Sugar: 0.6g Sodium: 425mg Fiber: 3.2g

16. Egg Casserole With Italian Cheeses, Sun-dried Tomatoes And Herbs

Servings: 8   Cooking Time: 4 Hours

Ingredients:

3 tablespoons sun-dried tomatoes, chopped

2 tablespoons onion, minced

2 tablespoons basil, chopped

2 tablespoons milk

1 tablespoon thyme leaves

Salt and pepper to taste

1 cup mixed Italian cheeses, grated

Directions:
Mix all ingredients in a bowl.   Place in a Ziploc bag and write the date when the recipe is made.   Place inside the freezer.   Once you are ready to cook the meal, allow to thaw on the countertop for at least 2 hours.   Place all ingredients in the crockpot. Cook on high for 2 hours or on low for 3 hours.

Nutrition Info: Calories: 140 Carbohydrates: 3.87g Protein: 10.93g Fat: 8.89g Sugar: 1.27g Sodium: 309mg Fiber: 0.3g

17. Sweet Pepper Hash

Servings: 10   Cooking Time: 3 Hours

Ingredients:

1 teaspoon of olive oil

1 ½ cups of sweet onion, sliced

2 teaspoons of fresh thyme

½ teaspoon of black pepper

¼ cup of chicken broth

10 eggs, beaten

1 ½ cups of diced green, red, and yellow sweet peppers

½ cup of Swiss cheese, shredded

2 teaspoons of fresh tarragon

¼ cup of cheddar cheese, shredded

Directions:
First, start by sautéing onion, and sausages separately in a greased skillet for 5 minutes.   Now begin by greasing the base of your Crockpot.   Add the sautéed onion, sausages, and other veggies to the Crockpot.   Whisk the egg with remaining Ingredients: except for cheese and pour into crockpot.   Sprinkle the cheese on top of this mixture.   Cover your Crockpot and select the high settings for 3 hours.   Remove the crockpot's lid. Slice and serve warm.

Nutrition Info: Calories 184 Total Fat 12.7 g Saturated Fat 7.3 g Cholesterol 35 mg Total Carbs 6.3 g Sugar 2.7 g Fiber 1.6 g Sodium 222 mg Protein 12.2 g

18. Homemade Vegetable Stock

Servings: 4   Cooking Time: 12 Hours

Ingredients:

12 whole peppercorns

3 peeled and chopped carrots

3 chopped celery stalks

4 smashed garlic cloves

2 bay leaves

1 large quartered onion

2 tablespoons apple cider vinegar

Any other vegetable scraps

Directions:
Put everything in your slow cooker and cover.   Do not turn on; let it sit for 30 minutes.   When that's done, cook on low for 12 hours.   Strain the broth and discard the solids.   Before using, keep the stock in a container in the fridge for 2-3 hours.

Stock will keep fresh for 4-5 days, or frozen indefinitely.
Nutrition Info: Total calories: 11 Protein: 0 Carbs: 3 Fat: 0 Fiber: 0

19. Sausage And Spinach

Servings: 6   Cooking Time: 6 Hours
Ingredients:

8 oz Italian sausages
1/3 cup spinach leaves, torn
1 tablespoon dried oregano
1 teaspoon sweet paprika
1 teaspoon salt
1 teaspoon black pepper
4 oz Cheddar cheese, shredded
1 tablespoon olive oil
1/3 cup coconut milk

Directions:
In the slow cooker, mix the sausage with the spinach, oregano and the other ingredients, toss and close the slow cooker lid.   Cook the casserole for 6 hours on Low.
Nutrition Info:calories 377, fat 16.4, fiber 4.5, carbs 6.4, protein 11.2

20. Pork Stew

Servings: 8   Cooking Time: 8 Hours
Ingredients:

1/2 tsp cumin
1 1/2 tsp oregano
1 tbsp. chili powder
2 garlic cloves
1/2 cup onion, chopped
1 1/2 cups rutabaga, peeled and cubed
15 oz. can tomatoes, diced
4 cups chicken broth, low-sodium
2 tbsp. olive oil
1/2 tsp black pepper
1 tsp kosher salt

Directions:
Add all ingredients to the slow cooker and stir well to mix.   Cover and cook on low for 8 hours. Remove pork from slow cooker and shred using a fork.   Return shredded pork to the slow cooker and stir well.   Season with pepper and salt. Serve and enjoy.
Nutrition Info: Calories 532 Fat 39.7 g Carbohydrates 7.1 g Sugar 4 g Protein 35.4 g Cholesterol 122 mg Fiber 2.2 g Net carbs 4.9 g

21. Chicken Chorizo Soup

Servings: 8   Cooking Time: 3 Hours And 50 Minutes
Ingredients:

4 lb. chicken thighs – no bones or skin
Hot sauce – ex. Frank's Red
Worcestershire – homemade or another keto replacement
2 tbsp. of each: Minced garlic
1 c. heavy cream
1 can stewed tomatoes
4 c. chicken stock
Garnish: Sour cream & parmesan

Directions:
Use a skillet to prepare the chorizo. When it's done, layer the fixings into the slow cooker. Set the timer for three hours on high.   Remove the chicken, shred, and add back to the cooker on low for 30 minutes longer.   Garnish as desired.

Nutrition Info: Calories: 659 Fat: 47 g Net Carbs: 5.0 g Protein: 52 g

22. The Better Quiche Lorraine

Servings: 8   Cooking Time: 4 Hours On Low
Ingredients:

10 eggs, beaten
1 cup Cheddar cheese, shredded
Pinch fresh ground black pepper
1 cup heavy cream
10 strips of bacon, crisped and crumbled
½ cup fresh spinach, chopped

Directions:
Butter the crock-pot.   In a large bowl, mix all the ingredients, except bacon crumbles.   Transfer mixture to the crock-pot, sprinkle bacon on top. Cover, cook on low for 4 hours. (In the last 15 minutes watch carefully, not to overcook it.)
Nutrition Info: Carbs: 2g Protein: 15g Fiber: 28g

23. Chicken Fajitas

Servings: 6   Cooking Time: 3 Hours
Ingredients:

½ cup salsa
8 oz. cream cheese
1 teaspoon cumin
1 teaspoon paprika
Salt and pepper to taste
1 onion, sliced
1 clove garlic, minced
1 red bell pepper, sliced
1 green bell pepper, sliced
1 teaspoon lime juice

Directions:
Combine all the ingredients except the lime wedges in your slow cooker.   Cover the pot.   Cook on high for 3 hours.   Shred the chicken.   Drizzle with lime juice.   Serve with toppings like sour cream and cheese.
Nutrition Info: Calories 276 Total Fat 17 g Saturated Fat 8 g Cholesterol 105 mg Sodium 827 mg Potassium 776 mg Total Carbohydrate 8 g Dietary Fiber 3 g Protein 25 g Total Sugars 2 g

24. Spicy Pepper Chicken Soup

Servings: 6   Cooking Time: 8 Hours
Ingredients:

8-ounces chicken stock
2 seeded and chopped jalapeno peppers
1 chopped poblano chili pepper
½ cup chopped green onions
3 minced garlic cloves
5 teaspoons 100% natural peanut butter
4 teaspoons coconut aminos
4 teaspoons lime juice
½ tablespoon+ crushed red pepper flakes
1 teaspoon ground ginger
Salt and pepper to taste

Directions:
The night before you plan on making the soup, put all the ingredients (minus green onions) in your slow cooker.   Marinate in the fridge overnight. When you're ready to cook, remove the slow cooker and wait 20 minutes before turning it on.   Turn to low and cook for 6-8 hours.   Taste and add more red pepper flakes if you want more heat.   Garnish with chopped green onions and serve!

Nutrition Info: Total calories: 102 Protein: 13
Carbs: 4 Fat: 4 Fiber: 0

25. Veggie Casserole

Servings: 6   Cooking Time: 4 Hours
Ingredients:

1 cup zucchinis, grated
½ cup broccoli, chopped
3 oz celery stalk, chopped
1 cup kale, chopped
1 tablespoon walnuts, chopped
1 teaspoon cream cheese
2 tablespoons butter
3 oz Mozzarella, shredded
1 tablespoon almond flour
1 teaspoon chili flakes
1 teaspoon salt
¼ teaspoon ground black pepper
½ cup of coconut milk

Directions:
Put the vegetables in the slow cooker.   Add coconut milk and the rest of the ingredients, toss and spread into the pot.   Close the lid, and cook the casserole for 4 hours on High. The cooked casserole should be very soft.
Nutrition Info:calories 296, fat 20.7, fiber 5.5, carbs 7.2, protein 11.2

26. Pork Breakfast Sausages

Servings: 3   Cooking Time: 7 Hours
Ingredients:

9 oz ground pork
1 oz onion, grated
1 tablespoon almond flour
1 teaspoon coconut flour
¼ teaspoon ground black pepper
¾ teaspoon chili flakes
1 teaspoon ghee

Directions:
Mix up together the ground pork and grated onion. Add almond flour and coconut flour.   Then add ground black pepper and chili flakes.   Stir the mixture well and form small sausages.   Place the sausages in the slow cooker and add the ghee. Cook the sausages for 7 hours on Low.   When the sausages are cooked, let them cool slightly.   Enjoy!
Nutrition Info:calories 188, fat 9.8, fiber 2.9, carbs 5.7, protein 25.1

27. Sausages And Peppers Hash

Servings: 3   Cooking Time: 2.5 Hour
Ingredients:

3 pork sausages, organic and sliced
2 red bell peppers, cubed
2 spring onions, chopped
2 tomatoes, cubed
2 oz bacon, sliced
1 teaspoon butter
¼ teaspoon ground black pepper

Directions:
Grease the slow cooker with the butter, combine the sausages with peppers and the other ingredients, toss and close the lid.   Cook the mix for 5 hours on High.
Nutrition Info:calories 308, fat 12.9, fiber 4.1, carbs 5.4, protein 9.6

28. Cheesy Turmeric Eggs

Servings: 4   Cooking Time: 1 Hour 30 Minutes
Ingredients:

4 eggs, beaten
¾ teaspoon turmeric
1 tablespoon butter, melted
3 tablespoons almond milk, unsweetened
2 oz Parmesan, grated

Directions:
Whisk the eggs and with the turmeric, butter, and almond milk.   Pour the mix into the slow cooker. Cook the eggs for 1 hours on High.   Scramble the eggs with a spatula and sprinkle with the grated cheese.   Cook the omelet for 30 minutes more on Low.   Enjoy!
Nutrition Info:calories 161, fat 13, fiber 0.3, carbs 5, protein 10.4

29. Cauliflower Hash Brown

Servings: 5   Cooking Time: 5 Hours
Ingredients:

10 oz cauliflower, chopped
2 tablespoons butter
1 garlic clove, chopped
2 eggs, beaten
1 teaspoon ground black pepper
3 oz Parmesan, grated

Directions:
Place the butter and cauliflower in the slow cooker. Add garlic clove and ground black pepper.   Add eggs and stir the mixture.   Sprinkle the mixture with the grated cheese and close the lid.   Cook the hash brown for 5 hours on Low.   Then stir the hash brown and serve!
Nutrition Info:calories 137, fat 10.1, fiber 1.5, carbs 4.2, protein 8.9

30. Ham & Cheese Broccoli Brunch Bowl

Servings: 6   Cooking Time: 8 Hours On Low.
Ingredients:

4 cups vegetable broth
2 Tablespoons olive oil
1 teaspoon mustard seeds, ground
2 cups ham, cubed
3 garlic cloves, minced
Salt and pepper to taste
2 cups Cheddar cheese, shredded
Pinch of paprika

Directions:
Add all ingredients to the crock-pot in order of the list.   Cover, cook on low for 8 hours.
Nutrition Info: Carbs: 8g Protein: 25g Fiber: 28g

31. Minced Pork Zucchini Lasagna

Servings: 4   Cooking Time: 8 Hours
Ingredients:

1 diced small onion
1 minced clove of garlic
2 cups of minced lean ground pork
2 cans of Italian diced tomatoes
2 tablespoons of olive oil
2 cups of shredded Mozzarella cheese
1 large egg
1 tablespoon of dried basil
Salt and pepper
2 tablespoons of butter

Directions:
Slice the zucchini lengthwise into 6 slices. Heat the olive oil in a saucepan, and sauté the garlic and onions for 5 minutes. Add the minced meat and cook for a further 5 minutes. Add the tomatoes and cook for a further 5 minutes. Add the seasoning and mix thoroughly. In a small bowl, combine the egg and cheese and whisk together. Use the butter to grease the Slow Cookerand then begin to layer the lasagna. First layer with the zucchini slices, add the meat mixture and then top with the cheese. Repeat and finish with the cheese. Cover and cook for 8 hours on low.
Nutrition Info: Carbohydrates: 10 grams Protein: 23 grams Fat: 30 grams Calories: 398

32. Egg Bars

Servings: 4   Cooking Time: 3 Hours
Ingredients:

1 green pepper, chopped	4 eggs, beaten
3 tablespoons almond milk	1/3 teaspoon cayenne pepper
1 tablespoon almond flour	1 teaspoon chili flakes
	1 tablespoon butter

Directions:
Mix together the whisked eggs and chopped green pepper. Add almond milk and almond flour. Then add cayenne pepper and chili flakes. Stir the mixture well. Then pour the egg mixture into the slow cooker and flatten it with a spatula. Close the lid and cook the meal for 3 hours on High. Let the cooked eggs chill to room temperature. Cut the eggs into bars and serve!
Nutrition Info:calories 161, fat 13.5, fiber 1.6, carbs 3.9, protein 7.6

33. Paprika Shrimp

Servings: 6   Cooking Time: 1 Hour
Ingredients:

1-pound shrimp, peeled	1 teaspoon paprika
1/4 teaspoon ground black pepper	1/4 teaspoon minced garlic
	3/4 cup chicken stock

Directions:
Sprinkle the peeled shrimp with the ground black pepper and paprika. Then sprinkle the shrimp with the minced garlic and stir well. Place the chicken stock in the slow cooker. Add the seasoned shrimp and close the lid. Cook the shrimp for 1 hour on High. Then transfer the shrimps to the serving plate and serve!
Nutrition Info:calories 92, fat 1.4, fiber 0.2, carbs 1.5, protein 17.4

34. Greek Crockpot Breakfast Casserole

Servings: 12   Cooking Time: 4 Hours
Ingredients:

1/2 c. milk	1 tsp. onion powder
1/4 tsp. black pepper	1/2 c. feta cheese, shredded
1/2 tsp. salt	
1 tsp. garlic powder	2 c. spinach

½ c. sun-dried tomatoes, soaked overnight

1 c. baby Bella mushrooms, sliced

Directions:
Lubricate the Crockpot with cooking spray. Mix everything in a bowl. Pour the mixture in the Crockpot. Cook on low for 4 hours.
Nutrition Info: Calories: 397 Carbohydrates: 7.5g Protein: 16.3g Fat: 20.3g Sugar: 1.2g Sodium: 347mg Fiber: 3.7 g

35. Crockpot Mediterranean Frittata

Servings: 8   Cooking Time: 3 Hours
Ingredients:

1/3 c. milk	1 ¼ c. red peppers, roasted and chopped
1 tsp. dried oregano	
Pepper and salt to taste	½ c. red onion, sliced thinly
4 c. baby arugula rockets, rinsed and drained	¾ c. goat cheese, crumbled

Directions:
Spray cooking oil inside the Crockpot. In a large bowl, mix the eggs, milk, and oregano. Season with pepper and salt. Take the arugula leaves at the bottom of the Crockpot. Add the red peppers, onions, and goat cheese. Pour over the egg mixture. Cook on low for 3 hours. Serve warm.
Nutrition Info: Calories: 416 Carbohydrates: 7.2g Protein: 18.3g Fat: 15.9g Sugar: 1.3g Sodium: 481mg Fiber: 4.8g

36. Turkey-stuffed Peppers

Servings: 2   Cooking Time: 8 Hours
Ingredients:

2 whole green bell peppers, top cut off and insides scraped off	12 oz. jar tomato sauce

Directions:
Mix turkey, 1 tbsp. tomato sauce and onion and garlic to taste in a bowl. Separate mixture into two parts and put them inside the peppers. Place the stuffed peppers in the crockpot and add the remaining tomato sauce. Add 1/4 cup of water. Cover and cook for 8 hours on low.
Nutrition Info: Calories: 422 Fat: 27.5 g Net carbs: 3.6 g Protein: 30.8 g

37. Creamy Asparagus Bake

Servings: 6   Cooking Time: 2.5 Hours
Ingredients:

1 cup asparagus, chopped	1 teaspoon olive oil
1 cup spring onions, chopped	½ teaspoon ground black pepper
½ cup heavy cream	½ teaspoon cayenne pepper
3 oz Swiss cheese, grated	1 teaspoon dill, chopped

Directions:
In the slow cooker, mix the asparagus with the spring onions and the other ingredients. Stir the bake mixture gently with the help of the wooden

spatula. Close the slow cooker lid and cook the casserole for 2.5 hours on High or until the broccoli is tender.
Nutrition Info:calories 250, fat 11.1, fiber 4.1, carbs 4.1, protein 9.5

38. Simple Ham And Egg Casserole

Servings: 6   Cooking Time: 3 Hours
Ingredients:

- ½ green bell pepper, diced
- ½ red bell pepper, diced
- 1 small onion, diced
- ½ c. ham, diced
- ½ c. cheese, shredded
- 6 eggs, beaten
- 1 tbsp. milk
- Pepper and salt to taste

Directions:
Spray the Crockpot with cooking spray.   Take melted butter in the Crockpot.   Add the bell peppers, onions, ham, and cheese in layers.   In a mixing bowl, mix the eggs and milk. Season with pepper and salt.   Pour over the layers of vegetables and ham.   Close the lid and cook for 3 hours on low or until a toothpick inserted in the middle comes out clean.
Nutrition Info: Calories: 379.1 Carbohydrates: 7.2g Protein: 15g Fat: 20.4g Sugar: 1.4g Sodium: 744mg Fiber: 3.9g

39. Sausage-stuffed Eggplants

Servings: 6   Cooking Time: 6 Hours
Ingredients:

- 2 cloves of garlic, minced
- 2 tablespoons rosemary, fresh
- Salt and pepper to taste
- 3 small eggplants, sliced
- 6 slices mozzarella cheese

Directions:
Mix all ingredients in a bowl.   Place in a Ziploc bag and write the date when the recipe is made.   Place inside the freezer.   Once you are ready to cook the meal, allow to thaw on the countertop for at least 2 hours.   Line the bottom of the crockpot with foil. Grease with cooking spray.   Pour into the crockpot and cook on low for 6 hours or on high for 4 hours.
Nutrition Info: Calories: 471 Carbohydrates: 6.3g Protein: 16.83g Fat: 38.9g Sugar: 0.4g Sodium: 1107mg Fiber: 3.8g

40. Superb Chicken, Bacon, Garlic Thyme Soup

Servings: 4   Cooking Time: 6 Hours
Ingredients:

- 1 chopped onion
- 1 chopped pepper
- 8 chicken thighs
- 8 slices of bacon
- 1 tablespoon of thyme
- 1 teaspoon of salt
- 1 tablespoon of minced garlic
- 1 tablespoon of coconut flour
- 1 teaspoon of pepper
- 3 tablespoons of lemon juice
- 1 cup of chicken stock
- ¼ cup of unsweetened coconut milk
- 3 tablespoons of tomato paste

Directions:
Spread the butter on the base of the slow cooker and arrange the peppers and onions on top of it.   Add the chicken thighs and then layer with the bacon. Add the remaining ingredients.   Cover and cook on low for 6 hours.   Cut the thighs into pieces, arrange in bowls and serve.
Nutrition Info: Calories: 396 Fat: 21 grams Carbohydrates: 7 grams Fiber: 2 grams Protein: 41 grams

41. Paprika And Shallots Omelet

Servings: 4   Cooking Time: 6 Hours
Ingredients:

- 4 eggs, beaten
- 4 tablespoons heavy cream
- ½ teaspoon sweet paprika
- ¾ teaspoon Pink salt
- 1 cup shallots, chopped
- 1 teaspoon curry powder
- Cooking spray

Directions:
Spray the slow cooker bottom with the cooking spray. Combine the eggs with shallots and the other ingredients and spread.   Close the slow cooker lid and cook the meal for 6 hours on Low or until the omelet is set.
Nutrition Info:calories 348, fat 11.1, fiber 5.9, carbs 17.7, protein 10.9

42. Breakfast Pie

Servings: 6   Cooking Time: 7 Hours
Ingredients:

- 1 eggs
- 4 tablespoons almond milk
- ½ cup coconut flour
- ¾ teaspoon salt
- 5 oz cauliflower, chopped
- ½ onion, chopped
- 1 teaspoon butter
- 1 tablespoon full-fat cream
- 1 teaspoon turmeric
- 4 oz Parmesan, grated
- 5 oz ground chicken

Directions:
Beat the egg in the bowl and whisk well.   Add almond milk and coconut flour.   Then add salt and butter.   Stir the mixture and knead into a smooth dough. Add more flour if needed.   Then place the dough in the slow cooker and push the dough along the bottom and halfway up the sides of the slow cooker bowl to make the pie crust.   Place the chopped cauliflower, onion, and grated parmesan on top of the pie crust.   Add full-fat cream and turmeric.   Then add ground chicken and close the lid.   Cook the pie for 7 hours on Low. Chill the cooked pie little and then cut into slices. Serve!
Nutrition Info:calories 199, fat 10.9, fiber 5.1, carbs 10.4, protein 16.1

43. Mexican Breakfast Casserole

Servings: 10   Cooking Time: 2 Hours And 30 Minutes
Ingredients:

- Garlic powder - ½ teaspoon
- Coriander – ½
- Pepper - ¼ teaspoon
- Eggs - 10

teaspoon
Cumin - 1 teaspoon
Salsa – 1 cup
Chili fine powder - 1
teaspoon
Salt - ¼ teaspoon

Milk low fat - 1 cup
Cheese (Pepper Jack
if available) - 1 cup
Toppings if required:
Avocado salsa, sour
cream, cilantro – as
per preference

Directions:
Put a pan on low flame and cook pork sausage until
it leaves its pink color.   Add all the spices given
and let it cool and set for some time.   Now take a
medium bowl and whisk eggs and milk together.
Add the pork to the eggs and stir well so that they get
mixed properly.   Take a Slow Cookerand grease
its bottom and pour the mixture you prepared.
Cook on high flame for 2 hours and 30 minutes.
You can put seasonal toppings on it according to
your taste.
Nutrition Info: Fat: 24 g Saturated fat: 8.5 g
Cholesterol: 231 g Sodium: 749 mg
Carbohydrates:5.2 g Protein: 17.9 g Dietary fiber:
2.6 g Potassium: 454 mg

44. Kale Muffins

Servings: 6   Cooking Time: 7 Hours
Ingredients:

2 cups kale, chopped
1 teaspoon oregano,
dried
½ teaspoon cayenne
pepper
1 teaspoon sweet
paprika

½ teaspoon salt
1 egg, beaten
1 teaspoon butter,
melted
3 spring onions,
chopped
½ cup of water

Directions:
In the bowl, combine the kale with oregano and the
other ingredients except the butter and the water
and stir.   Brush the muffin molds with melted
butter and divide the kale into the muffin molds.
Transfer the muffin molds in the slow cooker.
Add water in the slow cooker and close it.   Cook
the chicken muffins for 7 hours on Low.
Nutrition Info:calories 307, fat 6.8, fiber 4.1,
carbs 5.5, protein 14.5

45. Smoked Salmon Casserole

Servings: 2-3,   Cooking Time: 1 Hour And 10
Minutes
Ingredients:

1 tbsp. of cream
cheese
1 tbsp. of heavy
cream
⅓ Cup mozzarella
cheese

2 oz. of smoked
salmon slices,
roughly chopped
1 tsp of Dill
Salt
Pepper

Directions:
Whisk everything together in a bowl.   Set the slow
cooker to high heat, lightly grease the bottom inside,
and add the egg and salmon mixture.   Cook for an
hour prior scooping out and serving.
Nutrition Info: Calories: 68 Fat: 7g Carbs: 4 g
Protein: 6.2 g

46. Cheesy Green Omelet

Servings: 2   Cooking Time: Approximately 1
Hour
Ingredients:

2 cups fresh spinach,
chopped

4 eggs
½ cup grated
cheddar

Directions:
Rinse the spinach and place it in a microwave-proof
bow, cover the bowl and place in the microwave on
high for 1 minute, or until wilted.   Squeeze the
moisture out of the spinach and finely chop.   In a
medium-sized bowl, lightly beat the eggs, add the
spinach, cheese, salt and pepper, stir to combine.
Drizzle some olive oil into the Crock Pot.   Pour the
egg/spinach mixture into the pot.   Place the lid
onto the pot and set the temperature to LOW.
Cook for about 1 hour or until the egg has set to your
liking.   Serve with a side of bacon and a sprinkle
of fresh herbs!

47. Salmon And Avocado Breakfast Bake

Servings: 4   Cooking Time: 2 Hours
Ingredients:

1 avocado, pitted
7 oz salmon fillet
2 eggs
1 teaspoon ground
coriander

½ teaspoon salt
1 teaspoon butter
1 tablespoon almond
flour

Directions:
Peel the avocado and chop it.   Chop the salmon
fillet and sprinkle it with the ground coriander and
salt.   Beat the eggs in a separate bowl.   Add the
chopped fish and avocado to the whisked egg and
toss together.   Then transfer the ingredients to the
slow cooker bowl and sprinkle with the almond flour.
Stir the ingredients well.   Chop the butter and
place it in the slow cooker.   Close the lid and cook
the meal for 2 hours in High.   When the salmon
avocado bake is cooked, let it cool for 5 minutes and
serve!
Nutrition Info:calories 248, fat 19.5, fiber 4.1,
carbs 6, protein 14.9

48. Coconut Flour "porridge" With Blueberries And Cinnamon

Servings: 2   Cooking Time: 2 ½ Hours.
Ingredients:

⅓ Cup flaxseed flour
⅔ Cup unsweetened,
coconut cream
1 tbsp. of ghee

1 tsp of agave syrup
1 tbsp. of blueberries
1 tsp of cinnamon

Directions:
Place all the first four ingredients together in the
slow cooker to make a thick paste.   Set to cook on
low heat for 2 ½ hours to make a thick, creamy
porridge.   Transfer onto a big bowl (or two
smaller bowls) and drizzle with a bit of agave syrup.
Add the cinnamon and blueberries on top.
Nutrition Info: Calories: 453 Fat: 39g Carbs: 12g,
Protein: 14g

49. Full-flavored Pot Roast

Servings: 8   Cooking Time: 45 Minutes
Ingredients:

1 (4 pounds) beef pot roast, cut into large chunks
1 cup of beef broth
1 teaspoon of smoked paprika
1 teaspoon of onion powder
1 teaspoon of garlic powder
1 teaspoon of salt
1 teaspoon of black pepper
1 teaspoon of xanthan gum

Directions:
Press the "Sautee/Browning" button on the Crock-Pot Express and add the avocado oil.   Once hot, add the roast and brown on both sides. Remove and set aside.   Deglaze the Crock-Pot Express with the beef broth and scrape any browned bits from the bottom of the pot.   Return the roast to the Crock-Pot Express and season with salt, paprika, onion powder, garlic powder, salt, and black pepper. Lock the lid and ensure the valve is closed.   Press the "Meat/Stew" button and set the time to 35 minutes. Press start.   When the cooking is done, naturally release the pressure and remove the lid. Transfer the roast to a plate.   Sprinkle the xanthan gum to the liquid and stir until thickens. Return the roast to the liquid and stir until coated. Serve and enjoy!
Nutrition Info: Calories: 427 Fat: 14.6g Carbohydrates: 0.2g Dietary Fiber: 0.2g Protein: 68.2g

50. Egg Quiche

Servings: 6   Cooking Time: 4 Hours
Ingredients:

1 cup almond flour
¼ cup almond milk
½ teaspoon salt
4 eggs, beaten
3 oz cauliflower, chopped
1 tomato, chopped
1 teaspoon paprika
¾ teaspoon ground black pepper
½ teaspoon turmeric
1 tablespoon butter
5 oz ground chicken

Directions:
Mix together the almond flour and almond milk until smooth.   Add salt and beaten eggs.   Whisk the mixture until smooth.   Add chopped cauliflower, tomato, paprika, ground black pepper, turmeric, butter, and ground chicken. Mix well. Pour the quiche mixture into the slow cooker. Close the lid and cook the quiche for 4 hours on High. Let the cooked quiche cool slightly and serve!
Nutrition Info:calories 161, fat 11.4, fiber 1.4, carbs 3.4, protein 12.2

51. Cod Bites

Servings: 3   Cooking Time: 4 Hours
Ingredients:

2 tablespoons almond flour
1 teaspoon garlic powder
10 oz cod fillet
2 eggs, beaten
1 teaspoon ghee

Directions:
Cut the cod fillet into the medium squares. Sprinkle the cod fillets with the garlic powder. Then dip them in the beaten eggs.   Transfer the cod fillets onto a plate and coat the fillets on all sides with the almond flour.   Put the ghee in the slow cooker and add the cod fillets.   Cook the cod bites for 4 hours on Low.   When the cod bites are cooked, chill them a little and serve!
Nutrition Info:calories 240, fat 14.5, fiber 2.1, carbs 4.9, protein 24.7

52. Delightful Chicken-chorizo Spicy Soup

Servings: 10   Cooking Time: 3.5 Hours
Ingredients:

1 pound of chorizo
4 cups of chicken stock
1 can of stewed tomatoes
2 tablespoons of minced garlic
1 cup of heavy cream
2 tablespoons of Worcestershire sauce
2 tablespoons of red sauce
Parmesan and sour cream for garnish

Directions:
Heat a frying pan and brown the sausage.   Place the chicken into the slow cooker and add the remaining ingredients except the Parmesan and sour cream.   Cover and cook on high for 3 hours. Garnish with the Parmesan and the sour cream.
Nutrition Info: Calories: 659 Fat: 37 grams Carbohydrates: 6 grams Fiber: 1 gram Protein: 52 grams

53. Stuffed Breakfast Peppers(2)

Servings: 4   Cooking Time: 2 Hours
Ingredients:

3 eggs, lightly beaten
3 ounces feta cheese, cut into small chunks
2 cups baby spinach, roughly chopped
2 slices streaky bacon, chopped into small pieces

Directions:
In a small bowl, mix together the eggs, feta cheese, spinach, bacon pieces, salt, and pepper.   Prepare the peppers by cutting around the stalk and removing it, reach into the peppers and remove the seeds.   Carefully pour the egg mixture evenly into each pepper, (don't worry if they're only half filled). Drizzle some olive oil into the Slow Cooker   Place the filled peppers carefully into the pot, prop them up against each other so they stay upright while cooking.   Place the lid onto the pot and set the temperature to HIGH.   Cook for 2 hours. Remove the filled peppers from the Slow Cookerand serve while hot.
Nutrition Info: Calories: 200 Fat: 18 g Carbohydrates: 8 g Protein: 15 g

54. Ricotta Eggs

Servings: 4   Cooking Time: 5 Hours
Ingredients:

½ cup spring onions, chopped
1 teaspoon white pepper
1 teaspoon turmeric powder
3 oz Ricotta cheese
4 eggs, whisked
½ teaspoon butter, melted
1 tablespoon cilantro, chopped

Directions:
In the slow cooker, mix the eggs with Ricotta and the other ingredients and whisk. Close the lid and cook egg casserole on Low for 5 hours.
Nutrition Info:calories 179, fat 6.8, fiber 0.4, carbs 2.6, protein 6.3

55. Creamy Green Tea

Servings: 1   Cooking Time: 3 Hours
Ingredients:

1 teaspoon green tea powder	¾ teaspoon vanilla extract
1 cup heavy cream	½ cup walnuts, chopped
¼ teaspoon ground cinnamon	

Directions:
In the slow cooker, mix the cream with the green tea and the other ingredients and toss. Close the slow cooker lid and cook the mix for 3 hours on Low. Then strain the cooking liquid and transfer it into the serving cup.
Nutrition Info:calories 209, fat 11.8, fiber 4.3, carbs 2, protein 0.8

56. Green Beans Casserole

Servings: 6   Cooking Time: 9 Hours
Ingredients:

1-pound green beans, chopped	4 oz Mozzarella, sliced
4 oz Cheddar cheese, shredded	1 cup heavy cream
½ teaspoon curry powder	1 teaspoon chili flakes
1 teaspoon garam masala	1 teaspoon ground nutmeg
	1 teaspoon olive oil

Directions:
Spread the slow cooker bottom with the oil. Combine the green beans with the other ingredients except the Mozzarella and toss. Top the mix with Mozzarella slices and close the lid. Cook casserole for 9 hours on Low.
Nutrition Info:calories 362, fat 17.8, fiber 1.2, carbs 5, protein 12.5

57. Egg & Mushroom Breakfast

Servings: 4   Cooking Time: 6 Hours
Ingredients:

Bacon large - 3	Butter or ghee - 1 tablespoon
Eggs - 6	
Chopped shallots - 3 tablespoons	Pepper - ¼ spoon
Bell pepper, red - ½ cup	Salt to taste
	Spinach - for dressing
Shredded, kale leaves - 8 large	Avocado, sliced - for dressing
Parmesan cheese, shredded - 1 cup	Virgin olive oil - for dressing

Directions:
Wash, clean and slice the bacon   Wash, clean and remove the stem of the kale and chop it nicely. Take a pan and cook bacon until it becomes crispy. Add mushroom, pepper, and shallot and continue heating until it becomes soft.   Now add kale and switch off the stove and let the kale wilt.   Take a small mixing bowl and beat the eggs, with pepper and salt.   Put on the slow cooker and add some butter.   Grease the inside of the cooker properly with the butter.   Transfer the sautéed vegetables to the cooker.   Spread the cheese over it.   Add the beaten egg on top of the mixture.   Stir well and slow heat about 6 hours.   You may occasionally check the food after 4 hours.   Check with your finger to bounce back.   Serve it with sliced avocado, spread with spinach dressed in olive oil.
Nutrition Info: Total carbs 6.1 g Fiber 2.1 g Net carbs 4 g Fat 22.2 g Protein 22.9 g Saturated fat 9.8 g Energy313 kcal Magnesium 65 mg Potassium 503 mg

58. Coconut Avocado And Chicken Mix

Servings: 4   Cooking Time: 8 Hours
Ingredients:

1 avocado, pitted and roughly chopped	1 teaspoon olive oil
1/3 cup spring onions, chopped	½ teaspoon ground black pepper
3 oz Cheddar cheese, shredded	½ teaspoon salt
1 teaspoon turmeric powder	½ cup of coconut milk
	4 oz chicken fillet, chopped

Directions:
In the slow cooker, mix the avocado with spring onions and the other ingredients. Close the lid and cook avocado bake for 8 hours on Low.
Nutrition Info:calories 387, fat 22.1, fiber 4.5, carbs 7.9, protein 15.4

59. Avocado And Zucchini Bake

Servings: 2   Cooking Time: 2 Hours
Ingredients:

2 avocados, peeled, pitted and cubed	½ teaspoon almond extract
1 zucchini, grated	¾ teaspoon ground cinnamon
1 teaspoon turmeric powder	
1 teaspoon nutmeg, ground	1 tablespoon stevia extract
3 eggs, beaten	1 teaspoon butter
	¾ cup heavy cream

Directions:
In the slow cooker, mix the avocado with the zucchini, turmeric and the other ingredients, stir and spread into the slow cooker. Close the lid and cook egg Bake for 2 hours on High.
Nutrition Info:calories 214, fat 16.1, fiber 3.7, carbs 9.6, protein 10.5

60. Mexican Chicken Soup

Servings: 4   Cooking Time: 2 Hours
Ingredients:

One 28-ounce can of tomatoes	2 tablespoons no-sugar tomato paste
2 chopped cooked chicken breasts	1 handful of chopped parsley
2 seeded and diced	1 teaspoon cumin

jalapeno peppers
1 cup water
1 chopped red onion
4 minced garlic cloves

½ teaspoon chili powder
Drizzle of olive oil
Salt and pepper to taste

Directions:
Pour oil into a skillet and heat.   When hot, add ¼ cup broth, jalapenos, onion, garlic, salt, and pepper. When the onions and peppers are soft, pour into the slow cooker.   Pour in the rest of the ingredients, except parsley.   Close the lid.   Cook on low for 2 hours.   Chicken should be 165-degrees and very tender.   Shred chicken and serve!
Nutrition Info: Total calories: 135 Protein: 13 Carbs: 20 Fat: 3 Fiber: 2.5

61. Lovely Lentil Sausage Soup

Servings: 4   Cooking Time: 6-8 Hours
Ingredients:

2 tablespoons of butter
2 tablespoons of olive oil
5 cups of chicken stock
1 ½ cups of lentils
½ cup of diced carrots
4 minced cloves of garlic

1 cup of spinach
1 trimmed leek
1 diced celery rib
1 cup of heavy cream
½ cup of shredded Parmesan cheese
2 tablespoons of Dijon mustard
2 tablespoons of red wine vinegar
Salt and pepper

Directions:
Place the stock and the lentils into the slow cooker. In a saucepan, heat the olive oil and the butter and brown the sausage.   In the same saucepan, sauté the celery, pepper, salt, garlic, leek, spinach, onions and carrots for 10 minutes.   Pour the mixture into the slow cooker.   Cook on low for 6-8 hours. Spoon into bowls and serve.
Nutrition Info: Calories: 195 Fat: 14 g Carbohydrates: 4.9 gr Protein: 11 g

62. Chives And Sprouts Casserole

Servings: 4   Cooking Time: 7 Hours
Ingredients:

5 oz ham, chopped
1 cup Brussels sprouts, halved
3 eggs, beaten
¾ cup organic coconut milk

5 oz Parmesan, grated
1 tablespoon chives, chopped
1 teaspoon ground black pepper

Directions:
In the slow cooker, mix the sprouts with the ham and the other ingredients.   Close the lid and cook the casserole for 7 hours on Low.   When the casserole is cooked, open the lid and stir it one more time.
Nutrition Info:calories 304, fat 14.8, fiber 4.9, carbs 4.4, protein 19.4

63. Pork Chops With Cumin Butter And Garlic

Servings: 4   Cooking Time: 3-4 Hours
Ingredients:

3 tablespoons of butter
5 tablespoons of lime juice
½ teaspoon of ground cumin

½ cup of salsa
¾ teaspoon of garlic powder
¾ teaspoon of salt
¾ teaspoon of black pepper

Directions:
Combine the spices and season the pork chops. Melt the butter in a saucepan and brown the pork chops for 3 minutes on each side.   Place the chops into the slow cooker and pour the salsa over the top. Cover and cook on high for 3-4 hours.   Divide onto plates and serve.
Nutrition Info: Calories: 364 Fat: 17 grams Carbohydrates: 3 grams Fiber: 0 grams Protein: 51 grams

64. Ranch Chicken

Servings: 6   Cooking Time: 4 Hours And 5 Minutes
Ingredients:

3 tablespoons butter
4 oz. cream cheese

3 tablespoons ranch dressing mix

Directions:
Add the chicken to your slow cooker.   Place the butter and cream cheese on top of the chicken. Sprinkle ranch dressing mix.   Seal the pot. Cook on high for 4 hours.   Shred the chicken using forks and serve.
Nutrition Info: Calories 266 Total Fat 12.9 g Saturated Fat 8 g Cholesterol 102 mg Sodium 167 mg Potassium 450 mg Total Carbohydrate 8 g Dietary Fiber 0 g Protein 33 g Total Sugars 3 g

65. Baked Mushrooms With Pesto & Ricotta

Servings: 4   Cooking Time: 6 Hours
Ingredients:

16 large chestnut mushrooms
A 250-gram tub of ricotta
25 grams of freshly grated parmesan cheese

2 tablespoons of pesto
2 finely chopped cloves of garlic
2 tablespoons of fresh, chopped parsley

Directions:
Trim the mushroom stems level with the caps.   In a small bowl combine the garlic, pesto and ricotta, and spoon into the mushroom heads.   Place the mushroom caps in a slow cooker and cook on low for 4-6 hours.   In the last half-hour, sprinkle the parmesan cheese over the top of the mushrooms. Serve topped with the fresh parsley.
Nutrition Info: Calories: 400 grams Fat: 34 grams Carbohydrates: 2 grams Fiber: 1 gram Protein: 19 grams

66. Walnuts Yogurt

Servings: 3   Cooking Time: 12 Hours
Ingredients:

2 cups organic almond milk
1 cup walnuts, chopped
1 tablespoon yogurt starter
1 tablespoon stevia

Directions:
In the slow cooker, mix the milk with the other ingredients. Close the lid and cook yogurt on Low for 12 hours. When the time is over, the liquid should be thick. Pour yogurt into the serving ramekins.
Nutrition Info:calories 175, fat 3.4, fiber 3, carbs 8, protein 0.8

67. Chicken With Green Beans

Servings: 4   Cooking Time: 4 Hours
Ingredients:
2 cloves garlic, crushed and minced
2 tomatoes, diced
¼ cup dill, chopped
1 lb. green beans
1 tablespoon lemon juice
1 cup chicken broth
4 chicken thighs
Salt and pepper to taste
2 tablespoons olive oil

Directions:
Put the onion, garlic, tomatoes, dill and green beans in your slow cooker. Pour in the chicken broth and lemon juice. Season with salt and pepper. Mix well. Add the chicken on top of the vegetables. Drizzle chicken with oil. Cover the pot. Cook on high for 4 hours.
Nutrition Info: Calories 373 Total Fat 26 g Saturated Fat 6 g Cholesterol 111 mg Sodium 315 mg Potassium 726 mg Total Carbohydrate 14 g Dietary Fiber 4 g Protein 22 g Total Sugars 6 g

68. Sausage And Peppers

Servings: 8   Cooking Time: 6 Hours
Ingredients:
2 large yellow onions halved and thinly sliced
4 medium green bell peppers-halved from top to bottom, cleaned and thinly sliced
¼ cup of cold water
1 bay leaf
2 pounds uncooked Italian Sausage Links (about 6 to 8 sausages)) mild or spicy
28 ounces canned unsalted crushed tomatoes
1 tablespoon kosher salt
1 teaspoon Italian seasoning
¼ teaspoon dried oregano
½ teaspoon crushed red pepper flakes
Diced Italian parsley for serving- optional

Directions:
Thinly slice the garlic. Peel the onions and halve, then sliced. Add the chopped garlic and sliced onion into the crockpot insert. Remember to spray the crockpot with oil. Slice the bell peppers in half from top to bottom. Remove the ribs and any seeds in them. Then slice thinly. Add the sliced bell peppers to the crockpot as well as Italian seasoning, salt, crushed red pepper flakes, dried oregano, can have crushed tomatoes, and ¼ cup of water. Toss to coat and liquid is uniformly distributed. Take out almost half of the peppers and the onion mixture to a bowl. Immerse the uncooked sausage in the middle and then add the peppers and the onions back to the crockpot cover the sausage. Add the bay leaf. Cover, set to low, and cook for 6 hours. Top with some chopped parsley if desired. Serve hot.
Nutrition Info: Calories: 456 Fat: 36g Saturated Fat: 13g Cholesterol: 86mg Sodium: 1838mg Potassium: 746mg Carbs: 15g Fiber: 4g Sugar: 7g Protein: 19g

69. Thai-inspired Chicken Soup

Servings: 8   Cooking Time: 8 Hours
Ingredients:
One 14-ounce can of full-fat coconut milk
4-inch thumb of chopped ginger
1 chopped lemongrass stalk
Enough vegetable broth to cover chicken
Splash of Red Boat fish sauce
Salt to taste

Directions:
Put the whole chicken, ginger, and lemongrass in your slow cooker. Pour in coconut milk, and enough vegetable broth to cover chicken. Close the lid. Cook on low for 8-10 hours. When time is up, remove the chicken, and pull all the meat off the bones. Return meat to the soup. Taste, and season with salt and fish sauce as needed. Serve!
Nutrition Info: Total calories: 330 Protein: 22 Carbs: 2 Fat: 26 Fiber: 0

70. Delicious Bacon & Cheese Frittata

Servings: 8   Cooking Time: 2 Hours 30 Minutes
Ingredients:
2 tablespoons butter
8 oz. fresh spinach, packed down
1/2 cup heavy whipping cream
10 eggs
1/2 cup shredded cheese
Salt and pepper

Directions:
Butter or grease the inside of your slow-cooker. Loosely chop the spinach. Cut bacon into half inch pieces. Beat the eggs with the spices, cream, cheese and chopped spinach. Then everything will be blended smoothly. Line the bottom of the slow cooker with the bacon. Pour the egg mixture over the bacon. Cover the Slow Cookerand adjust the temperature to high Cook for 2 hours. Serve hot.
Nutrition Info: Calories: 392 Fat: 34g Carb: 4.5g Protein: 19g

71. Spinach Casserole

Servings: 2   Cooking Time: 3 Hours
Ingredients:
2 cups spinach
1 tablespoon spring onions, chopped
3 eggs, whisked
1/3 cup almond milk
½ teaspoon salt
½ teaspoon cayenne pepper
½ teaspoon olive oil
1 oz chorizo, chopped

Directions:
In the slow cooker, mix the spinach with spring onions, eggs and the other ingredients, stir and

spread into the pot.   Close the lid and cooked casserole for 3 hours on High.
Nutrition Info:calories 207, fat 13.9, fiber 5.1, carbs 6.1, protein 5.4

72. Ricotta Cheese And Almond Mini Pancakes

Servings: 2   Cooking Time: Approximately 2 Hours
Ingredients:

1 cup ricotta cheese	1 tsp vanilla extract
2 eggs	1 tsp cinnamon
½ cup ground almonds	

Directions:
In a medium-sized bowl, mix together the ricotta cheese, eggs, ground almonds, vanilla, cinnamon, and a small pinch of salt.   Drizzle some coconut oil into the Crock Pot.   Place dollops of pancake batter into the pot, don't worry if the pancakes run together a bit, you can simply detach them when you flip them.   Place the lid onto the pot and set the temperature to LOW.   Cook for 2 hours, flip the pancakes once, after the 1-hour mark.   Serve the pancakes warm, with a few fresh berries!.

73. Bacon And Spiced Egg Bake

Servings: 2   Cooking Time: Approximately 1 Hour
Ingredients:

4 eggs	4 slices streaky bacon
½ tsp mixed spices – paprika, chili powder, cumin	Fresh parsley, finely chopped

Directions:
Drizzle some olive oil into the Crock pot.   In a small bowl, lightly beat the eggs.   Add the spices to the eggs with a pinch of salt and pepper, stir to combine.   Lay the bacon slices on the bottom of the Crock Pot.   Pour the egg mixture over the bacon.   Place the lid onto the pot and set the temperature to LOW.   Cook for 1 hour or until the egg has set.   Heat some oil in a skillet or frying pan. Transfer the bacon and eggs in one piece to the pan and fry for 2 minutes until the bacon is crispy. Serve on 2 plates with a sprinkling of fresh parsley.

74. Rice & Shrimp Frittata

Servings: 4   Cooking Time: 2 Hours
Ingredients:

1/2 cup of shrimp, cooked, peeled, deveined and diced	Salt and black pepper- to taste
1/2 cup of baby spinach, chopped	1/2 cup of cauliflower rice, cooked
1/2 teaspoon of basil, dried	1/2 cup of Monterey jack cheese, grated
Cooking spray	

Directions:
Start by greasing the base of your Crockpot. Spread the shrimp and spinach at the base of the pot. Whisk the egg with remaining Ingredients: and pour into crockpot.   Cover your crockpot and select the Low settings for 2 hours.   Remove the crockpot's lid.   Serve warm.
Nutrition Info: Calories 399 Total Fat 17.4 g Saturated Fat 11.3 g Cholesterol 47 mg Total Carbs 9.9 g Sugar 5.5 g Fiber 4.3 g Sodium 192 mg Protein 12.4 g

75. Oozing Ground Beef Shawarma

Servings: 4   Cooking Time: 20 Minutes
Ingredients:

1 cup of onions, sliced	2 cups of cabbage, chopped
1 cup of red peppers, thickly sliced	2 tablespoons of shawarma mix
1 teaspoon of salt	

Directions:
Press the "Sautee/Browning" button on the Crock-Pot Express and add the ground beef. Cook until the beef is brown, breaking up the meat into smaller bits using a metal or wooden spoon.   Add the onions, red peppers, cabbage, shawarma mix, and salt to the Crock-Pot Express. Stir until well combined. Lock the lid and ensure the valve is closed.   Press the "Meat/Stew" button and set the time to 2 minutes.   When the cooking is done, naturally release the pressure for 5 minutes, then manually release the remaining pressure. Remove the lid. Serve and enjoy!
Nutrition Info: Calories: 191 Fat: 5g Carbohydrates: 8g Dietary Fiber: 2g Protein: 25g

76. Barbecue Beef Stew

Servings: 6   Cooking Time: 8 Hours
Ingredients:

1 jar/homemade (7 oz.) tomato paste	1 t. kosher salt
Balsamic vinegar	2 lb. extra-lean stew beef meat/boneless chuck roast
½ t. black pepper	
1 t. of each Smoked paprika	1 tbsp. olive oil
1 t. of kosher salt	½ t. black pepper
1 t. of Garlic powder	2 tbsp. cold tap water
2 tbsp. sweetener – ex. xylitol	1 tbsp. cornstarch or ½ t. konjac flour
For the Stew	14-inch skillet

Directions:
Chop the meat into one-inch pieces, and season it with pepper and salt.   Combine the barbecue sauce ingredients.   Prepare the skillet by adding the half of the oil using the med-high setting for three minutes.   Add half of the beef and cook about five minutes. Place in the slow cooker.   Add the rest of the oil and cook the second half of beef and add it also.   Empty the sauce over the prepared meat and stir. Place the top on the pot and cook for 7 ½ hours on low.   Whisk in the cornstarch and water together in a dish until smooth. Empty it into the beef juices. Set the slow cooker on high for 30 minutes.   When thickened to your liking, serve and enjoy.
Nutrition Info:445 Calories 10 g Net Carbs 30 g Protein 29 g Fat

77. Dill And Avocado Frittata

Servings: 4   Cooking Time: 2 Hours

Ingredients:

2 avocados, peeled, pitted and mashed	4 eggs, whisked
1 teaspoon green curry paste	1 teaspoon butter, softened
1 tablespoon fresh dill, chopped	2 oz Mozzarella, shredded

Directions:
Brush the slow cooker with softened butter from inside.   Combine the eggs with avocados and the other ingredients, stir and spread into the pot. Close the lid of the slow cooker and cook the frittata for 2 hours on High.
Nutrition Info:calories 324, fat 11.7, fiber 0.8, carbs 3.6, protein 10.7

78. Chicken Meatballs

Servings: 4   Cooking Time: 6.5 Hours
Ingredients:

1 ½ cup ground chicken meat	½ teaspoon salt
2 tablespoons oregano, chopped	2 red chilies, minced
1 teaspoon coriander, ground	1 teaspoon chili flakes
1 egg, beaten	¼ cup tomatoes, crushed
1 tablespoon coconut flour	¾ cup heavy cream
	1 teaspoon olive oil

Directions:
In a bowl, mix the chicken with the oregano and the other ingredients except the cream, oil and tomatoes, stir and make the medium-sized meatballs with the help of the fingertips.   Place the rest of the ingredients in the slow cooker.   Place the meatballs in the slow cooker to make 1 layer. Close the lid and cook meatballs for 6.5 hours on Low.
Nutrition Info:calories 303, fat 15.2, fiber 4.3, carbs 2.8, protein 13.3

79. Tasty Sausage & Eggplant Bake

Servings: 4   Cooking Time: 4 Hours
Ingredients:

1 tablespoon of olive oil	1 tablespoon of mustard
2 pounds of spicy pork sausage	2 cans of Italian diced tomatoes
1 tablespoon of Worcestershire sauce	2 cups of shredded mozzarella cheese
1 jar of tomato paste	

Directions:
Use the olive oil to grease the crock pot.   In a large bowl, combine the sausage, mustard and Worcestershire sauce and tomato paste; then add to the crock pot.   Add the eggplant on top of the sausage mixture.   Pour the tomatoes on top of the mixture; sprinkle the cheese over the top.   Cook the ingredients for 4 hours on low.
Nutrition Info: Carbohydrates: 6 grams Protein: 15 grams Calories: 210 grams Fat: 12 grams

80. Breakfast Ground Beef Casserole

Servings: 4   Cooking Time: 7 Hours
Ingredients:

8 oz ground beef	2 tablespoons butter
1 zucchini, chopped	1 teaspoon chili flakes
2 garlic cloves, chopped	1 teaspoon ground black pepper
3 oz mushrooms, chopped	½ teaspoon salt

Directions:
Place the chopped zucchini in the slow cooker. Sprinkle the zucchini with the chopped garlic cloves. Add chili flakes and ground black pepper.   Mix together salt and ground beef then add the butter and mix again.   Transfer the ground beef mixture to the slow cooker.   Add mushrooms and close the lid.   Cook for 7 hours on Low.   When the time is done, let the cooked casserole cool slightly.   Enjoy!
Nutrition Info:calories 172, fat 9.5, fiber 0.9, carbs 3.2, protein 18.7

81. Cilantro Pork Meatballs

Servings: 2   Cooking Time: 3 Hours
Ingredients:

½ cup ground pork	1 tablespoon cilantro, chopped
1 egg, beaten	1/2 cup coconut milk
1 teaspoon ground black pepper	1 teaspoon coconut oil
½ teaspoon salt	1 teaspoon chili flakes
½ teaspoon dried basil	1 jalapeno pepper, chopped
½ teaspoon oregano, dried	

Directions:
In a bowl, mix the pork with the egg and the other ingredients except the oil and the coconut milk, stir and shape medium meatballs.   Grease the slow cooker with the oil, add the milk and meatballs. Close the lid and cook meatballs for 3 hours on High. The time of cooking depends on meatballs size.
Nutrition Info:calories 202, fat 13.7, fiber 3.8, carbs 3, protein 12.2

82. Stuffed Peppers

Servings: 4   Cooking Time: 7 Hours
Ingredients:

2 yellow sweet peppers, deseeded and halved	½ teaspoon salt
1 cup ground turkey meat	1 tablespoon red curry paste
½ teaspoon ground black pepper	1 teaspoon oregano, dried
½ teaspoon garam masala	2 teaspoons butter
	2 oz Cheddar cheese, shredded
	¼ cup of water

Directions:
In the mixing bowl, mix up together the meat with salt, pepper and the other ingredients except the cheese and water, stir and stuff the peppers with this. Sprinkle the pepper halves with shredded Cheddar cheese.   Pour water in the slow cooker. Carefully add sweet pepper halves in the slow cooker and close the lid.   Cook the meal for 7 hours on Low.
Nutrition Info:calories 359, fat 10.9, fiber 4.3, carbs 5, protein 10.7

83. Creamy Chicken Soup

Servings: 4   Cooking Time: 8 Hours
Ingredients:

4 cups chicken stock	2 minced garlic cloves
1 cup heavy cream	1 teaspoon dried
2 chopped carrots	thyme
2 chopped celery	Salt and pepper to
stalks	taste
1 diced sweet onion	

Directions:
Put all the ingredients (except cream) into your slow cooker.   Cook on low for 8 hours.   When there are thirty minutes left to go, add cream.   When time is up, taste and season more with salt and pepper if needed.   Serve hot!
Nutrition Info: Total calories: 123 Protein: 16 Carbs: 10 Fat: 3 Fiber: 1

84. Vanilla Pancakes(2)

Servings: 6   Cooking Time: 2 Hours
Ingredients:

1 cup almond flour	½ cup almond milk
¼ cup coconut flour	4 tablespoons water
1 teaspoon stevia	1 teaspoon olive oil
extract	1 teaspoon vanilla
4 eggs, beaten	extract

Directions:
Mix together the almond flour and coconut flour. Add stevia extract and beaten eggs and stir well. Add almond milk and water and blend.   Add the vanilla extract and olive oil and mix until smooth. Pour the pancake batter into the slow cooker and cover.   Cook the pancake for 2 hours on High. Let the cooked pancake cool a little.   Enjoy!
Nutrition Info:calories 143, fat 11.3, fiber 2.9, carbs 5.8, protein 5.8

85. Zucchini Quiche

Servings: 6   Cooking Time: 7.5 Hours
Ingredients:

2 oz zucchinis, grated	4 eggs, beaten
1 cup spring onions,	½ teaspoon salt
chopped	1 teaspoon curry
1 teaspoon ground	powder
black pepper	1 teaspoon oregano,
	dried

Directions:
In the bowl, combine the eggs with the zucchinis and the other ingredients, toss, pour into the slow cooker and spread.   Close the lid and cook the quiche for 7.5 hours on Low.   Chill the cooked quiche well and then slice it into the servings.
Nutrition Info:calories 271, fat 5.7, fiber 4.4, carbs 11.2, protein 8.4

86. Onion Zucchini Hash

Servings: 2   Cooking Time: 3 Hours
Ingredients:

2 teaspoon of olive oil	1 yellow onion, diced
2 eggs, room	1 green bell pepper,
temperature	diced
1/2 teaspoon of	Salt and black
thyme, dried	pepper- to taste

Directions:
Start by greasing the base of your Crockpot with cooking spray.   Whisk the egg with all other Ingredients: and pour into crockpot.   Cover your crockpot and select the Low settings for 3 hours. Remove the crockpot's lid.   Serve warm.
Nutrition Info: Calories 212 Total Fat 15.7 g Saturated Fat 9.7 g Cholesterol 49 mg Total Carbs 46 g Sugar 3.4 g Fiber 1.5 g Sodium 141 mg Protein 8.5 g

87. Cinnamon Eggs

Servings: 4   Cooking Time: 8 Hours / 2.5 Hours
Ingredients:

1 teaspoon almond	1 tablespoon stevia
extract	4 eggs, beaten
½ teaspoon ground	1/3 cup coconut
cinnamon	cream
	Cooking spray

Directions:
In the mixer bowl, combine the eggs with the other ingredients except the coking spray.   Mix the mixture until homogenous.   Then spray the slow cooker pot with cooking spray.   Transfer the sweet egg mixture in the slow cooker and close the lid. Cook the breakfast bake for 8 hours on Low or 2.5 hours on High.
Nutrition Info:calories 216, fat 11.5, fiber 4.3, carbs 4.9, protein 4.8

88. Mushroom Spinach Breakfast

Servings: 4   Cooking Time: 3 Hours
Ingredients:

7 oz. baby spinach	4 eggs, room
8 chestnuts	temperature
mushrooms, halved	4 bacon strips, diced
8 tomatoes, halved	Salt and black
1 garlic clove, minced	pepper- to taste
	Cooking spray

Directions:
Start by greasing the base of your Crockpot. Whisk spinach with all other Ingredients: and spread into the crockpot.   Make four wells into this mixture and crack on egg into each well. Cover your crockpot and select the Low settings for 3 hours.   Remove the crockpot's lid.   Serve.
Nutrition Info: Calories 393 Total Fat 15.8 g Saturated Fat 10.3 g Cholesterol 47 mg Total Carbs 4.1 g Sugar 0.4 g Fiber 0.4 g Sodium 421 mg Protein 12.6 g

89. Mediterranean Meatloaf

Servings: 6   Cooking Time: 6 Hours
Ingredients:

2 large eggs	2 Tablespoons olive
2 small zucchini,	oil
shredded and drained	1 Tablespoon dry
1 red onion, cut small	oregano
1 red bell pepper, cut	Salt and pepper to
in small cubes	taste
1 cup hard cheese of	Topping:
your preference –	¼ cup of ketchup
Parmesan or	2 Tablespoons
Cheddar, shredded	shredded cheese

Directions:
Place all ingredients, except topping, in a mixing bowl and combine well by hand.   Make 4 folded strips of aluminum foil and lay across bottom of crock-pot in a crisscross pattern.   Sprinkle olive oil across the foil, bottom of the crock-pot and sides. Form one meat loaf from meat mixture, place on top of foil grid.   Cover, cook on low for 6 hours or on high for 3 hours.   Remove the lid, spread the ketchup on top of meatloaf. Sprinkle with cheese, cook for an additional 5 minutes to melt the cheese.
Nutrition Info: Carbs 8g Protein 23g Fiber 39g

90. Mouth-watering Cauliflower & Cheese Bake

Servings: 4   Cooking Time: 4 Hours
Ingredients:

½ cup of cream cheese	½ teaspoon of ground black pepper
¼ cup of whipping cream	½ cup of shredded cheddar cheese
3 tablespoons of butter or lard, divided	6 slices of crispy bacon, crumbled
1 teaspoon of salt	

Directions:
Use 1 tablespoon of butter or lard to grease the crock-pot.   Add the remaining ingredients to the crock-pot except the bacon and cheddar cheese. Cook for 3 hours on low.   Remove the lid and add the cheddar cheese. Cover and cook for another hour. Sprinkle the bacon over the top. Divide onto plates and serve.
Nutrition Info: Carbohydrates: 3 grams Protein: 11 grams Fat: 20 grams Calories: 232

91. Green Chile Chicken Soup

Servings: 6   Cooking Time: 8 Hours
Ingredients:

4 cups chicken broth	1 bell pepper, diced
1/2 lime juice	1 onion, diced
1 tsp paprika	2 jalapeno peppers, minced
1 tsp oregano	
1 tsp cumin	5 garlic cloves, minced
7 oz. can green chilies, diced	1 tsp salt

Directions:
Add all ingredients to the slow cooker and stir well to mix.   Cover and cook on low for 8 hours. Shred the chicken using a fork and stir well.   Serve hot and enjoy.
Nutrition Info: Calories 198 Fat 6.8 g Carbohydrates 6.9 g Sugar 3.7 g Protein 25.9 g Cholesterol 67 mg Fiber 1.2 g Net carbs 5.7 g

92. Berry Pudding

Servings: 6   Cooking Time: 3 Hours
Ingredients:

2 cups of almond milk	1/3 cup chia seeds
2 tablespoons strawberry, sliced	2 tablespoons blueberries
2 tablespoons blackberries	2 tablespoons stevia

Directions:
In the slow cooker, mix the berries with the milk and the rest of the ingredients.   Close the slow cooker lid and cook the pudding for 3 hours on Low. When the pudding is cooked, transfer it into the serving ramekins and serve.
Nutrition Info:calories 131, fat 5.2, fiber 5.1, carbs 3.7, protein 3.4

93. Roasted Chicken With Lemon & Parsley Butter

Servings: 2   Cooking Time: 8 Hours
Ingredients:

1 whole lemon, sliced	1 tbsp. parsley, chopped
2 tbsp. butter or ghee	

Directions:
Rub chicken all over with salt and pepper to taste. Put it in the crockpot and pour 1 cup of water. Cover and cook for 3 hours on high.   When cooked, add the lemon slices butter and parsley to the crockpot.   Cook and cover for another 10 minutes.
Nutrition Info: Calories: 300 Fat: 18 g Net carbs: 1 g Protein: 29 g

94. Breakfast Shredded Pork

Servings: 5   Cooking Time: 10 Hours
Ingredients:

1-pound pork chops	1 teaspoon salt
1 cup chicken stock	1 teaspoon full-fat cream
1 teaspoon thyme	
1 garlic clove	

Directions:
Sprinkle the pork chops with the thyme and salt. Chop the garlic clove and place it in the slow cooker. Add full-fat cream and pork chops.   Then add the chicken stock and close the lid.   Cook the pork chops for 10 hours on low.   When the time is done, transfer all the content of the slow cooker to a big bowl.   Shred the pork with forks and serve it!
Nutrition Info:calories 295, fat 22.8, fiber 0.1, carbs 0.5, protein 20.6

95. Breakfast Meatloaf

Servings: 5   Cooking Time: 3 1/2 Hours
Ingredients:

1 red onion, chopped	2 eggs, beaten
1 garlic clove	1 tbsp. of almond flour
1 tbsp. of coconut oil	
1 tbsp. of fresh sage or chives, chopped	⅔ cup cheddar cheese
1 tsp of paprika	Salt
	Pepper

Directions:
Combine all the ingredients together in a bowl. Lightly grease the bottom of the slow cooker, form the mixture into a meatloaf, and carefully place inside the slow cooker, making sure it doesn't touch the sides.   Set on high heat and cook for 3 hours. Pour the cheddar cheese during the last 20 minutes of cooking to melt.   Remove from the slow cooker and let sit for at least 10 minutes prior cutting and serving.
Nutrition Info: Calories: 280 Fat: 22g Carbs: 7g Protein: 15g.

96. Basil Sprouts And Eggs

Servings: 6   Cooking Time: 7 Hours

Ingredients:

1 cup Brussels sprouts, trimmed and shredded	1 teaspoon ground black pepper
1 tablespoon basil, chopped	1 teaspoon butter
1 tablespoon yellow curry paste	½ cup of coconut milk
½ teaspoon salt	3 eggs, beaten
	½ teaspoon chili powder

Directions:

Spread the slow cooker bottom with the butter. Combine the sprouts with the basil and the other ingredients.   Close the slow cooker lid.   Cook the meal for 7 hours on Low.

Nutrition Info:calories 321, fat 7.9, fiber 3.8, carbs 12.6, protein 4.6

97. Cheesy Chicken Pot

Cooking Time: 8 Hours

Ingredients:

2 tablespoons / 28 gr of white onion, chopped	2 tablespoons / 28 gr of ghee
2 tablespoons / 28 gr of carrots, finely chopped	1 pinch of oregano
	1 pinch of time
1 tablespoon / 14 gr of Cheddar cheese, diced	1 tablespoon / 14 gr of cocoa butter
	¼ cup / 100 gr of sour cream

Directions:

Pour all of your ingredients in the Slow Cooker pot, except for the sour cream, cocoa butter, and Cheddar and ghee   Cover and cook on LOW for 8 hours and pour the sour cream, cheddar and ghee in Cook for another half an hour without the lid

Nutrition Info: Calories: 590 Fat: 50 g Total carbs: 5.5 Net carbs: 5.5 Protein 35 g

98. Chili Tomatoes Bowls

Servings: 4   Cooking Time: 1.15 Hour

Ingredients:

4 eggs, beaten	4 tomatoes, chopped
1 chili pepper, minced	2 shallots, chopped
1 teaspoon curry powder	1 tablespoon butter
	½ teaspoon salt
1 teaspoon sweet paprika	1 teaspoon dried parsley

Directions:

Put butter in the slow cooker.   Add the eggs, tomatoes and all the other ingredients.   Stir gently and close the lid. Cook on High for 1 hour and 15 minutes.   Divide into bowls and serve.

Nutrition Info:calories 201, fat 7.5, fiber 1.4, carbs 6.3, protein 6.5

99. Coconut Chip Rice Pudding

Servings: 2   Cooking Time: 2.5 Hours

Ingredients:

1/2 cup of coconut chips	2 cups of water
	1/4 cup of raisins
1 cup of almond milk	1/4 cup of almonds
1/2 cup of maple syrup	A pinch Cinnamon powders

Directions:

Start by throwing all the Ingredients: into the Crockpot.   Cover your crockpot and select the Low settings for 2 1/2 hours.   Remove the crockpot's lid.   Serve fresh.

Nutrition Info: Calories 432 Total Fat 42.3 g Saturated Fat 26.7 g Cholesterol 144 mg Total Carbs 47 g Sugar 5.6 g Fiber 4.5 g Sodium 148 mg Protein 4.2 g

100.   Veggie Pot Pie

Servings: 6   Cooking Time: 4 Hours

Ingredients:

½ cup of diced onions	¼ cup of cornstarch
4 cloves of minced garlic	¼ cup of heavy cream
Fresh thyme, finely chopped	Salt and pepper
½ cup of flour	1 thawed frozen puff pastry sheet
2 cups of chicken broth	2 tablespoons of butter

Directions:

Add the chopped veggies to the slow cooker as well as the garlic and onions.   Add the flour.   Add the broth and stir until everything is well blended. Cover and cook for 3-4 hours on high.   In a small bowl, combine the cornstarch and ¼ cup of water and whisk together thoroughly. Add the cornstarch mix to the slow cooker.   Add the cream, cover and continue to cook until the mixture thickens, approximately 15 minutes.   Transfer the vegetable mixture into a baking dish.   Lay the puff pastry over the top.   Melt the butter and brush it over the top of the pastry.   Bake at 350 degrees for 10 minutes until the pastry turns fluffy and golden. Divide onto dishes and serve

Nutrition Info: Calories: 325 Fat: 0.8 grams Protein: 4.5 grams Carbohydrates: 6.7 grams

101.Avocado Boats

Servings: 2   Cooking Time: 2 Hours

Ingredients:

1 avocado, pitted, halved	2 eggs, whisked
¾ teaspoon ground black pepper	¾ teaspoon salt
	2 teaspoons butter

Directions:

Place the avocado halves in the slow cooker.   Put the butter in both holes of the avocado halves. Then pour the eggs into the avocado holes. Sprinkle the eggs with the ground black pepper and salt.   Close the lid and cook the boats for 2 hours on High.   When the eggs are cooked, serve the avocado boats hot.

Nutrition Info:calories 304, fat 27.8, fiber 6.9, carbs 9.5, protein 7.6

102.   Breakfast Sausage Casserole

Servings: 6   Cooking Time: 3 Hours 10 Minutes

Ingredients:

½ cup chopped green bell pepper
½ cup chopped red bell pepper
1 tablespoon ghee
12 large eggs
1 tablespoon nutritional yeast
1 teaspoon dry rubbed sage
½ cup of coconut milk
1 teaspoon dried thyme
½ teaspoon garlic powder
½ teaspoon ground black pepper
½ teaspoon salt
½ cup sliced red onion

Directions:
Heat a medium cast-iron skillet over medium heat for 2 minutes. Add the pork sausage; then break it into small crumbles. Cook for 3 minutes. Stir in the black pepper, sea salt, thyme, sage, and garlic powder. Cook for an additional 5 minutes. Turn the heat off. Stir in the bell peppers and the chopped onion. Coat the bowl of the crockpot with ghee. Add the pork and vegetable mixture into the bottom of the crockpot. Whisk the coconut milk, nutritional yeast, and the eggs until the eggs are well incorporated together in a large bowl. Pour it into the crockpot on top of the pork mixture. Cover and cook on low for 2 to 3 hours, until the eggs are cooked through. Chop into 6 servings. Serve hot.

103.	Feta Eggs

Servings: 2   Cooking Time: 2 Hours
Ingredients:
4 eggs, beaten
1 tablespoon chives, chopped
1 tablespoon coconut cream
1 tablespoon Ricotta cheese
2 oz Feta, crumbled
1/3 teaspoon salt
½ teaspoon white pepper
1 teaspoon butter, melted

Directions:
In the slow cooker, mix the eggs with cream, chives and the other ingredients and toss. Close the lid and cook egg mix for 2 hours on high.
Nutrition Info:calories 266, fat 16.5, fiber 4.5, carbs 4.7, protein 15.4

104.	Pork Shoulder Roast

Servings: 6.   Cooking Time: 8 Hours
Ingredients:
1 can Italian diced tomatoes
1 sweet onion, diced
3 garlic cloves, diced
4 Tablespoons lard
1 cup water
1 bay leaf
¼ teaspoon ground cloves
Salt and pepper to taste

Directions:
Place meat in crock-pot, pour water and tomatoes over it, so the liquid covers 1/3 of the meat. Add remaining ingredients. Cover, cook on low for 8 hours.
Nutrition Info: Carbs: 10g Protein: 43g Fiber: 36g

105.	Coconut Sausage Mix

Servings: 3   Cooking Time: 4 Hours
Ingredients:
6 oz sausages, chopped
½ cup coconut cream
1 teaspoon turmeric powder
½ teaspoon cayenne pepper
2 egg, whisked
1/2 cup Parmesan, grated
¼ teaspoon ground black pepper
1 tablespoon fresh parsley, chopped

Directions:
In the slow cooker, mix the sausages with the cream and the other ingredients and toss. Close the lid. Cook casserole for 4 hours on High.
Nutrition Info:calories 403, fat 29.5, fiber 1.9, carbs 5.9, protein 14.4

106.	Beef Meatloaf

Servings: 8   Cooking Time: 5 Hours
Ingredients:
2 cups beef meat, ground
1 egg
2 tablespoons chives, chopped
½ cup tomatoes, cubed
1 teaspoon smoked paprika
1 teaspoon salt
1 teaspoon chili flakes
2 tablespoon fresh basil, chopped
1 teaspoon keto tomato sauce
1 teaspoon Ricotta cheese

Directions:
Line the slow cooker bottom with the baking paper. In a bowl, mix the beef with the egg and the other ingredients except the cheese and tomato sauce Mix up together Ricotta cheese and tomato sauce in the shallow bowl. Spread the uncooked meatloaf with the tomato spread. Close the slow cooker lid and cook meatloaf for 5 hours on High. Cool down, slice and serve.
Nutrition Info:calories 269, fat 11.8, fiber 4.3, carbs 8.6, protein 14.3

107.	Cream Of Zucchini Soup

Servings: 4   Cooking Time: 2 Hours
Ingredients:
2 pounds chopped zucchini
2 minced garlic cloves
¾ cup chopped onion
¼ cup basil leaves
1 tablespoon extra-virgin olive oil
Salt and pepper to taste

Directions:
Heat olive oil in a skillet. When hot, cook garlic and onion for about 5 minutes. Pour into your slow cooker with the rest of the ingredients. Close the lid. Cook on low for 2 hours. When time is up, puree the soup with an immersion blender, or in batches in a regular blender. Taste and season more if needed!
Nutrition Info: Total calories: 96 Protein: 7 Carbs: 11 Fat: 5 Fiber: 2.3

108. Crack Chicken(2)

Servings: 2   Cooking Time: 8 Hours
Ingredients:

1 packet of Ranch dressing	2 slices bacon, cooked and crumbled
4 oz. cream cheese	

Directions:
Put the chicken breast in the crockpot.   Pour the dressing in and add the cream cheese.   Cover and cook for 8 hours on low.   Mix in the crumbled bacon when cooked.
Nutrition Info: Calories: 410 Fat: 32 g Net carbs: 4 g Protein: 28 g

109. Mushroom And Brie "melters"

Servings: 6 As A Starter   Cooking Time: Approximately 2 Hours
Ingredients:

12 medium-sized brown mushrooms (Swiss Browns are ideal)	1/3 lb wheel of brie, cut or torn into 12 pieces
3 garlic cloves, crushed	2 tsp chopped fresh or dried parsley

Directions:
Drizzle some olive oil into the Crock Pot.   Lay the mushrooms on a board and rub them with olive oil. Sprinkle the crushed garlic, herbs, salt, and pepper evenly over the mushrooms.   Place a piece of brie on top of each mushroom.   Very carefully transfer the mushrooms to the Slow Cookerand lay in a single layer.   Place the lid onto the pot and set the temperature to HIGH.   Cook for 2 hours.   Heat a small drizzle of olive oil on a fry pan or skillet. Transfer the cooked mushrooms to the skillet and sauté for about 1 minute to get the mushrooms golden on the bottom (you can skip this step if you prefer softer mushrooms, but I like the slightly charred flavor) .   Serve on a platter with a sprinkling of grated parmesan cheese if you want to get extra fancy!

110. Lovely Sausage Casserole Breakfast

Servings: 4   Cooking Time: 4-5 Hours
Ingredients:

1 ½ cups of low fat milk	1 chopped red bell pepper
1 pound of cooked bulk sausage, drained	¾ cup sliced green onions
1 seeded and chopped jalapeño	2 cups of low fat Mexican blend cheese
9 corn tortillas	½ cup of salsa

Directions:
In a large bowl, whisk together the eggs, jalapeño and milk.   In another large bowl combine the cheese, green onions, sausage and red bell pepper. Arrange 3 tortillas on the base of a greased slow cooker.   Spread a layer of the sausage mixture over the tortillas.   Repeat the layering and then pour the egg mixture over the top.   Cover and cook on low for 4-5 hours.   Divide onto plates and serve with the salsa.
Nutrition Info: Calories: 386 Fat: 24 g Fiber: 2.6 g Protein: 24.7 g

111. Puff Spinach Salmon

Cooking Time: 4 Hours
Ingredients:

1 clove / 3 gr of garlic, minced	2 tablespoons / 28 gr of fresh spinach, chopped
2 tablespoons / 28 gr of kitchen cream	1 tablespoon / 4 gr of powdered saffron
2 tablespoons / 28 gr of ghee	1 pinch of salt and pepper
2 tablespoons / 28 gr of olive oil	

Directions:
Clean wash and chop the fresh spinach   Pour the spinach on the bottom of your Slow Cooker pot and sprinkle with ghee and minced garlic. Place over the some slices of salmon   Adjust the dressing. Repeat the operation by forming layers   Mix the cream with the saffron in a small bowl   Pour over the cream mixed with saffron, sprinkle it over the fish layers   Cover the Slow Cooker and cook on LOW for 3 hours
Nutrition Info: Calories: 883 Fat: 61.2 g Total carbs: 4.28 Net carbs: 4.28 Protein 42.36 g

112. Sesame Ginger Chicken

Servings: 4   Cooking Time: 5 Hours
Ingredients:

½ cup tomato sauce	2 cloves garlic, minced
¼ cup low-sugar peach jam	¼ cup onion, minced
¼ cup chicken broth	
2 tablespoons coconut aminos	¼ teaspoon red pepper flakes, crushed
1 ½ tablespoons sesame oil	2 tablespoons red bell pepper, chopped
1 tablespoon honey	
1 teaspoon ground ginger	1 ½ tablespoons green onion, chopped
	2 teaspoons sesame seeds

Directions:
Combine all the ingredients except green onion and sesame seeds in your slow cooker.   Mix well. Cover the pot and cook on high for 4 hours. Garnish with the green onion and sesame seeds.
Nutrition Info: Calories 220 Total Fat 13 g Saturated Fat 8 g Cholesterol 100 mg Sodium 246 mg Potassium 550 mg Total Carbohydrate 7 g Dietary Fiber 1 g Protein 26 g Total Sugars 2 g

113. Eggplant Parmesan

Servings: 12   Cooking Time: 8 Hours
Ingredients:

1 tablespoon of salt	2 teaspoons of Italian seasoning
3 large eggs	4 cups of marinara sauce
¼ cup of milk	
1 ½ cup of breadcrumbs	16 ounces of mozzarella cheese

3 ounces of parmesan
cheese
Directions:
Peel the eggplant and cut it into 1/3 inch-rounds.
Layer the eggplant in a colander and sprinkle each
layer with salt. Let sit for 30 minutes and then rinse
and pat dry.   Spread ½ cup of sauce on the bottom
of the slow cooker.   In a small bowl, whisk
together the milk and eggs.   In another small bowl,
whisk together the Italian seasoning, Parmesan
cheese and breadcrumbs.   Dip the eggplant into
the egg mixture and then into the breadcrumb
mixture.   Layer 1/3 of the slices in the slow cooker.
Pour 1 cup of sauce and the mozzarella cheese over
the top.   Repeat twice, cover and cook for 8 hours.
Divide onto plates and serve.
Nutrition Info: Calories: 258 Carbohydrates: 23
grams Fiber: 6 grams Fat: 6 grams Protein: 16
grams

114. Salmon And Asparagus With Herb Butter

Servings: 4   Cooking Time: Approximately 2
Hours
Ingredients:

20 asparagus spears, (5 spears per person)	2 garlic cloves, crushed
2 tsp fresh herbs, finely chopped – use any herbs you have, I like rosemary, mint, oregano, thyme and sage	1 tsp dried chili flakes
	3 tbsp butter
	3 ounces smoked salmon

Directions:
Drizzle some olive oil into the Crock Pot.   Lay the
asparagus into the Slow Cookerand sprinkle the
garlic, chili, salt, and pepper over the top, toss the
asparagus to combine.   Drizzle some more olive
oil over the asparagus.   Place the lid onto the pot
and set the temperature to HIGH.   Cook for 2
hours.   While the asparagus cooks, prepare the
herb butter by mixing the butter, herbs, salt, and
pepper together and store in the fridge until needed.
Once the asparagus has finished cooking, place on
plates while hot, with a dollop of herb butter on top.
Drape the smoked salmon over the asparagus and
serve immediately.

115. Ham And Kale Bake

Servings: 2   Cooking Time: 2 Hours
Ingredients:

2 ounces Mozzarella, shredded	½ teaspoon salt
½ cup kale	½ teaspoon smoked paprika
1 cup ham, chopped	½ teaspoon olive oil
1 egg, whisked	

Directions:
Brush the slow cooker with the oil from inside.
Combine the kale with ham and the other
ingredients and spread into the pan.   Close the
slow cooker lid and cook the meal for 2 hours on
High.
Nutrition Info:calories 235, fat 12.3, fiber 0.9,
carbs 4.6, protein 20.3

116. Salmon Cutlets

Servings: 2   Cooking Time: 2 Hours
Ingredients:

8 oz salmon fillet, chopped	1 tablespoon coconut flour
1 garlic clove, chopped	1/3 teaspoon ground black pepper
1 oz onion, chopped	¾ teaspoon salt
1 tablespoon almond flour	1 tablespoon butter

Directions:
Mix up together the chopped salmon fillet, garlic,
and onion.   Add ground black pepper and salt
then stir the mixture well.   Add the almond flour
and coconut flour.   Stir the mixture well.   Form
medium cutlets from the fish mixture.   Put the
butter in the slow cooker then place the fish cutlets
in the slow cooker as well.   Close the lid and cook
the cutlets for 2 hours on High.   Then transfer the
cooked salmon cutlets to a serving plate and enjoy!
Nutrition Info:calories 305, fat 20.2, fiber 3.4,
carbs 7.6, protein 25.9

117. Keto Porridge

Servings: 3   Cooking Time: 2 Hours
Ingredients:

1 tablespoon flaxseed meal	1 cup almond milk
3 tablespoons coconut flour	1 teaspoon stevia
	1 teaspoon vanilla extract

Directions:
Place the flaxseed meal, coconut flour, vanilla
extract, and stevia in the slow cooker.   Stir the
mixture gently.   Then add the almond milk and
stir the mixture until homogenous.   Close the lid
and cook the porridge for 2 hours on Low.   Stir the
cooked porridge and serve it immediately!
Nutrition Info:calories 260, fat 21.8, fiber 7.4,
carbs 13.3, protein 4.3

118. Warm Ricotta, Cream, Berry And Macadamia Whip

Servings: 6   Cooking Time: Approximately 2
Hours
Ingredients:

1 cup fresh berries, chopped (strawberries and raspberries are wonderful)	2 cups ricotta cheese
	1 tsp cinnamon
	1 tsp coconut oil, melted
½ cup toasted macadamia nuts, chopped	1 cup cream, lightly whipped

Directions:
In a medium-sized bowl, mix together the ricotta
cheese, berries, cinnamon, and macadamia nuts.
Rub the bottom of the Slow Cookerwith the melted
coconut oil.   Pour the ricotta mixture into the
Crock Pot.   Place the lid onto the pot and set the
temperature at LOW.   Cook for 2 hours.
Remove the mixture from the pot and place into a
bowl, leave to cool.   Add the whipped cream and
fold through, with a few more fresh berries.   Store
in the fridge, covered.

119. Breakfast Cream And Egg Soufflé

Servings: 4   Cooking Time: 2 Hours

Ingredients:

4 tablespoons of heavy cream

2 tablespoons of parsley, chopped

2 tablespoons of chives, diced

A pinch of red chili pepper, crushed

Salt and black pepper- to taste

Directions:

Start by adding and whisking all the Ingredients: in a mixing bowl.   Divide the souffle mixture into four ramekins.   Place these ramekins in the Crockpot and pour ¼ cup of water into its base. Cover your Crockpot and select the high settings for 2 hours.   Remove the crockpot's lid.   Serve fresh.

Nutrition Info: Calories 224 Total Fat 22.4 g Saturated Fat 17 g Cholesterol 30 mg Total Carbs 5.4 g Sugar 1.2 g Fiber 2.8 g Sodium 206 mg Protein 14.3 g

120.   Chicken Muffins

Servings: 2   Cooking Time: 5 Hours

Ingredients:

5 oz ground chicken

1 tablespoon coconut flour

1 teaspoon minced garlic

½ teaspoon chili flakes

1 tablespoon butter

1 egg, beaten

Directions:

Mix the ground chicken and coconut flour.   Add minced garlic and chili flakes.   Stir the mixture gently and add the egg.   Mix until homogenous. Then transfer the mixture into individual muffin molds and put a small amount of the butter in every muffin.   Put the muffins in the slow cooker and cook for 5 hours on Low.   Cool the cooked muffins. Enjoy!

Nutrition Info:calories 234, fat 13.6, fiber 1.5, carbs 3.2, protein 23.9

121. Coconut Sausages

Servings: 4   Cooking Time: 3 Hours

Ingredients:

1 tablespoon butter, softened

1/2 teaspoon coriander, ground

1 teaspoon cumin, ground

½ cup coconut cream

¾ teaspoon salt

4 sausages, organic and sliced

1 tablespoon coconut oil

Directions:

Spread the slow cooker pot with the coconut oil, add the cream, sausages and the other ingredients and toss.   Close the lid and cook the breakfast for 3 hours on High.

Nutrition Info:calories 209, fat 11.7, fiber 5.4, carbs 8.1, protein 3.3

122.   Egg Hash Browns

Servings: 4   Cooking Time: 3 Hours

Ingredients:

1 egg, whisked

16 oz. hash browns

1/2 teaspoon of paprika

1/2 teaspoon of garlic powder

1/4 cup of olive oil

1 cup of cheddar, shredded

Salt and black pepper- to taste

Directions:

Start by greasing the base of your Crockpot. Spread the hash browns at the base of the pot. Whisk the egg with all other Ingredients: and pour into crockpot.   Cover your crockpot and select the Low settings for 3 hours.   Remove the crockpot's lid.   Slice and serve warm.

Nutrition Info: Calories 228 Total Fat 20.2 g Saturated Fat 12.5 g Cholesterol 54 mg Total Carbs 26 g Sugar 2.3 g Fiber 2.4 g Sodium 250 mg Protein 23.7 g

123.   Egg, Kale, And Mozzarella Casserole

Servings: 6   Cooking Time: 4 Hours

Ingredients:

1 ½ cup mozzarella cheese, grated

1/3 cup green onions, sliced

2 teaspoons olive oil

8 eggs, beaten

Salt and pepper to taste

Directions:

Mix all ingredients in a bowl and stir to combine all ingredients.   Place in a Ziploc bag and write the date when the recipe is made.   Place inside the freezer.   Once you are ready to cook the meal, allow to thaw on the countertop for at least 2 hours. Place in the crockpot.   Close the lid and cook on low for 4 hours or on high for 2 hours.

Nutrition Info: Calories: 284 Carbohydrates: 3.2g Protein: 28.1g Fat: 31.4g Sugar: 0.3g Sodium: 318mg Fiber: 1.8g

124.   Bacon And Spinach Frittata

Servings: 5-6   Cooking Time: 55 Minutes

Ingredients:

2 cups of fresh spinach leaves, washed and drained

8 large eggs, whisked

¼ cup heavy cream

1 cup of mozzarella cheese

1 tsp of Dill

Salt

Pepper

Directions:

Whisk all the ingredients together in a bowl. Lightly grease the bottom of your slow cooker with butter and add all the ingredients.   Set and cook on high heat for 50 minutes.

Nutrition Info: Calories: 270 Fat: 20 g Carbs: 9 g Protein: 15g

125.   French Onion Meatloaf

Servings: 8   Cooking Time: 1 Hour And 30 Minutes

Ingredients:

2 onions, thinly sliced

4 tablespoons of unsalted butter

French Onion Meatloaf Ingredients:

2 pounds of ground

2 teaspoons of salt

1 teaspoon of black pepper

½ teaspoon of red pepper flakes

beef
1 tablespoon of olive oil
½ cup of crushed saltines
½ cup of caramelized onions
1 large egg
1 tablespoon of fresh thyme

½ cup of beef stock
Gruyere Gravy
Ingredients:
2 tablespoons of almond or coconut flour
¾ cup of beef stock
1 tablespoon of fresh thyme
½ cup of gruyere cheese, shredded

Directions:
Press the "Sautee/Browning" button on the Crock-Pot Express and add the butter.   Once the butter is melted, add the onions and cook until brown and caramelized, stirring constantly.   Turn off "Sautee/Browning" button on the Crock-Pot Express and transfer to a plate. Allow to cool and set aside.   In a large bowl, add all the meatloaf ingredients EXCEPT for the olive oil and beef stock and stir until well combined. Form into one or two loaves.   Press the "Sautee/Browning" button on the Crock-Pot Express and add the olive oil.   Once hot, add the loaves and sauté until brown.   Once hot, add the loaf(s) and brown on all sides. Add the beef stock to the Crock-Pot Express. Lock the lid and ensure the valve is closed.   Press the "Meat/Stew" button on the Crock-Pot Express and set the time to 18 minutes. Press start.   When the cooking is done, naturally release the pressure and remove the lid. Remove the meatloaf.   Press "Sautee/Browning" button on the Crock-Pot Express and add the almond or coconut flour to the Crock-Pot Express. Add the reserved caramelized onions, fresh thyme, cheese, and beef stock to the Crock-Pot Express. Ladle the sauce over the meatloaf. Serve and enjoy!
Nutrition Info: Calories: 421 Fat: 32g
Carbohydrates: 9g Dietary Fiber: 1g Protein: 24g

126.	**Onion Broccoli Cream Cheese Quiche**

Servings: 8   Cooking Time: 2 Hours 30 Minutes
Ingredients:

2 cups cheese, shredded and divided
8 oz. cream cheese
1/4 Tsp onion powder

3 cups broccoli, cut into florets
1/4 Tsp pepper
3/4 Tsp salt

Directions:
Add broccoli into the boiling water and cook for 3 minutes. Drain well and set aside to cool.   Add eggs, cream cheese, onion powder, pepper, and salt in mixing bowl and beat until well combined. Spray slow cooker from inside using cooking spray. Add cooked broccoli into the slow cooker then sprinkle half cup cheese.   Pour egg mixture over broccoli and cheese mixture.   Cover slow cooker and cook on high for 2 hours and 15 minutes. Once it done then sprinkle remaining cheese and cover for 10 minutes or until cheese melted.   Serve warm and enjoy.
Nutrition Info: Calories 296 Fat 24.3 g Carb 3.9 g Protein 16.4 g

127.	**Mushroom Casserole**

Servings: 3   Cooking Time: 3 Hours 5 Minutes
Ingredients:

2 ½ oz. cremini mushrooms, diced
5 oz. cauliflower florets, diced
½ leek, sliced
1/4 teaspoon of salt

Black pepper to taste
6 sausage links, cooked and sliced
½ (8 oz.) package cheddar cheese

Directions:
Start by greasing the base of your Crockpot. Spread all the veggies, sausages, and mushrooms. Whisk the egg with remaining Ingredients: except for cheese and pour them over the veggies.   Cover your Crockpot and select the medium settings for 3 hours.   Remove the crockpot's lid.   Drizzle the reserved cheese on top and then cover again. Cook for another 5 minutes on High setting. Serve warm.
Nutrition Info: Calories 244 Total Fat 11.5 g Saturated Fat 1.5 g Cholesterol 61 mg Total Carbs 5 g Sugar 0.4 g Fiber 0.2 g Sodium 246 mg Protein 12.5 g

128.	**Lemon Thyme Chicken**

Servings: 4   Cooking Time: 4 Hours
Ingredients:

2 sliced lemons
½ teaspoon of ground pepper

1 teaspoon of thyme
3 ½-pound whole chicken

Directions:
Arrange the lemon and garlic on the base of a slow cooker.   Mix the spices and use them to season the chicken.   Put the chicken in the slow cooker. Cover and cook on low for 4 hours.   Remove the chicken, let it stand for 15 minutes and then serve.
Nutrition Info: Calories: 120 Fat: 8 grams Carbohydrates: 1 gram Fiber: 0 grams Protein: 12 grams

129.	**Bacon Topped Hash Browns**

Servings: 4   Cooking Time: 3 Hours
Ingredients:

1 cup of milk
1 cup of cheddar cheese, shredded
6 green onions, diced
6 eggs, room temperature

8 bacon strips, diced
9 oz. cream cheese
1 yellow onion, diced
Salt and black pepper- to taste
Cooking spray

Directions:
Start by greasing the base of your Crockpot. Spread the hash brown at the base of the pot. Whisk the egg with all other Ingredients: and pour into crockpot.   Cover your crockpot and select the Low settings for 3 hours.   Remove the crockpot's lid.   Slice and serve warm.
Nutrition Info: Calories 382 Total Fat 36.5 g Saturated Fat 5.5 g Cholesterol 0 mg Total Carbs 54.6 g Sugar 3.4 g Fiber 5.5 g Sodium 73 mg Protein 6.3 g

130.	**Balsamic Pot Roast**

Servings: 10   Cooking Time: 4 Hours

Ingredients:

2 tablespoons of olive oil	1 tablespoon of salt
1 teaspoon of black pepper	2 cups of water
1 teaspoon of garlic powder	½ cup of onions, chopped
¼ cup of balsamic vinegar	¼ teaspoon of xanthan gum
	1 tablespoon of fresh parsley, chopped

Directions:
Season the chuck roast with salt, black pepper, and garlic powder. Press the "Saute/Browning" button on the Crock-Pot Express and add the olive oil. Once hot, add the chuck roast and cook until brown. Deglaze the Crock-Pot Express with the balsamic vinegar and cook for an additional minute. Add the water and onions to the Crock-Pot Express and bring to a boil. Lock the lid and ensure the valve is closed. Press the "Slow Cook" button and set the time to 4 hours. When the cooking is done, manually release the pressure and remove the lid. Transfer the meat to a large bowl and shred or cut into pieces. Add the xanthan gum to the broth inside the Crock-Pot Express and return the meat. Stir the parsley and allow to heat through. Serve and enjoy!
Nutrition Info: Calories: 393 Fat: 28g Carbohydrates: 4g Dietary Fiber: 1g Protein: 30g

131. Reuben Soup With Thousand Island Dressing(1)

Servings: 12   Cooking Time: 7 Hours
Ingredients:

8 c. beef broth/stock	Coriander seeds
3 minced cloves of garlic	1 Hour before serving:
2 tbsp. butter	8 oz. shredded Swiss cheese
2 lbs. diced corned beef	2 c. heavy cream
1 lb. Sauerkraut	For the Topping:
1 tbsp. mustard seeds	Thousand Island dressing
1 t. of each:	
Dill seeds	

Directions:
Use the medium heat setting to brown the onion and garlic using one tablespoon of butter. Sautee for two minutes. Stir in the beef broth, remaining butter, garlic, onions, mustard seeds, sauerkraut, corned beef, and beef broth. Prepare the soup using the high setting for 5 hrs. or 7 hrs. on low. Approximately one hour before dinner, add the whipping cream, and Swiss cheese. Top if off with the Thousand Island dressing as desired.
Nutrition Info: Calories: 343 Net Carbs: 1.3 g Fat: 25.6 g Protein: 22.8 g

132.   Brussel Sprouts Eggs

Servings: 2   Cooking Time: 4 Hours
Ingredients:

7 oz Brussel Sprouts	1 tablespoon butter
½ teaspoon salt	2 eggs
1 teaspoon paprika	

Directions:
Wash Brussel sprouts well then sprinkle them with the salt and paprika. Transfer Brussel sprouts into the slow cooker. Add the butter. Beat the eggs and pour over Brussel sprouts then close the slow cooker. Cook the meal for 4 hours on Low. When the meal is cooked, transfer it to serving plates and enjoy!
Nutrition Info:calories 160, fat 10.6, fiber 4.1, carbs 10, protein 9.1

133.   Shallot Parmesan Zucchini Asparagus Frittata

Servings: 6   Cooking Time: 1 Hour 40 Minutes
Ingredients:

1/4 cup fresh basil, chopped	1 medium zucchini, sliced
1 cup parmesan cheese, grated	2 medium shallots, chopped
8 oz. asparagus, trimmed and cut into 2-inch pieces	3 tbsp. olive oil
	Pepper
	Salt

Directions:
Heat olive oil in a pan over medium-high heat. Add zucchini, asparagus, and shallots into the pan and cook until asparagus is tender. Remove pan from heat and set aside for 10 minutes to cool. Spray slow cooker from inside using cooking spray. Add cooked vegetables into the slow cooker. In a bowl, whisk together eggs, basil, parmesan, pepper, and salt. Pour egg mixture into the slow cooker over vegetables. Cover slow cooker with lid and cook on high for 1 hour or until frittata is set. Cut into pieces and serve immediately.
Nutrition Info: Calories 366 Fat 26.6 g Carb: 7.6 g Protein 28.6 g

134.   Steak And Salsa

Servings: 6   Cooking Time: 8 Hours
Ingredients:

2 big beef tomatoes, diced	1 onion, sliced in semi-circles
1 Tablespoon olive oil	4 Tablespoons butter
1 small red onion finely diced	2 Tablespoons of mixed dry seasoning:
½ bunch of cilantro, chopped	1 teaspoon ground cumin
Salt and pepper to taste	½ teaspoon sweet paprika
2 pounds stewing beef, sliced in strips	½ teaspoon paprika flakes
2 bell peppers, sliced in strips	1 teaspoon garlic salt
	½ teaspoon fresh ground black pepper

Directions:
Cover bottom of crock-pot with the salsa. Add remaining ingredients and mix well. Cover, cook on low for 6-8 hours.
Nutrition Info: Carbs 6g Protein 38g Fiber 22g

135.   Peppers And Eggs Mix

Servings: 5   Cooking Time: 8 Hours
Ingredients:

1 tablespoon smoked paprika
2 red bell peppers, chopped
2 green bell peppers, chopped
1 tablespoon Mozzarella, shredded
1 teaspoon salt
1 teaspoon turmeric powder
½ teaspoon cayenne pepper
5 eggs, whisked
½ cup heavy cream
1 tablespoon chives, chopped
1 teaspoon olive oil

Directions:
Grease the slow cooker with the oil and combine the peppers with the Mozzarella, eggs and the other ingredients inside.   Close the lid, cook on Low for 8 hours, divide between plates and serve.
Nutrition Info:calories301, fat 12.6, fiber 2.2, carbs 8, protein 14.6

136.   Avocado Tuna Balls

Servings: 4   Cooking Time: 2 Hours
Ingredients:
1 avocado, pitted, peeled
2 tablespoons coconut flour
1 teaspoon salt
6 oz tuna
1 egg
1 teaspoon olive oil
1 tablespoon coconut flakes, unsweetened

Directions:
Chop tuna into tiny pieces.   Mash the avocado and combine it with the chopped tuna.   Beat the egg into the mixture and add the salt. Stir well.   Make small balls and sprinkle them with the coconut flakes and coconut flour.   Pour the olive oil in the slow cooker.   Add the tuna balls and close the lid. Cook the meal for 2 hours on High.   Serve the cooked meal hot!
Nutrition Info:calories 242, fat 16.9, fiber 6, carbs 8.6, protein 14.7

137.Summery Bell Pepper + Eggplant Salad

Servings: 4   Cooking Time: 8 Hours
Ingredients:
2 sliced yellow bell peppers
2 small eggplants (smaller ones tend to be less bitter)
1 sliced red onion
1 tablespoon paprika
2 teaspoons cumin
Salt and pepper to taste
Squeeze of lime juice

Directions:
Mix all the ingredients in your slow cooker.   Close the lid.   Cook on low for 7-8 hours.   When time is up, serve warm, or chill in the fridge for a few hours before eating.
Nutrition Info: Total calories: 128 Protein: 5 Carbs: 27 Fat: 1 Fiber: 9.7

138.   Tuscan Garlic Chicken

Servings: 6   Cooking Time: 3 Hours
Ingredients:
6 cloves garlic, crushed and minced
½ cup chicken broth
1 cup heavy cream
¾ cup Parmesan
4 chicken breasts
Salt and pepper to taste
½ cup sundried tomatoes, chopped
cheese, grated
1 tablespoon Italian seasoning
2 cups spinach, chopped

Directions:
Pour the oil into your pan over medium heat. Cook the garlic for 1 minute.   Stir in the broth and cream.   Simmer for 10 minutes.   Stir in the Parmesan cheese and remove from heat.   Put the chicken in your slow cooker.   Season with the salt, pepper and Italian seasoning.   Place the tomatoes on top of the chicken.   Pour the cream mixture on top of the chicken.   Cover the pot.   Cook on high for 3 hours.   Take the chicken out of the slow cooker and set aside.   Add the spinach and stir until wilted.   Pour the sauce over the chicken and serve with the sun-dried tomatoes and spinach.
Nutrition Info: Calories 306 Total Fat 18.4g Saturated Fat 7.5g Cholesterol 115mg Sodium 287mg Potassium 482mg Total Carbohydrate 4.9g Dietary Fiber 0.8g Protein 30.1g Total Sugars 2g

139.   Chili Frittata

Servings: 4   Cooking Time: 2 Hours
Ingredients:
1 red chili, minced
1 teaspoon chili powder
1 cup chives, chopped
1 zucchini, cubed
½ bell pepper, chopped
4 eggs, beaten
¾ teaspoon salt
Cooking spray

Directions:
Grease the slow cooker with the cooking spray and combine the eggs with the other ingredients inside. Close the lid.   Cook frittata for 2 hours on High.
Nutrition Info:calories 232, fat 4.6, fiber 4.4, carbs 7.1, protein 5.8

140.   Almond Avocado Mix

Servings: 4   Cooking Time: 2 Hours
Ingredients:
3 eggs, whisked
1 teaspoon almond extract
1 avocado, peeled, pitted and mashed
1 tablespoon stevia
1 cup heavy cream
¾ teaspoon ground cardamom

Directions:
In the slow cooker, mix the eggs with the avocado and the other ingredients and toss.   Close the lid and cook cream bake for 2 hours on High.
Nutrition Info:calories 207, fat 7.9, fiber 4.1, carbs 6.6, protein 3.2

141.Mini Mushroom & Sausage Quiche

Servings: 6   Cooking Time: 3 Hours
Ingredients:
2 large eggs
4 ounces mushrooms, sliced
1 teaspoon extra virgin olive oil
2 tablespoons Swiss cheese, shredded
Freshly ground pepper to taste
Salt to taste
1 scallion, thinly sliced
2 small egg whites
1 cup milk
Directions:

Place a pan over medium heat. Add oil. When the oil is heated, add mushrooms and sauté until golden brown. Transfer into a bowl.   Place the pan back on heat. Add sausage and sauté until brown. Break it simultaneously as it cooks. Remove with a slotted spoon and place in the bowl along with the mushroom. Cool for a while.   Add cheese, and pepper.   Grease muffin molds with butter or oil. Whisk together eggs, whites and milk in a bowl. Divide and pour the mixture into the muffin molds. Place about a tablespoon of mushroom mixture into each cup.   Place crumpled aluminum foil at the bottom of the cooker (this step can be avoided if your cooking pot is ceramic). Place the muffin molds inside the cooker.   Close the lid. Set cooker on 'High' option and timer for 2-3 hours. Check after 2 hours of cooking. If it is not looking done, then cook for some more time.   If you like the top to be dry, then uncover and cook during the last 40-60 minutes of cooking.   For medium top, you can place a chopstick on the top of the cooker before closing the lid.   Let it cool in the cooker for a while. Cool slightly. Run a knife around the edges. Invert on to a plate and serve immediately.
Nutrition Info: Calories 104 Fat 7 grams Carbohydrate 3 grams Protein 8 grams

142.	Kale Frittata

Servings: 3   Cooking Time: 2 Hours
Ingredients:

3 oz Italian dark leaf kale, chopped	¾ cup almond milk
2 eggs	1 tablespoon butter
	1 teaspoon paprika

Directions:
Beat the eggs in a mixing bowl.   Add paprika and almond milk.   Stir well then add the chopped kale. Place the butter in the slow cooker and add the egg mixture.   Close the lid and cook frittata for 2 hours on High.   Chill the cooked frittata slightly and serve!
Nutrition Info:calories 230, fat 21.2., fiber 2, carbs 6.9, protein 6.1

143.	Bone Broth

Servings: 6-8 Cups   Cooking Time: 6 Hours To 10 Hours
Ingredients:

1 tbsp. pink Himalayan salt	2 med. of Celery stalks
1 med. of Parsnip	2 med. of Carrots
1 med. of White onion – skin on	2 tbsp. apple cider vinegar or lemon juice
5 peeled garlic cloves	8 c. of water

Directions:
Peel and slice the vegetables with roots into 1/3-inch pieces. Slice the onion in half. Chop the celery into thirds. Add the bay leaves into the slow cooker. Toss in the chosen bones (can also be pork). Pour the water up to ¾ capacity – along with the juice/vinegar, and bay leaves. Sprinkle with the salt. Secure the lid. Choose either low (ten hours) or high (six hours). You can simmer up to 48 hours.   Use a strainer to remove the bits of veggies. Set the bones aside to chill. Shred the meat and use as desired. Refrigerate the broth overnight. Scrape away the fat (greasy layer) if desired.   Use within five days or freeze. You can also keep it in the canning jars for up to 45 days.
Nutrition Info:72 Calories 6 g Fat 0.7 g Net Carbs 3.6 g Protein

144.	Herb Chicken & Mushroom Stew

Servings: 5   Cooking Time: 3-4 Hours
Ingredients:

24 oz. whole white button mushrooms	Pepper & Salt
½ t. dried of Oregano	2 tbsp. butter
½ t. dried of Basil	¼ c. heavy whipping cream
3 garlic cloves	
¼ t. dried thyme	8 bacon slices – chopped & cooked
1 c. chicken broth	
2 bay leaves	¼ c. freshly chopped parsley

Directions:
Cut away the stems on the larger mushrooms and wash.   Dice into bite-sized pieces and place in the slow cooker.   Arrange the chicken in the pot next along with the spices, (garlic, basil thyme, oregano, and bay leaves) and broth.   Give it a shake of the pepper and salt.   Set the timer for three to four hours using the low-temperature setting. Combine the butter and whipping cream. Jazz it up with some salt and pepper to your liking.   Serve with the parsley and bacon bits.
Nutrition Info:297.2 Calories 4.42 g Net Carbs 17.5 g Fat 29.99 g Protein

145.	Chia Seeds Pudding

Servings: 4   Cooking Time: 1 Hour
Ingredients:

½ cup chia seeds	1 teaspoon vanilla extract
1 cup almond milk	
1 teaspoon stevia extract	1 teaspoon butter

Directions:
Place the chia seeds, almond milk, stevia extract, and vanilla extract in the slow cooker.   Add butter and stir gently.   Close the lid and cook the meal for 1 hour on Low.   Stir the pudding and serve immediately.   Enjoy!
Nutrition Info:calories 253, fat 21.8, fiber 8.6, carbs 12.4, protein 4.9

146.	Cheese & Cauliflower Bake

Servings: 6   Cooking Time: 4 Hours On Low.
Ingredients:

½ cup cream cheese	¼ cup whipping cream
2 Tablespoons lard (or butter, if you prefer)	1 teaspoon salt
1 Tablespoon lard (or butter, if you prefer) to grease the crock-pot	½ teaspoon fresh ground black pepper
	½ cup yellow cheese, Cheddar, shredded

6 slices of bacon,
crisped and crumbled

Directions:
Grease the crock-pot. Add all the ingredients, except the cheese and the bacon. Cook on low for 3 hours. Open the lid and add cheese. Re-cover, cook for an additional hour. Top with the bacon and serve.
Nutrition Info: Carbs: 3g Protein: 11g Fiber: 25g

147. Cauliflower Breakfast Cake With Capsicum And Chorizo

Servings: 6   Cooking Time: Approximately 4 Hours
Ingredients:

½ head of cauliflower, roughly chopped
2 red capsicums, seeds and core removed, roughly chopped
2 zucchinis, sliced
3 garlic cloves, crushed
2 chorizo sausages, cut into chunks
½ cup grated cheddar cheese
Fresh parsley, finely chopped

Directions:
Drizzle the Slow Cookerwith olive oil. Add the garlic, cauliflower, capsicums, zucchinis, and chorizo to the pot, sprinkle with salt and pepper. Drizzle some more olive oil over the vegetables, then sprinkle the grated cheese over the top. Place the lid onto the pot and set the temperature to LOW. Cook for 4 hours. If you like, you can transfer the whole dish from the Slow Cookerto a hot skillet or fry pan to finish off once it has cooked in the Crock Pot, this will ensure a crispy, golden finish. Serve on a plate with a poached egg, and a healthy sprinkling of fresh parsley.

148. Healthy Slow Cooker Frittata

Servings: 8   Cooking Time: 1 Hour
Ingredients:

1 ½ cups artichoke hearts, chopped
½ cup yellow bell pepper, chopped
½ cup low fat cheddar cheese, grated
Salt to taste
Pepper to taste
1 tomato, deseeded, chopped
½ cup green onion, chopped
Cooking spray

Directions:
Spray the bottom of the slow cooker with cooking spray. Add all the ingredients except cheese into a bowl and mix well. Pour into the slow cooker. Close the lid. Select 'Low' and set the timer for 1-2

hours or until well set. Sprinkle cheese on top. Cover and let it sit for some time. Chop into 8 wedges and serve. Left overs can be stored in an airtight container in the refrigerator.
Nutrition Info: Calories: 141 Fat: 9 g Carbohydrate: 3 g Protein: 12 g

149. Oriental Lamb

Servings: 4   Cooking Time: 4 Hours On High
Ingredients:

2 Tablespoons almond flower
2 cups fresh spinach
4 small red onions, halved
2 garlic cloves, minced
¼ cup yellow turnip, diced
2 Tablespoons dry sherry
2-3 bay leaves
1 teaspoon hot mustard
¼ teaspoon ground nutmeg
1 teaspoon chopped fresh thyme
1 teaspoon chopped fresh rosemary
5-6 whole pimento berries
1 ⅓ cups broth of your choice – beef, chicken, or lamb
Salt and pepper to taste
8 baby zucchini, halved
2 Tablespoons olive oil

Directions:
Preheat the crock-pot on high. Place the lamb in the crock-pot, cover with almond flour. Add the remaining ingredients to crock-pot. Cover, cook on high for 4 hours.
Nutrition Info: Carbs 24g Protein 50g Fiber 57g

150. Warming Bean And Veg Soup

Servings: 4   Cooking Time: 10 Hours
Ingredients:

1 medium sized potato, diced
2 carrots, peeled and sliced
2 celery stalks, diced
A handful of frozen broad beans
Paprika
2 tins of butter beans
Worcestershire sauce
Chili
Salt and pepper
Parmesan cheese
Fresh herbs of your choice

Directions:
Add all the ingredients except the Parmesan cheese and the fresh herbs to the slow cooker. Cook on low for 8-10 hours. Spoon onto dishes, top with Parmesan cheese and fresh herbs and serve.
Nutrition Info: Carbohydrates: 5.2 grams Fat: 8 grams Protein: 3.7 grams Fiber: 7.4 grams Calories: 527

Side Dishes Recipes

151. Mushroom Stew

Servings: 8   Cooking Time: 6 Hours

Ingredients:

10 oz white mushrooms, sliced	1 garlic clove, diced
2 eggplants, chopped	1 cup water
1 onion, diced	1 tablespoon butter
2 bell peppers, chopped	½ teaspoon salt
	½ teaspoon ground black pepper

Directions:

Place the sliced mushrooms, chopped eggplant, and diced onion into the slow cooker.   Add garlic clove and bell peppers.   Sprinkle the vegetables with salt and ground black pepper.   Add butter and water and stir it gently with a wooden spatula. Close the lid and cook the stew for 6 hours on Low. Stir the cooked stew one more time and serve!

Nutrition Info: calories 71, fat 1.9, fiber 5.9, carbs 13, protein 3

152.   Zucchini Pasta

Servings: 4   Cooking Time: 1 Hour

Ingredients:

1 teaspoon dried oregano	2 zucchini
1 teaspoon dried basil	2 tablespoons butter
	¼ teaspoon salt
	5 tablespoons water

Directions:

Peel the zucchini and spiralize it with a veggie spiralizer.   Melt the butter and mix it together with the dried oregano, dried basil, salt, and water. Place the spiralized zucchini in the slow cooker and add the spice mixture.   Close the lid and cook the meal for 1 hour on Low.   Let the cooked pasta cool slightly.   Serve it!

Nutrition Info: calories 68, fat 6, fiber 1.2, carbs 3.5, protein 1.3

153.   Brussel Sprouts With Parmesan

Servings: 3   Cooking Time: 4 Hours 30 Minutes

Ingredients:

9 oz Brussel sprouts	¾ cup water
3 oz Parmesan, sliced	1 teaspoon dried oregano
¼ teaspoon minced garlic	

Directions:

Place Brussel sprouts in the slow cooker.   Add the minced garlic and dried oregano.   Add the water and cook the vegetables for 4 hours on Low. Strain the Brussel sprouts and place them back in the slow cooker.   Add the sliced cheese and cook it for 30 minutes more on High.   Enjoy!

Nutrition Info: calories 130, fat 6.4, fiber 3.4, carbs 9.1, protein 12.1

154.   Garlic Artichoke

Servings: 4   Cooking Time: 2 Hours

Ingredients:

8 oz artichoke, trimmed, chopped	2 teaspoons butter
1 garlic clove, peeled	¼ cup water
	½ teaspoon ground black pepper

Directions:

Chop the garlic clove.   Melt the butter and mix it with the chopped garlic.   Add the ground black pepper and stir the mixture.   Place the artichoke in the slow cooker and cover it with the butter mixture.   Add water and close the lid.   Cook the artichoke for 2 hours on High.   Transfer the cooked artichoke to a platter and serve!

Nutrition Info: calories 45, fat 2, fiber 3.2, carbs 6.4, protein 2

155. Broccoli & Cauliflower & Blue Cheese Casserole

Servings: 10.   Cooking Time: 6 Hours On Low.

Ingredients:

Alfredo sauce:	4 cups cauliflower florets, fresh or frozen
4 Tablespoons butter	
2 crushed garlic cloves	1 red onion, diced
2 cups heavy cream	1 teaspoon dry oregano, thyme, or basil
½ cup grated Parmesan cheese	
Main Dish:	¾ cup any blue cheese, crumbled
4 cups broccoli florets, fresh or frozen	Salt and pepper to taste

Directions:

In a small pot, combine ingredients for Alfredo sauce. Simmer for 10 minutes.   Add remaining ingredients to the crock-pot.   Pour the warm Alfredo sauce over mixture in crock-pot.   Cover, cook on low for 6 hours.

Nutrition Info: net C 6g; P 9g; 29F g

156.   Broccoli Stew

Servings: 3   Cooking Time: 6 Hours

Ingredients:

6 oz broccoli, chopped	1 cup spinach
¾ cup almond milk, unsweetened	1 tablespoon butter
	1 teaspoon salt
2 oz white cabbage, shredded	1 teaspoon white pepper
	2 cups water

Directions:

Chop the spinach and place it in the slow cooker. Add chopped broccoli, almond milk, shredded cabbage, butter, salt, water and white pepper.   Stir the ingredients and close the lid.   Cook the stew for 6 hours on Low.   Stir the stew gently and transfer to serving bowls.   Enjoy!

Nutrition Info: calories 200, fat 18.4, fiber 3.7, carbs 9, protein 3.6

157. Swiss Chard Mix

Servings: 4   Cooking Time: 2.5 Hours

Ingredients:
- 11 oz Swiss chard, chopped
- 5 oz bacon, chopped
- 1 tablespoon butter
- 1 teaspoon turmeric powder
- 1 teaspoon coriander, ground
- ½ cup of water
- ½ teaspoon ground black pepper

Directions:
In the slow cooker, mix the chard with the bacon and the other ingredients, Close the slow cooker lid and cook the casserole for 5 hours on High.

Nutrition Info:calories 283, fat 14.7, fiber 1.4, carbs 4.5, protein 14.2

158. Red Cabbage Sauté

Servings: 4   Cooking Time: 7 Hours

Ingredients:
- 1-pound red cabbage, shredded
- 1 teaspoon sweet paprika
- 1 teaspoon curry powder
- ½ cup of veggie stock
- 1 teaspoon black pepper
- 1 bay leaf
- 1 teaspoon salt

Directions:
In the slow cooker, mix all the ingredients and toss. Close the lid and cook red cabbage for 7 hours on Low.   Mix up the cabbage well before serving.

Nutrition Info:calories 200, fat 7.1, fiber 4.3, carbs 9.9, protein 3.2

159. Oregano Green Beans

Servings: 4   Cooking Time: 6 Hours

Ingredients:
- 2 cups green beans, trimmed and halved
- ½ cup coconut cream
- 1 teaspoon turmeric powder
- 1 teaspoon rosemary, dried
- 1 teaspoon salt
- ¾ teaspoon dried oregano

Directions:
In the slow cooker, mix the peas with the cream and the other ingredients.   Close the slow cooker lid and cook for 6 hours on Low.   Divide between plates and serve.

Nutrition Info:calories 167, fat 4.5, fiber 4, carbs 10.9, protein 5.2

160. Red Cabbage Slices

Servings: 4   Cooking Time: 1 Hour

Ingredients:
- 4 tablespoons olive oil
- 1 teaspoon dried oregano
- 14 oz red cabbage
- 1 teaspoon dried dill
- 4 tablespoons water
- 1 teaspoon salt

Directions:
Slice the red cabbage and sprinkle it with the olive oil, dried oregano, dried dill, and salt. Stir well. Transfer the red cabbage mix into the slow cooker. Add the water and close the lid.   Cook the red cabbage for 1 hour on High.   Serve the cabbage immediately!

Nutrition Info:calories 147, fat 14.2, fiber 2.7, carbs 6.1, protein 1.4

161. Garlicky Mashed Cauliflower

Servings: 6.   Cooking Time: 3 Hours On High.

Ingredients:
- 1 good-sized head of cauliflower, cut into florets
- 1 small head of garlic, peeled
- 4 cups vegetable broth
- ⅓ cup sour cream
- 3 Tablespoons of butter
- 4 Tablespoons combined fresh chopped herbs: chives, parsley or spring onions
- Salt and pepper

Directions:
Place the cauliflower, garlic in the crock-pot. Pour in broth until cauliflower is covered. Add more liquid, if needed.   Cover, cook on high for 3 hours. Drain the liquid, reserving for later.   Mash the vegetables with a fork or a potato masher.   Add the cream and butter and mash again until smooth. If necessary, add some of the reserved cooking liquid to soften the mash.   Mix in chopped herbs, add salt and fresh ground pepper. Stir to combine thoroughly.

Nutrition Info:net C 7g; P 13g; F 6g

162. Party Sausages

Servings: 16   Cooking Time: 2 Hours

Ingredients:
- 1 bottle (8 oz.) Catalina salad dressing
- 1 bottle (8 oz.) Russian salad dressing
- 1/2 cup of packed brown swerve
- 1/2 cup of apple cider
- Sliced green onions, optional

Directions:
Start by throwing all the Ingredients: into the Crockpot.   Cover its lid and cook for 2 hours on Low setting.   Once done, remove its lid of the crockpot carefully.   Mix well and garnish as desired.   Serve warm.

Nutrition Info: Calories 190 Total Fat 17.25 g Saturated Fat 7.1 g Cholesterol 20 mg Total Carbs 5.5 g Sugar 2.8 g Fiber 3.8 g Sodium 28 mg Potassium 47 mg Protein 23 g

163. Moroccan Eggplant Mash

Servings: 4   Cooking Time: 7 Hours

Ingredients:
- 1 eggplant, peeled
- 1 jalapeno pepper
- 1 teaspoon curry powder
- ½ teaspoon salt
- 1 teaspoon paprika
- ¾ teaspoon ground nutmeg
- 2 tablespoons butter
- ¾ cup almond milk
- 1 teaspoon dried dill

Directions:
Chop the eggplant into small pieces.   Place the eggplant in the slow cooker.   Chop the jalapeno pepper and combine it with the eggplant.   Then sprinkle the vegetables with the curry powder, salt, paprika, ground nutmeg, and dried dill.   Add almond milk and butter.   Close the lid and cook the vegetables for 7 hours on Low.   Cool the vegetables and then blend them until smooth with a hand blender.   Transfer the cooked eggplant mash into the bowls and serve!

Nutrition Info:calories 190, fat 17, fiber 5.6, carbs 10, protein 2.5

164.   Pumpkin Nut Bread

Servings: 10.   Cooking Time: 3 Hours On Low.
Ingredients:

- 1 ½ cup ground almonds (2 cups, if you reduce the sweetener; see below)
- ¾ cup sweetener, Swerve (½ cup, if you prefer not so sweet breakfast version)
- ½ cup coconut flour
- ¼ cup unsweetened whey protein powder
- 2 teaspoons baking powder
- 1 ½ teaspoon cinnamon
- 1 teaspoon turmeric
- 1 teaspoon ground ginger
- ¼ teaspoon ground cloves
- Pinch of salt
- 1 cup pumpkin, mashed
- 4 large eggs
- ¼ cup butter, melted
- 1 teaspoon vanilla extract

Directions:
Butter the crock-pot.   In a bowl, combine the walnuts with dry ingredients.   Stir in the pumpkin, eggs, butter, and vanilla. Mix well.   Pour the batter in the buttered crock-pot.   Cover the crock-pot with a paper towel to absorb the water.   Cover, cook on low for 3 hours.
Nutrition Info:net C 5g; P 6g; F 13g

165.   Paprika Green Beans

Servings: 2   Cooking Time: 1 Hour
Ingredients:

- 2 teaspoons sweet paprika
- 7 oz green beans, halved
- 1 tablespoon butter
- ¼ cup of water
- 1 teaspoon salt
- ½ teaspoon cumin, ground
- 1 teaspoon black pepper
- 1 teaspoon apple cider vinegar

Directions:
In the slow cooker, mix the green beans with the paprika and the other ingredients, toss and close the lid.   Cook the green beans on High for 1 hour. Divide between plates and serve.
Nutrition Info:calories 200, fat 7.9, fiber 4.9, carbs 7.1, protein 6.3

166.   Cauliflower Garlic Bread

Servings: 8.   Cooking Time: 4 Hours On High.
Ingredients:

- 1 head of cauliflower, cut into florets
- 2 large eggs
- 2 cups shredded cheese, your choice
- 3 Tablespoons coconut flakes
- ½ teaspoon salt
- ½ teaspoon fresh ground black pepper
- 2 cloves garlic, minced
- 4 Tablespoons fresh basil, coarsely chopped

Directions:
Chop the cauliflower to a rice-like consistency. Place in a bowl.   Stir in 1 cup cheese, eggs, coconut flakes, salt and pepper. Combine well.   Butter bottom of the crock-pot. Press mixture to bottom of the crock-pot to form a crust.   Sprinkle with garlic and remaining cheese.   Cover, cook on high for 4 hours.   Sprinkle with chopped basil.
Nutrition Info:net C 2g; P 10g; F 10g

167.Oregano Beans And Cucumber

Servings: 4   Cooking Time: 2 Hours
Ingredients:

- 1 ½ cup green beans, trimmed and halved
- 1 cup cucumber, sliced
- ½ cup chicken stock
- 1 teaspoon mint, dried
- 1 tablespoon dried oregano
- 1 teaspoon salt

Directions:
In the slow cooker, mix the green beans with all the other ingredients.   Close the slow cooker lid and cook the side dish for 2 hours on Low.   Serve the snap beans right away.
Nutrition Info:calories 117, fat 2.2, fiber 1.9, carbs 3.8, protein 1

168.   Zucchini And Radish Mix

Servings: 4   Cooking Time: 2 Hours
Ingredients:

- 2 zucchinis, trimmed and sliced
- 1 cup radishes, halved
- ¼ cup of veggie stock
- 1 tablespoon butter
- ½ teaspoon salt
- ½ teaspoon ground black pepper
- 1 tablespoon chives, chopped

Directions:
In the slow cooker, combine all the ingredients and toss gently.   Close the slow cooker lid and cook a meal for 2 hours on Low.
Nutrition Info:calories 157, fat 6.1, fiber 1.2, carbs 3.7, protein 6.5

169.   Pesto Spaghetti Squash

Servings: 4   Cooking Time: 6 Hours
Ingredients:

- 1 cup spinach
- 2 tablespoons olive oil
- 1 oz pumpkin seeds, crushed
- 1-pound spaghetti squash
- 1 teaspoon butter
- ¾ cup water

Directions:
Chop the spaghetti squash and put it in the slow cooker.   Add butter and water.   Close the lid and cook for 6 hours on Low.   Meanwhile, chop the spinach and place it in the blender.   Add olive oil and pumpkin seeds.   Blend the mixture until smooth.   When the spaghetti squash is cooked, transfer it into the serving bowls and sprinkle with the spinach (pesto) mixture.   Serve it!
Nutrition Info:calories 144, fat 11.9, fiber 0.5, carbs 9.4, protein 2.7

170.   Cabbage And Tomatoes

Servings: 4   Cooking Time: 2 Hours
Ingredients:

- 1-pound white cabbage, shredded
- ½ pound cherry
- 1 teaspoon coriander, ground
- 1 teaspoon garlic,

tomatoes, halved
½ cup keto tomato sauce
½ jalapeno pepper
1 teaspoon cumin, ground
diced
1 teaspoon chili flakes
1 teaspoon salt
½ teaspoon olive oil

Directions:
In the slow cooker, mix the cabbage with the tomatoes and the other ingredients.   Close the lid and cook it for 2 hours on High.
Nutrition Info:calories 129, fat 1.2, fiber 3.8, carbs 4.1, protein 4.5

171. Slow Cooker Spaghetti Squash

Servings: 5   Cooking Time: 4 Hours
Ingredients:
1-pound spaghetti squash
1 tablespoon butter
¼ cup water
1 teaspoon ground black pepper
¼ teaspoon ground nutmeg

Directions:
Peel the spaghetti squash and sprinkle it with the ground black pepper and ground nutmeg.   Pour water in the slow cooker.   Add butter and spaghetti squash.   Close the lid and cook for 4 hours on Low.   Chop the spaghetti squash into small pieces and serve!
Nutrition Info:calories 50, fat 2.9, fiber 6.6, carbs 0.1, protein 0.7

172. Cauliflower Croquettes

Servings: 4   Cooking Time: 2 Hours
Ingredients:
1 egg
8 oz cauliflower, grated
3 tablespoons almond flour
1 teaspoon salt
1 tablespoon butter
½ teaspoon cayenne pepper

Directions:
Beat the egg in a bowl.   Add grated cauliflower, salt, and cayenne pepper to the whisked egg and stir. Then make small balls from the mixture and coat them with the almond flour.   Toss the butter in the slow cooker.   Add the cauliflower croquettes to the slow cooker as well and cook them for 2 hours on High.   Let the cooked croquettes cool for at least 10 minutes.   Serve!
Nutrition Info:calories 176, fat 14.6, fiber 3.7, carbs 7.7, protein 7.1

173. Masala Broccoli

Servings: 4   Cooking Time: 6 Hours
Ingredients:
2 cups broccoli florets
1 tablespoon garam masala
2 spring onions, chopped
1 teaspoon curry powder
½ teaspoon chili pepper
½ cup organic almond milk

Directions:
In the slow cooker, mix the broccoli with the masala and the other ingredients.   Close the lid and cook

korma for 6 hours on low.   Divide between plates and serve.
Nutrition Info:calories 102, fat 8, fiber 2.9, carbs 7.4, protein 2.3

174. Flax Meal Coffeecake

Servings: 8.   Cooking Time: 2.5 Hours On Low.
Ingredients:
1 Tablespoon butter for the crock-pot
10 eggs
¾ cup coconut flour
1 tablespoon gelatin
1 cup butter, divided
½ teaspoon baking soda
½ cup flax seed meal
¾ cup powdered Swerve, divided (or suitable substitute)
2 teaspoons vanilla extract, divided
2 teaspoons cinnamon
½ cup of warm water

Directions:
Butter the crock-pot.   In a blender, mix the eggs, flour, ½ cup butter, sweetener, gelatin and vanilla. Blend for 20 seconds.   In a small bowl, mix flax meal and baking soda. Add to mixture in blender. Blend for 10 seconds.   Combine ½ cup melted butter, sweetener, water, and cinnamon to make a syrup; add a bit of water, if not liquid enough. Pour 1 layer of batter in the buttered crock-pot. Sprinkle with ¼ of the syrup.   Repeat two more times, finishing with ½ of the syrup.   Cover the crock-pot with a paper towel to absorb the water. Cover, cook on low for 2.5 hours.
Nutrition Info:net C 4g; P 9g; F 24g

175. Paprika Spaghetti Squash

Servings: 3   Cooking Time: 4.5 Hours
Ingredients:
1-pound spaghetti squash, shredded
1 teaspoon ground paprika
1 teaspoon smoked paprika
1 tablespoon rosemary, chopped
1 teaspoon salt
½ teaspoon curry powder
1 teaspoon onion powder
1 teaspoon garlic powder
1/3 cup chicken stock

Directions:
In the slow cooker, mix the squash with paprika and the other ingredients, toss and close the lid.   Cook it for 4.5 hours on Low.   Divide between plates and serve.
Nutrition Info:calories 186, fat 5.1, fiber 2.8, carbs 6.5, protein 7.4

176. Soft Keto Kale Salad

Servings: 4   Cooking Time: 30 Minutes
Ingredients:
6 oz bacon, chopped, cooked
1 oz almond, chopped
1 cup Italian dark-leaf kale, chopped
1 tablespoon olive oil
¾ cup almond milk, unsweetened
1 cucumber, chopped
1 garlic clove, diced

Directions:
Place the chopped kale, almond milk, and diced garlic in the slow cooker.   Close the lid and cook

the kale for 30 minutes on High. Meanwhile, place the chopped cucumbers in the salad bowl. Add olive oil, bacon, and chopped almond. When the kale is cooked, transfer it immediately to the salad bowl and stir. Serve it warm!
Nutrition Info:calories 423, fat 35.6, fiber 2.8, carbs 8.4, protein 19.3

177. Coconut Celery

Servings: 2   Cooking Time: 2 Hours
Ingredients:

7 oz celery stalks, roughly chopped	1 teaspoon fresh parsley
1/3 cup coconut cream	½ teaspoon salt

Directions:
In the slow cooker, mix the celery stalks with the other ingredients. Then close the lid and cook the vegetable for 2 hours on High. Divide between plates and serve.
Nutrition Info:calories 67, fat 2.8, fiber 2.8, carbs 9.7, protein 2

178.   Spiced Fennel Slices

Servings: 5   Cooking Time: 2 Hours
Ingredients:

1-pound fennel bulb	1 oz butter
1 teaspoon cumin	1 tablespoon olive oil
1 teaspoon thyme	
1 teaspoon salt	

Directions:
Mix the cumin, thyme, salt, and olive oil. Slice the fennel bulb and sprinkle it with the spice mixture. Place the fennel in the slow cooker and add butter. Close the lid and cook for 2 hours on High. Serve the meal hot!
Nutrition Info:calories 95, fat 7.7, fiber 2.9, carbs 6.9, protein 1.3

179. Green Bean And Avocado Salad

Servings: 4   Cooking Time: 2 Hours
Ingredients:

1 avocado, peeled, pitted	1 teaspoon salt
8 oz green beans	1 cucumber, chopped
1 cup water	1 teaspoon butter
1 teaspoon ground black pepper	1 oz walnuts, chopped
	1 tablespoon olive oil

Directions:
Put the green beans in the slow cooker. Add the water, ground black pepper, and salt. Close the lid and cook the green beans for 2 hours on High. Meanwhile, chop the avocado and put it in a salad bowl. Add the chopped cucumber, walnuts, and olive oil to the salad bowl as well Add the cooked warm green beans and stir the salad. Enjoy it!
Nutrition Info:calories 216, fat 18.6, fiber 6.3, carbs 12.1, protein 4.3

180.   Garlic Peppers

Servings: 4   Cooking Time: 4 Hours
Ingredients:

4 green peppers	2 tablespoons water
1 tablespoon olive oil	1 teaspoon ground
1 teaspoon minced garlic	nutmeg
	1 tablespoon butter

Directions:
Remove the seeds from the green peppers and cut them into the strips. Sprinkle the green peppers with the minced garlic, ground nutmeg, and olive oil. Place the peppers in the slow cooker. Add butter and water. Close the lid and cook on Low for 4 hours. Let the cooked green peppers cool slightly. Serve!
Nutrition Info:calories 83, fat 6.8, fiber 2.1, carbs 6, protein 1.1

181. Glazed Spiced Carrots

Servings: 6   Cooking Time: 8 Hours
Ingredients:

1/2 cup of peach preserves	1/4 teaspoon of salt
1/2 cup of butter, melted	1/8 teaspoon of ground nutmeg
1/4 cup of packed brown swerve	2 tablespoons of xanthan gum
1 teaspoon of vanilla extract	2 tablespoons of water
1/2 teaspoon of cinnamon, ground	Toasted diced pecans, optional

Directions:
Start by throwing all the Ingredients: into the Crockpot. Cover its lid and cook for 8 hours on Low setting. Once done, remove its lid of the crockpot carefully. Mix well and garnish as desired. Serve warm.
Nutrition Info: Calories 220 Total Fat 20.1 g Saturated Fat 7.4 g Cholesterol 132 mg Total Carbs 63 g Sugar 0.4 g Fiber 2.4 g Sodium 157 mg Potassium 42 mg Protein 6.1 g

182.   Artichoke And Broccoli Mix

Servings: 4   Cooking Time: 5 Hours
Ingredients:

4 tablespoons lemon juice	½ teaspoon sweet paprika
2 artichokes, trimmed and halved	3 tablespoons olive oil
1 cup broccoli florets	
1 teaspoon tahini paste	½ teaspoon salt
	½ garlic clove, minced
	1/4 cup water

Directions:
In the slow cooker, mix the artichokes with the broccoli and the other ingredients and close the lid. Cook the vegetable for 5 hours on Low. Divide between plates and serve.
Nutrition Info:calories 142, fat 11.2, fiber 4.6, carbs 9.5, protein 3

183.   Herbed Mushrooms

Servings: 4   Cooking Time: 2 Hours
Ingredients:

1 cup white mushrooms, halved	1 tablespoon oregano, chopped
4 tablespoons lemon juice	1 tablespoon basil, chopped

1 tablespoon chives, chopped
½ teaspoon salt
½ teaspoon peppercorns
1/4 cup veggie stock
Directions:
In the slow cooker, mix the mushrooms with the lemon juice and the other ingredients.   Cook on High for 2 hours.
Nutrition Info:calories 212, fat 4.2, fiber 3.6, carbs 7.2, protein 0.6

184.   Rosemary Bok Choy

Servings: 4   Cooking Time: 8 Hours
Ingredients:
8 oz bok choy, chopped
1 cup spring onions, chopped
1 teaspoon curry powder
½ cup chicken stock
½ jalapeno pepper, chopped
1 tablespoon keto tomato sauce
1 teaspoon almond butter
1 tablespoon rosemary

Directions:
In the slow cooker, mix the bok choy with the spring onions and the other ingredients.   Close the slow cooker lid and cook the mix for 8 hours on Low. Divide between plates and serve.
Nutrition Info:calories 49, fat 2.6, fiber 2, carbs 5.4, protein 2.7

185.   Pumpkin Cubes

Servings: 2   Cooking Time: 5 Hours
Ingredients:
8 oz pumpkin
1 teaspoon ground cinnamon
1 teaspoon liquid stevia
1 teaspoon butter
2 tablespoons water
1 teaspoon ground ginger

Directions:
Peel the pumpkin and chop it.   Place the chopped pumpkin in the slow cooker.   Add ground cinnamon, liquid stevia, and ground ginger.   Stir it gently and add water and butter.   Close the lid and cook the pumpkin for 5 hours on Low.   When the pumpkin is cooked, it will be nice and tender. Let it rest for 10 minutes.   Enjoy!
Nutrition Info:calories 61, fat 2.3, fiber 4, carbs 10.7, protein 1.4

186.   Collard Greens And Mushrooms

Servings: 4   Cooking Time: 3.5 Hours
Ingredients:
9 oz collard greens, trimmed, chopped
2 spring onions, chopped
1 cup white mushrooms, sliced
1 cup of water
1 teaspoon salt
1 teaspoon chili powder
1 teaspoon olive oil

Directions:
In the slow cooker, mix the greens with mushrooms and the other ingredients and close the slow cooker lid.   Cook the greens for 3.5 hours on High. Divide into bowls and serve.

Nutrition Info:calories 184, fat 7.5, fiber 4.8, carbs 7.6, protein 5.8

187.   Eggplant Hash

Servings: 6   Cooking Time: 3 Hours
Ingredients:
2 eggplants, peeled, chopped
1 onion, diced
5 oz white mushrooms, chopped
½ cup water
1 oz butter
1 teaspoon cayenne pepper

Directions:
Place the eggplants and onion in the slow cooker. Sprinkle the vegetables with the chopped mushrooms, water, butter, and cayenne pepper. Stir the vegetable gently and close the lid.   Cook the eggplants hash for 3 hours on High.   When the eggplants hash is cooked, let it chill for 10 minutes. Serve it!
Nutrition Info:calories 93, fat 4.3, fiber 7.2, carbs 13.4, protein 2.8

188.   Garlic Eggplant Mix

Servings: 4   Cooking Time: 3 Hours
Ingredients:
8 oz eggplant, roughly cubed
1 teaspoon garlic powder
2 garlic cloves, diced
1 tablespoon apple cider vinegar
2 shallots, chopped
3 tablespoons avocado oil
1 teaspoon capers
½ teaspoon salt
¼ cup of vegetable stock

Directions:
In the slow cooker, mix the eggplant with the shallots and eth other ingredients, stir, close the slow cooker lid and cook for 3 hours on high. Open the lid and mix up the cooked meal one more time.
Nutrition Info:calories 129, fat 4.5, fiber 3.6, carbs 8.3, protein 1.5

189.   Garlic Green Beans With Gorgonzola

Servings: 6   Cooking Time: 4 Hours
Ingredients:
1 can (8 oz.) sliced chestnuts, drained
4 green onions, diced
5 bacon strips, cooked and crumbled, divided
1/3 cup of white wine
2 tablespoons of minced fresh thyme
4 garlic cloves, minced
1 1/2 teaspoons of seasoned salt
1 cup of (8 oz.) sour cream
3/4 cup of crumbled Gorgonzola cheese

Directions:
Start by throwing all the Ingredients: into the Crockpot except cheese and bacon.   Cover its lid and cook for 4 hours on Low setting.   Once done, remove its lid of the crockpot carefully.   Mix well and garnish with bacon and cheese.   Serve warm.
Nutrition Info: Calories 331 Total Fat 32.9 g Saturated Fat 6.1 g Cholesterol 10 mg Total Carbs

9.1 g Sugar 2.8 g Fiber 0.8 g Sodium 18 mg
Potassium 37 mg Protein 4.4 g

190. Mushroom And Kale

Servings: 2   Cooking Time: 3 Hours
Ingredients:

1 tablespoon chives, chopped
1 cup kale, chopped
1 cup mushrooms, sliced
1/3 cup coconut milk
1 tablespoon almond butter
½ teaspoon salt
1 teaspoon curry powder

Directions:
In the slow cooker, mix the kale with mushrooms and the other ingredients.   Close the lid and cook for 3 hours on Low.   Divide between plates and serve.
Nutrition Info:calories 225, fat 11.5, fiber 5.1, carbs 9.1, protein 11.2

191. Zucchini Spaghetti

Servings: 16
Ingredients:

2 cups of water
Cilantro to serve

Directions:
Start by throwing all the Ingredients: except cilantro into the Crockpot.   Cover its lid and cook for 2 hours on Low setting.   Once done, remove its lid of the crockpot carefully.   Garnish this spaghetti with cilantro.   Serve warm.
Nutrition Info: Calories 139 Total Fat 4.6 g Saturated Fat 0.5 g Cholesterol 1.2 mg Total Carbs 7.5 g Sugar 6.3 g Fiber 0.6 g Sodium 83 mg Potassium 113 mg Protein 3.8 g

192. Lime Cauliflower

Servings: 2   Cooking Time: 4 Hours
Ingredients:

1 ½ cup cauliflower, shredded
1 teaspoon sweet paprika
½ teaspoon chili flakes
½ teaspoon salt
½ teaspoon ground black pepper
1/2 cup coconut cream
1 teaspoon lime juice
1 teaspoon lime zest, grated
1 teaspoon butter

Directions:
In the slow cooker, mix the cauliflower with the paprika, chili and the other ingredients   Close the lid and cook for 4 hours on High.
Nutrition Info:calories 158, fat 4, fiber 2.5, carbs 5.4, protein 6.9

193. Brussels Sprouts

Servings: 6   Cooking Time: 4 Hours
Ingredients:

1 pinch salt and black pepper
2 teaspoons of sweet paprika
1 lb. Brussels sprouts halved
1 yellow onion, diced
2 tablespoons of stevia
7 bacon strips, diced
2 tablespoon of olive oil

Directions:

Start by throwing all the Ingredients: into the Crockpot.   Cover its lid and cook for 4 hours on Low setting.   Once done, remove its lid of the crockpot carefully.   Mix well and garnish as desired.   Serve warm.
Nutrition Info: Calories 285 Total Fat 27.3 g Saturated Fat 14.5 g Cholesterol 175 mg Total Carbs 3.5 g Sugar 0.4 g Fiber 0.9 g Sodium 165 mg Potassium 83 mg Protein 7.2 g

194. Garlic Green Beans

Servings: 4   Cooking Time: 3.5 Hours
Ingredients:

1-pound green beans, trimmed and halved
4 teaspoons minced garlic
4 teaspoons olive oil
1 tablespoon salt
1 teaspoon chili powder
1 teaspoon dried oregano
1/2 cup veggie stock

Directions:
In the slow cooker, mix the green beans with the garlic and the other ingredients and close the lid. Cook the artichokes on High for 3.5 hours.
Nutrition Info:calories 217, fat 4.9, fiber 7.4, carbs 7.6, protein 4.5

195. Keto Leeks

Servings: 3   Cooking Time: 2 Hours
Ingredients:

8 oz leek, sliced
1 tablespoon butter
1 tablespoon full-fat cream cheese
1 teaspoon ground black pepper
¼ teaspoon minced garlic

Directions:
Place the sliced leek, butter, cream cheese, ground black pepper, and minced garlic in the slow cooker. Stir the ingredients and close the lid.   Cook the leeks for 2 hours on High.   Stir the cooked leeks and serve!
Nutrition Info:calories 52, fat 2.5, fiber 0.9, carbs 6.9, protein 1.2

196. Swiss Chard Saute

Servings: 2   Cooking Time: 2 Hours
Ingredients:

2 cups Swiss chard, trimmed, chopped
¼ cup cream cheese
1 teaspoon butter
½ teaspoon salt
½ teaspoon turmeric
1 teaspoon garlic powder
1 teaspoon white pepper
1 teaspoon basil, dried

Directions:
In the slow cooker, mix the chard with the cream cheese and the other ingredients.   Close the lid. Cook the side dish for 2 hours on High.
Nutrition Info:calories 225, fat 12.4, fiber 0.8, carbs 3.9, protein 7.5

197. Zucchini And Cabbage

Servings: 3   Cooking Time: 1 Hour And 30 Minutes
Ingredients:

10 oz zucchini, trimmed
1 cup cabbage, shredded
1 teaspoon chili powder

¼ cup heavy cream
½ teaspoon turmeric
½ teaspoon butter
1 teaspoon garam masala

Directions:
In the slow cooker, mix the zucchinis with the cabbage and the other ingredients. Close the lid and cook side dish for 1 hour and 30 minutes on High.
Nutrition Info:calories 164, fat 8.1, fiber 2.2, carbs 5.3, protein 4.1

198. Quinoa Brussels Sprout Salad

Servings: 4   Cooking Time: 6 Hours
Ingredients:
½ cup of quinoa, rinsed
½ carrot, peeled and shredded
¾ cup of water
¼ teaspoon of salt
1 cup of Brussels sprout, diced
½ cup of red onions, sliced
1 tablespoon of brown swerve

2 tablespoons, balsamic vinegar
1 tablespoon of vegetable oil
1 tablespoon of sunflower seeds
1 teaspoon of ginger, grated
1 garlic clove, minced
Black pepper, to taste

Directions:
Start by putting quinoa and water into the Crockpot. Cover its lid and cook for 6 hours on Low setting. Once done, remove its lid of the crockpot carefully. Strain the cooked quinoa and add to a salad bowl. Toss in all other Ingredients: and give it a stir. Mix well and garnish as desired. Serve warm.
Nutrition Info: Calories 195 Total Fat 14.3 g Saturated Fat 10.5 g Cholesterol 175 mg Total Carbs 4.5 g Sugar 0.5 g Fiber 0.3 g Sodium 125 mg Potassium 83 mg Protein 3.2 g

199. Brussels Sprouts Au Gratin

Servings: 6.   Cooking Time: 6 Hours On Low.
Ingredients:
2.2 pounds Brussels sprouts, washed, dried, trimmed and halved
1 cup cream
Zest of 1 lemon
1 teaspoon black pepper

1 teaspoon salt
4 Tablespoons butter
1 cup Parmesan cheese, grated
½ cup almond meal
Salt and pepper to taste

Directions:
Butter the crock-pot. Place the trimmed Brussels sprouts in the crock-pot. Sprinkle with seasoning. Pour the cream over the Brussel sprouts. Toss to cover them. In a bowl, cut the butter into small pieces. Add ½ cup of the Parmesan cheese, almond meal, salt and pepper. Stir until combined. Mix with sprouts. Add the remaining Parmesan cheese. Pour over the Brussel sprouts in the crock-pot. Cover, cook on low for 6 hours.
Nutrition Info:net C 5g; P 10g; F 25g

200. Nutmeg Artichokes

Servings: 2   Cooking Time: 2.5 Hours
Ingredients:
2 artichokes, trimmed and halved
3 tablespoons coconut cream
1 teaspoon ground cinnamon

¾ teaspoon ground nutmeg
½ teaspoon salt
1/3 cup organic almond milk

Directions:
In the slow cooker, mix the artichokes with the cream and the other ingredients. Close the lid and cook the pudding on High for 5 hours.
Nutrition Info:calories 202, fat 5.2, fiber 4.7, carbs 9.2, protein 7.4

201. Cauliflower Puree With Parmesan

Servings: 5   Cooking Time: 6 Hours
Ingredients:
1-pound cauliflower
1 cup water

2 tablespoons butter
2 oz Parmesan, grated

Directions:
Chop the cauliflower and place it in the slow cooker. Add the water and close the lid. Cook the cauliflower for 6 hours on Low. Strain the cauliflower and place it in the blender. Add the butter and blend it until you get a smooth puree. Transfer the cauliflower puree to serving plates and sprinkle with grated Parmesan. Serve it!
Nutrition Info:calories 100, fat 7.1, fiber 2.3, carbs 5.2, protein 5.5

202. Kale Mash With Blue Cheese

Servings: 3   Cooking Time: 5 Hours
Ingredients:
3 oz Blue cheese
1 cup Italian dark-leaf kale
¾ cup almond milk, unsweetened

1 tablespoon butter
1 teaspoon salt
1 teaspoon ground black pepper

Directions:
Chop the kale and place it in the slow cooker. Add almond milk, salt, and ground black pepper. Close the lid and cook the kale for 5 hours on Low. Meanwhile, chop Blue cheese and butter. Combine the cooked kale with the butter and stir it until butter is melted. Add the Blue cheese and stir it gently. Serve!
Nutrition Info:calories 285, fat 26.3, fiber 1.8, carbs 6.8, protein 8.2

203. Rutabaga Wedges

Servings: 3   Cooking Time: 2 Hours
Ingredients:
8 oz rutabaga
1 tablespoon olive oil
1 teaspoon butter
1 teaspoon dried dill

1 teaspoon minced garlic
4 tablespoons almond milk, unsweetened
½ teaspoon salt

Directions:

Mix the olive oil, butter, dried dill, minced garlic, almond milk, and salt. Whisk the mixture until homogenous. Then slice the rutabaga into wedges. Sprinkle the rutabaga wedges with the olive oil mixture from each side and place them in the slow cooker. Close the lid and cook the side dish for 2 hours on High. Enjoy!
Nutrition Info:calories 127, fat 10.9, fiber 2.4, carbs 7.8, protein 1.5

204. Saucy Beans

Servings: 4   Cooking Time: 2 Hours
Ingredients:

- ½ cup of bacon, diced
- ¼ medium onion, diced
- ½ teaspoon of salt
- ½ teaspoon of dry mustard
- ½ tablespoon of Worcestershire sauce
- ½ tablespoon of balsamic vinegar
- ½ teaspoon of pepper
- 1 tablespoon of tomato paste
- 3 tablespoons of dark brown swerve
- ½ cup of chicken stock
- ½ cup of water

Directions:
Start by throwing all the Ingredients: into the Crockpot. Cover its lid and cook for 2 hours on Low setting. Once done, remove its lid of the crockpot carefully. Mix well and garnish as desired. Serve warm.
Nutrition Info: Calories 151 Total Fat 14.7 g Saturated Fat 1.5 g Cholesterol 13 mg Total Carbs 1.5 g Sugar 0.3 g Fiber 0.1 g Sodium 53 mg Potassium 131 mg Protein 0.8 g

205. Okra Stew

Servings: 4   Cooking Time: 5 Hours
Ingredients:

- 10 oz okra, chopped
- 1 onion, diced
- 5 oz cauliflower, chopped
- 1 cup water
- 1 teaspoon butter
- 1 teaspoon paprika
- ½ teaspoon ground black pepper
- 1 teaspoon dried dill

Directions:
Mix the chopped okra, diced onion, cauliflower, and spices. Stir the mixture and place it in the slow cooker. Add water and butter and close the lid. Cook the stew for 5 hours on Low. Transfer the dish into serving bowls and serve!
Nutrition Info:calories 59, fat 1.3, fiber 4.1, carbs 10.3, protein 2.5

206. Seasoned Carrots

Servings: 8   Cooking Time: 4 Hours
Ingredients:

- 3 lbs. carrots, sliced
- 1 teaspoon of onion powder
- 2 teaspoons of garlic powder
- 2 teaspoons of salt
- ½ teaspoon of paprika
- ½ teaspoon of black pepper
- 2 cups of chicken broth

Directions:

Start by throwing all the Ingredients: into the Crockpot. Cover its lid and cook for 4 hours on Low setting. Once done, remove its lid of the crockpot carefully. Mix well and garnish as desired. Serve warm.
Nutrition Info: Calories 252 Total Fat 17.3 g Saturated Fat 11.5 g Cholesterol 141 mg Total Carbs 7.2 g Sugar 0.3 g Fiber 1.4 g Sodium 153 mg Potassium 73 mg Protein 5.2 g

207. Broccoli Cheese Florets

Servings: 4   Cooking Time: 4 Hours
Ingredients:

- 2 broccoli heads, florets separated
- 4 garlic cloves, minced
- 1 cup of mozzarella, shredded
- ½ cup of parmesan, grated
- 1 cup of coconut cream
- 2 tablespoons of parsley, chopped

Directions:
Start by throwing all the Ingredients: into the Crockpot. Cover its lid and cook for 4 hours on Low setting. Once done, remove its lid of the crockpot carefully. Mix well and garnish as desired. Serve warm.
Nutrition Info: Calories 175 Total Fat 16 g Saturated Fat 2.1 g Cholesterol 0 mg Total Carbs 2.8 g Sugar 1.8 g Fiber 0.4 g Sodium 8 mg Potassium 81 mg Protein 9 g

208. Green Bean Casserole

Servings: 8.   Cooking Time: 3 Hours On High.
Ingredients:

- 8 bacon strips, crisped and crumbled
- 1 yellow onion, sliced
- ¼ cup chicken broth
- 2.2 pounds fresh green beans, trimmed
- Salt and pepper to taste
- 3 sprigs fresh thyme

Directions:
In a pan, fry the bacon. Set aside. In the same pan, add some olive oil, sauté the onion 3-4 minutes. Add the beans, cook for 2 minutes. Transfer to crock-pot, add the remaining ingredients. Stir. Cover, cook on high for 3 hours. Open the lid, sprinkle the crumbled bacon. Serve warm.
Nutrition Info:net C 8g; P 9g; F 6g

209. Bacon Wrapped Cauliflower

Servings: 4   Cooking Time: 7 Hours
Ingredients:

- 11 oz cauliflower head
- 3 oz bacon, sliced
- 1 teaspoon salt
- 1 teaspoon cayenne pepper
- 1 oz butter, softened
- ¾ cup water

Directions:
Sprinkle the cauliflower head with the salt and cayenne pepper then rub with butter. Wrap the cauliflower head in the sliced bacon and secure with toothpicks. Pour water in the slow cooker and add the wrapped cauliflower head. Cook the cauliflower head for 7 hours on Low. Then let the cooked cauliflower head cool for 10 minutes. Serve it!

210. Paprika Peppers

Servings: 4   Cooking Time: 3 Hours
Ingredients:

1 cup red bell peppers, cut into strips	1 teaspoon hot paprika
1 cup green bell peppers, cut into strips	1 teaspoon salt
1 teaspoon keto tomato sauce	2 spring onions, chopped
	½ teaspoon ground black pepper
	½ cup of coconut milk

Directions:
In the slow cooker, mix the peppers with the paprika and the other ingredients and close the lid.   Cook the peppers for 3 hours on Low.
Nutrition Info:calories 206, fat 7.4, fiber 3.7, carbs 10.2, protein 4.5

211. Creamy Eggplant Salad

Servings: 5   Cooking Time: 3 Hours
Ingredients:

1 eggplant, peeled	1 teaspoon salt
2 bell peppers, chopped	¾ cup coconut milk, unsweetened
1 jalapeno pepper, chopped	1 tablespoon almond flour
1 tablespoon almond milk, unsweetened	1 tablespoon dried dill

Directions:
Chop the eggplant and place it in the slow cooker. Add chopped jalapeno pepper, almond milk, coconut milk, almond flour, and dried dill.   Stir the vegetables gently and close the lid.   Cook the vegetables for 3 hours on High.   Transfer cooked vegetable mixture into the salad bowl.   Add chopped bell peppers and stir well.   Serve the salad!
Nutrition Info:calories 123, fat 8.9, fiber 4.8, carbs 11.5, protein 2.4

212. Creamy Green Beans

Servings: 4   Cooking Time: 2 Hours
Ingredients:

2 cups green beans, trimmed and halved	1 teaspoon turmeric powder
1 tablespoon tahini paste	½ teaspoon salt
1 red chili, minced	1 teaspoon olive oil
	1/3 cup heavy cream

Directions:
Put green beans in the slow cooker.   Add the rest of the ingredients and put the lid on.   Cook the mix for 2 hours on High.   Put in the serving bowls.
Nutrition Info:calories 134, fat 5.9, fiber 3.1, carbs 6.3, protein 6.7

213. Spinach Mix

Servings: 4   Cooking Time: 4 Hours
Ingredients:

3 cups spinach, chopped	4 oz Parmesan, grated
1 cup organic coconut milk	1 teaspoon olive oil
	1 cup fresh cilantro, chopped

Directions:
In the slow cooker, mix the spinach with the milk and the other ingredients, toss and close the lid. Cook the dip on Low for 4 hours.
Nutrition Info:calories 241, fat 7.5, fiber 2.4, carbs 5.5, protein 5.4

214. Layered Mushrooms

Servings: 6   Cooking Time: 6 Hours
Ingredients:

7 oz white mushrooms, sliced	1 teaspoon cayenne pepper
1 eggplant, peeled, sliced	1 onion, grated
1 tablespoon dried dill	5 tablespoons almond milk, unsweetened
	1 oz butter

Directions:
Mix the dried dill, cayenne pepper, and butter. Stir the mixture until smooth.   Melt the butter mixture.   Make a layer of the slice eggplant in the slow cooker.   Brush it with some of the butter mixture.   Make the layer of the mushrooms and top it with the grated onion.   Add all the remaining butter mixture and almond milk. Close the lid and cook the meal for 6 hours on Low. Let the cooked mushrooms rest for 15-20 minutes. Serve!
Nutrition Info:calories 98, fat 7.1, fiber 3.8, carbs 8.4, protein 2.5

215. Asparagus And Onion Mix

Servings: 4   Cooking Time: 3 Hours
Ingredients:

1 cup spring onions, chopped	1 teaspoon salt
12 oz asparagus, chopped	1 teaspoon ground black pepper
½ cup heavy cream	1 tablespoon chives, chopped

Directions:
In the slow cooker, mix the asparagus with the spring onions and the other ingredients, toss and close the lid.   Cook the casserole for 3 hours on High.
Nutrition Info:calories 233, fat 7, fiber 2.6, carbs 7.3, protein 4.7

216. Eggplant Gratin

Servings: 7   Cooking Time: 5 Hours
Ingredients:

1 tablespoon butter	1 teaspoon salt
1 teaspoon minced garlic	4 oz Parmesan, grated
2 eggplants, chopped	4 tablespoons water
1 tablespoon dried parsley	1 teaspoon chili flakes

Directions:
Mix the dried parsley, chili flakes, and salt together. Sprinkle the chopped eggplants with the spice mixture and stir well.   Place the eggplants in the

slow cooker.   Add the water and minced garlic. Add the butter and sprinkle with the grated Parmesan.   Close the lid and cook the gratin for 5 hours on Low.   Open the lid and cool the gratin for 10 minutes.   Serve it.
Nutrition Info:calories 107, fat 5.4, fiber 5.6, carbs 10, protein 6.8

217.Lime Zucchini Noodles

Servings: 4   Cooking Time: 1 Hour And 30 Minutes
Ingredients:
7 oz zucchini noodles
1 tablespoon balsamic vinegar
1 tablespoon lime juice
¼ teaspoon sweet paprika
½ teaspoon salt
1/3 cup water
1 teaspoon butter
Directions:
In the slow cooker, mix the noodles with the vinegar and the other ingredients.   Put the lid on and cook noodles for 1.5 hours on Low.   Divide between plates and serve.
Nutrition Info:calories 120, fat 5.1, fiber 5.3, carbs 0.1, protein 3.4

218.   Peanut Butter & Chocolate Cake

Servings: 12.   Cooking Time: 4 Hours On Low.
Ingredients:
1 Tablespoon butter for greasing the crock-pot
2 cups almond flour
¾ cup sweetener, your choice
¼ cup coconut flakes
¼ cup whey protein powder
1 teaspoon baking powder
¼ teaspoon salt
¾ cup peanut butter, room temperature
4 large eggs
1 teaspoon vanilla extract
½ cup water
3 Tablespoons sugarless dark chocolate, melted
Directions:
Grease the crock-pot well.   In a bowl, mix the dry ingredients. One item at a time, stir in the wet ingredients.   Spread about 2/3 of batter in the crock-pot, add half the chocolate. Swirl with a fork. Top up with the remaining batter and chocolate. Swirl with fork again.   Cover, cook on low for 4 hours. Switch off. Let it set covered for 30 minutes.
Nutrition Info:net C 5g; P 6g; F 20g

219.   Grated Zucchini With Cheese

Servings: 4   Cooking Time: 30 Minutes
Ingredients:
2 oz Parmesan cheese, grated
1 zucchini, grated
1 teaspoon ground black pepper
1 tablespoon olive oil
1 teaspoon dried dill
4 tablespoons water
Directions:
Mix the grated zucchini, ground black pepper, and dried dill.   Stir the mixture and transfer it to the slow cooker.   Add water and olive oil.   Then sprinkle a layer of Parmesan cheese over the zucchini and close the lid.   Cook the meal for 30 minutes on High.   Serve the dish hot!
Nutrition Info:calories 85, fat 6.7, fiber 0.7, carbs 2.6, protein 5.3

220.   Rosemary Cauliflower

Servings: 7   Cooking Time: 3 Hours
Ingredients:
1-pound cauliflower florets
1 teaspoon turmeric powder
1 tablespoon rosemary, chopped
1 teaspoon curry powder
2 tablespoons butter
3 tablespoons almond milk
Directions:
In the slow cooker, mix the cauliflower with the turmeric and the other ingredients, toss and put the lid on.   Cook the vegetables for 3 hours on High. Divide between plates and serve.
Nutrition Info:calories 111, fat 4.5, fiber 1.7, carbs 4.3, protein 1.2

221.   Cilantro Cauliflower Rice

Servings: 2   Cooking Time: 3 Hours
Ingredients:
Juice of 1 lime
salt and black pepper to taste
½ cup of cauliflower rice
2/3 cup of vegetable broth
½ tablespoon of cilantro, diced
Directions:
Start by throwing all the Ingredients: into the Crockpot.   Cover its lid and cook for 2 3 hours on Low setting.   Once done, remove its lid of the crockpot carefully.   Mix well and garnish as desired.   Serve warm.
Nutrition Info: Calories 288 Total Fat 25.3 g Saturated Fat 6.7 g Cholesterol 23 mg Total Carbs 9.6 g Sugar 0.1 g Fiber 3.8 g Sodium 74 mg Potassium 3 mg Protein 7.6 g

222.   Cauliflower Casserole

Servings: 5   Cooking Time: 7 Hours
Ingredients:
2 tomatoes, chopped
11 oz cauliflower chopped
5 oz broccoli, chopped
1 cup water
1 teaspoon salt
1 tablespoon butter
5 oz white mushrooms, chopped
1 teaspoon chili flakes
Directions:
Mix the water, salt, and chili flakes.   Place the butter in the slow cooker.   Add a layer of the chopped cauliflower.   Add the layer of broccoli and tomatoes.   Add the mushrooms and pat down the mix to flatten.   Add the water and close the lid. Cook the casserole for 7 hours on Low.   Cool the casserole to room temperature and serve!
Nutrition Info:calories 61, fat 2.6, fiber 3.2, carbs 8.1, protein 3.4

223.   Cranberry Brussels Sprouts Mix

Servings: 8   Cooking Time: 3 Hours

Ingredients:

4 tablespoon of olive oil	2 teaspoons of thyme, diced
2 teaspoons of rosemary, diced	1 cup of cranberries, dried
2 tablespoons of balsamic vinegar	

Directions:
Start by throwing all the Ingredients: into the Crockpot. Cover its lid and cook for 3 hours on Low setting. Once done, remove its lid of the crockpot carefully. Mix well and garnish as desired. Serve warm.
Nutrition Info: Calories 198 Total Fat 19.2 g Saturated Fat 11.5 g Cholesterol 123 mg Total Carbs 4.5 g Sugar 3.3 g Fiber 0.3 g Sodium 142 mg Potassium 34 mg Protein 3.4 g

224. Mozzarella Zucchinis And Leeks

Servings: 5   Cooking Time: 5 Hours
Ingredients:

1 cup zucchinis, roughly cubed	1 tablespoon chives, chopped
1 cup leeks, sliced	½ teaspoon ground black pepper
1 oz Mozzarella, shredded	¾ cup coconut cream

Directions:
In the slow cooker, mix the zucchinis and leeks with the other ingredients, toss and close the lid. Cook the squash cubes for 5 hours on Low.
Nutrition Info:calories 162, fat 10.6, fiber 1, carbs 5.6, protein 3.9

225. Glazed Leeks

Servings: 2   Cooking Time: 1.5 Hours
Ingredients:

3 leeks, roughly sliced	1 teaspoon butter, melted
1 teaspoon sweet paprika	½ teaspoon ground nutmeg
1 teaspoon stevia	

Directions:
In the slow cooker, mix the leeks with paprika and the other ingredients and close the lid. Cook the parsnip for 1.5 hours on High.
Nutrition Info:calories 115, fat 4.2, fiber 2.7, carbs 4.4, protein 4.4

226. Tomato And Radish

Servings: 4   Cooking Time: 4 Hours
Ingredients:

2 cups radish, trimmed and halved	1 teaspoon oregano, dried
2 cups cherry tomatoes, halved	1 teaspoon salt
½ cup of water	1 teaspoon butter

Directions:
In the slow cooker, mix the radishes with the tomatoes and the other ingredients. Close the lid and cook radish on Low for 4 hours. Divide between plates and serve.

Nutrition Info:calories 109, fat 3.2, fiber 1.2, carbs 2.4, protein 0.4

227. Bok Choy And Radishes

Servings: 2   Cooking Time: 5 Hours
Ingredients:

1 cup bok choy, chopped	3 tablespoons coconut cream
1 tablespoon balsamic vinegar	1 teaspoon salt
1 cup radishes, halved	1 tablespoon lime juice
1 teaspoon olive oil	1 teaspoon paprika

Directions:
In the slow cooker, mix the bok choy with the radishes and the other ingredients, toss and close the lid. Cook the side dish for 5 hours on Low. Divide between plates and serve.
Nutrition Info:calories 121, fat 3.6, fiber 1.5, carbs 3.7, protein 1.5

228. Chard And Radishes

Servings: 4   Cooking Time: 4 Hours
Ingredients:

2 cups red chard, torn	¼ cup butter
1 cup radishes, halved	1 teaspoon salt
1 teaspoon sweet paprika	¼ teaspoon ground ginger
	1/4 cup veggie stock

Directions:
In the slow cooker, mix the chard with radishes and the other ingredients   Close the slow cooker lid and cook the beet greens for 4 hours on High. Mix up the mix carefully before serving.
Nutrition Info:calories 122, fat 4.7, fiber 2.1, carbs 6.5, protein 4.5

229. Dill Broccoli

Servings: 4   Cooking Time: 1.5 Hour
Ingredients:

2 cups broccoli florets	2 tablespoons butter
2 tablespoons fresh dill, chopped	1 teaspoon oregano, dried
1 teaspoon basil, dried	½ cup heavy cream
	¼ teaspoon ground nutmeg

Directions:
In the slow cooker, mix the broccoli with the dill and the other ingredients. Close the lid and cook the vegetables on High for 1.5 hours on High. When the time is over, divide between plates and serve.
Nutrition Info:calories 120, fat 6.5, fiber 1.5, carbs 4, protein 4.7

230. Curry Mushrooms

Servings: 2   Cooking Time: 4 Hours
Ingredients:

1-pound white mushrooms, halved	1 cup of coconut milk
1 teaspoon curry paste	1 teaspoon coriander, ground
1 teaspoon garam masala	1 teaspoon dill, chopped
	1 teaspoon olive oil

Directions:
In the slow cooker, mix the mushrooms with coconut milk, curry paste and the other ingredients, toss and close the lid. Cook the side dish for 4 hours on High.
Nutrition Info:calories 213, fat 7.9, fiber 4.1, carbs 7.5, protein 4.5

231.	Zucchini Gratin

Servings: 3   Cooking Time: 5 Hours
Ingredients:

1 zucchini, sliced	3 oz Parmesan, grated
1 teaspoon ground black pepper	1 tablespoon butter
	½ cup almond milk

Directions:
Sprinkle the sliced zucchini with the ground black pepper. Chop the butter and place it in the slow cooker. Transfer the sliced zucchini to the slow cooker to make the bottom layer. Add the almond milk. Sprinkle the zucchini with the grated cheese and close the lid. Cook the gratin for 5 hours on Low. Then let the gratin cool until room temperature. Serve it!
Nutrition Info:calories 229, fat 19.6, fiber 1.8, carbs 5.9, protein 10.9

232.	Tomato Gratin With Bell Pepper

Servings: 4   Cooking Time: 4 Hours
Ingredients:

2 tomatoes, sliced	1 tablespoons dried parsley
6 oz bell pepper, sliced	¼ teaspoon ground coriander
4 oz Parmesan, grated	1 teaspoon butter
¼ cup almond milk, unsweetened	1 garlic clove, diced

Directions:
Chop the butter and place it in the slow cooker. Make a layer of the sliced tomatoes in the bottom of the slow cooker on top of the butter. Next, make a layer of the bell peppers. Sprinkle the vegetables with the almond milk, dried parsley, ground coriander, and diced garlic clove. Place the grated cheese over the vegetables and close the lid. Cook the gratin for 4 hours on Low. Serve the side dish immediately!
Nutrition Info:calories 204, fat 1.2, fiber 3.5, carbs 18, protein 11.9

233.	Vegetable Stew

Servings: 5   Cooking Time: 7 Hours
Ingredients:

1 cup spinach	2 cups water
5 oz white cabbage, chopped	1 garlic clove, peeled
5 oz white mushrooms, chopped	1 teaspoon white pepper
6 oz cauliflower, chopped	1 teaspoon chili flakes
½ cup almond milk, unsweetened	1 teaspoon turmeric
	1 teaspoon butter

Directions:
Chop the spinach roughly and place it in the slow cooker. Add white cabbage, mushrooms, and cauliflower. Add almond milk, water, garlic clove, white pepper, chili flakes, and turmeric. Stir the vegetables with a spoon. Add butter and close the lid. Cook the stew for 7 hours on Low. Let the stew cool for 15 minutes. Serve it!
Nutrition Info:calories 89, fat 6.7, fiber 2.7, carbs 6.7, protein 2.8

234.	Mayo Salad

Servings: 8   Cooking Time: 5 Hours
Ingredients:

3 media eggplant, peeled and cubed	1/8 cup of diced onion
3 large eggs, boiled, peeled and cubed	½ tablespoon of dill pickle juice
½ cup of mayonnaise	½ tablespoon of mustard
1 tablespoon of finely fresh parsley, chopped	Salt and black pepper-to taste

Directions:
Start by putting eggplant and water into the Crockpot. Cover its lid and cook for 5 hours on Low setting. Once done, remove its lid of the crockpot carefully. Toss the slow-cooked eggplant with the remaining Ingredients: in a salad bowl. Mix well and garnish as desired. Serve warm.
Nutrition Info: Calories 114 Total Fat 9.6 g Saturated Fat 4.5 g Cholesterol 10 mg Total Carbs 3.1 g Sugar 1.4 g Fiber 1.5 g Sodium 155 mg Potassium 93 mg Protein 3.5 g

235.	Tomato And Eggplant Salad

Servings: 3   Cooking Time: 2 Hours
Ingredients:

1 large eggplant, roughly sliced	¼ teaspoon salt
1-pound cherry tomatoes, halved	½ teaspoon black pepper
1 teaspoon balsamic vinegar	¼ teaspoon turmeric
1 teaspoon fresh basil, chopped	3 tablespoons heavy cream
	1 teaspoon butter

Directions:
Spread the slow cooker bottom with butter and combine all the ingredients inside. Close the slow cooker lid and cook the eggplant slices for 2 hours on High.
Nutrition Info:calories 206, fat 7.1, fiber 5.7, carbs 6.3, protein 7

236.	Coconut Cauliflower Mash

Servings: 4   Cooking Time: 4 Hours
Ingredients:

1/6 cup of coconut cream	½ tablespoon of chives, diced
1/6 cup of coconut milk	Salt and black pepper- to taste

Directions:

Start by throwing all the Ingredients: into the Crockpot. Cover its lid and cook for 4 hours on Low setting. Once done, remove its lid of the crockpot carefully. Puree the slow-cooked cauliflower using an immersion blender. Mix well and garnish as desired. Serve warm.

Nutrition Info: Calories 192 Total Fat 17.44 g Saturated Fat 11.5 g Cholesterol 125 mg Total Carbs 2.2 g Sugar 1.4 g Fiber 2.1 g Sodium 135 mg Potassium 53 mg Protein 4.7 g

237. Greens Mix

Servings: 6   Cooking Time: 8 Hours

Ingredients:
- 2 cups of kale, chopped
- 1 lb. ham shanks, sliced
- 4 pickled jalapeno peppers, diced
- black pepper to taste
- 1/2 teaspoon of baking soda
- 1 teaspoon of olive oil
- garlic powder to taste

Directions:
Start by throwing all the Ingredients: into the Crockpot. Cover its lid and cook for 8 hours on Low setting. Once done, remove its lid of the crockpot carefully. Mix well and garnish as desired. Serve warm.

Nutrition Info: Calories 77.8 Total Fat 7.13 g Saturated Fat 4.5 g Cholesterol 15 mg Total Carbs 0.8 g Sugar 0.2 g Fiber 0.3 g Sodium 15 mg Potassium 33 mg Protein 2.3 g

238. Chinese Broccoli

Servings: 4   Cooking Time: 1 Hour

Ingredients:
- 1 tablespoon sesame seeds
- 1 tablespoon olive oil
- 1 teaspoon chili flakes
- 10 oz broccoli
- 1 tablespoon apple cider vinegar
- 3 tablespoons water
- ¼ teaspoon garlic powder

Directions:
Cut the broccoli into the florets and sprinkle with the olive oil, chili flakes, apple cider vinegar, and garlic powder. Stir the broccoli and place it in the slow cooker. Add water and sesame seeds. Cook the broccoli for 1 hour on High. Transfer the cooked broccoli to serving plates and enjoy!

Nutrition Info:calories 69, fat 4.9, fiber 2.1, carbs 5.4, protein 2.4

239. Coconut Radish Mix

Servings: 2   Cooking Time: 4 Hours

Ingredients:
- 1 cup radishes, halved
- ½ cup coconut cream
- 1 tablespoon dried rosemary
- 1 tablespoon butter
- 1 teaspoon black pepper
- ½ teaspoon salt

Directions:
In the slow cooker, mix the radishes with the cream and the other ingredients. Close the lid and cook the mix for 4 hours on Low.

Nutrition Info:calories 82, fat 6.2, fiber 2.5, carbs 6.8, protein 1

240. Tofu And Green Beans

Servings: 6   Cooking Time: 7.5 Hours

Ingredients:
- 1 teaspoon cumin seeds
- ½ teaspoon sweet paprika
- 1 teaspoon keto tomato sauce
- 1 teaspoon chili flakes
- 1 teaspoon rosemary, dried
- 1 teaspoon salt
- 7 oz firm tofu, cubed
- 7 oz green beans, halved
- ½ cup crushed tomatoes
- 1 chili pepper, chopped
- 1 tablespoon almond butter

Directions:
In the slow cooker, combine the tofu with green beans and the other ingredients. Close the lid and cook for 7.5 hours on Low.

Nutrition Info:calories 132, fat 3.3, fiber 3.5, carbs 7.4, protein 5.3

241. Sesame Snow Peas

Servings: 4   Cooking Time: 1 Hour

Ingredients:
- 1 tablespoon sesame seeds
- 1 teaspoon cayenne pepper
- 1-pound snow peas
- 1 teaspoon butter
- 1 cup water

Directions:
Place the snow peas in the slow cooker. Add the cayenne pepper, sesame seeds, and butter. Add water and close the lid. Cook the snow peas for 1 hour on High. Strain the vegetables and serve them immediately!

Nutrition Info:calories 70, fat 2.4, fiber 3.6, carbs 8.8, protein 4.2

242. Ginger Peppers

Servings: 2   Cooking Time: 1 Hour

Ingredients:
- 4 red bell peppers, cut into strips
- 1 teaspoon ground ginger
- 1/2 cup veggie stock
- 1 teaspoon sweet paprika
- 1 teaspoon butter
- ½ teaspoon salt

Directions:
In the slow cooker, mix the peppers with the ginger and the other ingredients. Close the lid and cook for 1 hour on High.

Nutrition Info:calories 162, fat 3.9, fiber 0.1, carbs 4.3, protein 2.3

243. Zucchini Slices With Mozzarella

Servings: 4   Cooking Time: 1 Hour

Ingredients:
- 3 oz Mozzarella, sliced
- 1 zucchini, sliced
- 1 tablespoon olive oil
- 1 teaspoon butter
- 1 tablespoon coconut flakes, unsweetened
- 1 teaspoon minced garlic

Directions:
Sprinkle the zucchini slices with the olive oil, coconut flakes, and minced garlic. Place the zucchini slices in a flat layer on the bottom of the slow cooker along with the butter. Place a piece of mozzarella on top of each zucchini slice. Close the lid and cook the meal for 1 hour on High. Serve hot!
Nutrition Info:calories 112, fat 8.7, fiber 0.7, carbs 2.8, protein 6.7

244.   Sautéed Bell Peppers

Servings: 6   Cooking Time: 5 Hours
Ingredients:

8 oz bell peppers	¾ cup coconut milk, unsweetened
7 oz cauliflower, chopped	1 teaspoon butter
2 oz bacon, chopped	1 teaspoon thyme
1 teaspoon salt	1 onion, diced
1 teaspoon ground black pepper	1 teaspoon turmeric

Directions:
Remove the seeds from the bell peppers and chop them roughly. Place the bell peppers, cauliflower, and bacon in the slow cooker. Add the salt, ground black pepper, coconut milk, butter, milk, and thyme. Stir well then add the diced onion. Add the turmeric and stir the mixture. Close the lid and cook 5 hours on Low. When the meal is cooked, let it chill for 10 minutes and serve it!
Nutrition Info:calories 195, fat 12.2, fiber 4.2, carbs 13.1, protein 6.7

245.   Celery Puree

Servings: 3   Cooking Time: 3 Hours
Ingredients:

1 cup celery stalks, chopped	2 tablespoons butter
1 teaspoon sweet paprika	1 teaspoon chives, chopped
	½ cup of water

Directions:
Put celery and water in the slow cooker. Close the lid and cook it for 3 hours on High. Then drain water and mash until you get soft mash. Add the rest of the ingredients, whisk and serve.
Nutrition Info:calories 151, fat 6.8, fiber 2.2, carbs 8, protein 0.6

246.   Spicy Kale

Servings: 3   Cooking Time: 2.5 Hours
Ingredients:

2 cups kale, chopped	1/3 cup coconut cream
4 oz Mozzarella balls, sliced	1 teaspoon keto tomato sauce

Directions:
In the slow cooker, mix the kale with the remaining ingredients. Close the lid and cook spinach on Low for 5 hours.
Nutrition Info:calories 202, fat 8.5, fiber 0.5, carbs 1.5, protein 6.6

247.   Tender Green Cabbage

Servings: 4   Cooking Time: 1 Hour

Ingredients:

¼ cup almond milk, unsweetened	1 oz almonds, chopped
11 oz green cabbage, shredded	1 teaspoon butter
	4 tablespoons water

Directions:
Place the shredded green cabbage in the slow cooker. Add butter, water, and almond milk. Stir gently and close the lid. Cook the cabbage for 1 hour on High. Transfer the cooked side dish into the serving bowls. Sprinkle with the chopped almonds and serve!
Nutrition Info:calories 103, fat 8.2, fiber 3.2, carbs 6.9, protein 2.9

248.   Bbq Smokies

Servings: 6   Cooking Time: 2 Hours
Ingredients:

1 cup of sugar-free tomato sauce	1/3 cup of diced onion
1 tablespoon of Worcestershire sauce	2 (16 ounce) packages little wieners

Directions:
Start by throwing all the Ingredients: into the Crockpot. Cover its lid and cook for 2 hours on Low setting. Once done, remove its lid of the crockpot carefully. Mix well and garnish as desired. Serve warm.
Nutrition Info: Calories 251 Total Fat 24.5 g Saturated Fat 14.7 g Cholesterol 165 mg Total Carbs 4.3 g Sugar 0.5 g Fiber 1 g Sodium 142 mg Potassium 80 mg Protein 51.9 g

249.   Cheesy Spaghetti Squash

Servings: 2   Cooking Time: 4 Hours
Ingredients:

10 oz spaghetti squash, peeled and seeded	½ teaspoon thyme
1 tablespoon butter	1 teaspoon paprika
	1/3 cup water
	2 oz Parmesan, sliced

Directions:
Grate the spaghetti squash and place it in the slow cooker. Add the butter, thyme, paprika, and water. Stir the mixture gently with a spoon. Then cover the squash with the sliced cheese and close the lid. Cook the meal for 4 hours on Low. Let the cooked squash rest for 15 minutes. Serve it!
Nutrition Info:calories 190, fat 12.8, fiber 0.5, carbs 11.6, protein 10.3

250.   Thyme Mushrooms

Servings: 4   Cooking Time: 2 Hours
Ingredients:

10 oz mushrooms, halved	1 teaspoon black pepper
1 tablespoon thyme	½ teaspoon salt
½ cup chicken stock	

Directions:
In the slow cooker, mix all the ingredients, toss and close the lid. Cook the mix for 2 hours on High. When the side dish is cooked, shake it well.
Nutrition Info:calories 158, fat 3.3, fiber 1, carbs 2.9, protein 1

| **251.** | **Garlicky Cauliflower Florets** |

Servings: 6   Cooking Time: 6 Hours
Ingredients:

2 tablespoon of sweet chili sauce	Juice of 1 lime
1 pinch salt and black pepper	3 Garlic cloves, minced
1 teaspoon of Cilantro, diced	1 Cauliflower head, florets separated

Directions:
Start by throwing all the Ingredients: into the Crockpot.   Cover its lid and cook for 6 hours on Low setting.   Once done, remove its lid of the crockpot carefully.   Mix well and garnish as desired.   Serve warm.
Nutrition Info: Calories 167 Total Fat 35.1 g Saturated Fat 10.1 g Cholesterol 12 mg Total Carbs 8.9 g Sugar 3.8 g Fiber 2.1 g Sodium 48 mg Potassium 87 mg Protein 6.3 g

| **252.** | **Hot Green Beans** |

Servings: 5   Cooking Time: 1 Hour
Ingredients:

1-pound green beans, chopped	1 teaspoon curry powder
1 teaspoon chili powder	1 tablespoon sesame oil
1 teaspoon hot paprika	1 tablespoon Erythritol
1 cup of water	

Directions:
In the slow cooker, mix the green beans with chili powder and the other ingredients, close the lid and cook on High for 1 hour.   Divide between plates and serve.
Nutrition Info:calories 56, fat 3.1, fiber 3.2, carbs 9.6, protein 1.8

| **253.** | **Rhubarb And Zucchini Mix** |

Servings: 4   Cooking Time: 6 Hours
Ingredients:

2 cups rhubarb, chopped	7 oz Cheddar cheese, shredded
1 cup zucchini, sliced	4 tablespoons coconut cream
1 teaspoon coriander, ground	1 teaspoon butter
1 teaspoon curry powder	1 teaspoon olive oil
1 teaspoon garam masala	½ teaspoon salt
	¼ cup fresh cilantro, chopped

Directions:
In the slow cooker, mix the rhubarb with the zucchini and the other ingredients, toss and close the slow cooker lid.   Cook the mix for 6 hours on Low.
Nutrition Info:calories 200, fat 10.2, fiber 1.2, carbs 4.3, protein 7.6

| **254.** | **Curry Cauliflower** |

Servings: 2   Cooking Time: 5 Hours
Ingredients:

10 oz cauliflower	½ teaspoon dried cilantro
1 teaspoon curry paste	1 oz butter
1 teaspoon curry powder	¾ cup water
	¼ cup chicken stock

Directions:
Chop the cauliflower roughly and sprinkle it with the curry powder and dried cilantro.   Place the chopped cauliflower in the slow cooker.   Mix the curry paste with the water.   Add chicken stock and transfer the liquid to the slow cooker.   Add butter and close the lid.   Cook the cauliflower for 5 hours on Low.   Strain ½ of the liquid off and discard. Transfer the cauliflower to serving bowls.   Serve it!
Nutrition Info:calories 158, fat 13.3, fiber 3.9, carbs 8.9, protein 3.3

| **255.** | **Cowboy Mexican Dip** |

Servings: 24   Cooking Time: 2 Hours
Ingredients:

1 (15 oz.) can chili	1 (1 lb.) loaf processed cheese, cubed
1 (14.5 oz.) can tomatoes and green chilis	

Directions:
Start by throwing all the Ingredients: into the Crockpot.   Cover its lid and cook for 2 hours on Low setting.   Once done, remove its lid of the crockpot carefully.   Mix well and garnish as desired.   Serve warm.
Nutrition Info: Calories 107 Total Fat 29 g Saturated Fat 14g Cholesterol 111 mg Total Carbs 7 g Sugar 1 g Fiber 3 g Sodium 122 mg Potassium 78 mg Protein 6 g

| **256.** | **Artichoke Spinach** |

Servings: 4   Cooking Time: 4 Hours
Ingredients:

salt and black pepper to taste	Juice of a ½ lemon
1 cup of baby spinach	¼ cup of chicken stock
1 tablespoon of parsley, chopped	garlic clove, minced
½ cup of mozzarella, shredded	1 tablespoon of butter, melted
2/3 cup of coconut milk	1/2 pinch red pepper flakes

Directions:
Start by throwing all the Ingredients: into the Crockpot.   Cover its lid and cook for 4 hours on Low setting.   Once done, remove its lid of the crockpot carefully.   Mix well and garnish as desired.   Serve warm.
Nutrition Info: Calories 215 Total Fat 20 g Saturated Fat 7 g Cholesterol 38 mg Total Carbs 8 g Sugar 1 g Fiber 6 g Sodium 12 mg Potassium 30 mg Protein 5 g

| **257.** | **Marinated Mushrooms** |

Servings: 12   Cooking Time: 12 Hours
Ingredients:

4 cubes beef bouillon	1 cup of dry red wine
2 cups of boiling	1 teaspoon of garlic

water | powder
1 teaspoon of dill weed | 4 lbs. fresh mushrooms
1 teaspoon of Worcestershire sauce | 1/2 cup of butter, or more as needed

Directions:
Start by throwing all the Ingredients: into the Crockpot. Cover its lid and cook for 12 hours on Low setting. Once done, remove its lid of the crockpot carefully. Mix well and garnish as desired. Serve warm.
Nutrition Info: Calories 159 Total Fat 34 g Saturated Fat 10.3 g Cholesterol 112 mg Total Carbs 8.5 g Sugar 2 g Fiber 1.3 g Sodium 92 mg Protein 7.5 g

258. Radish And Tomato Salad

Servings: 4   Cooking Time: 1 Hour
Ingredients:

1 cup cherry tomatoes, halved | 1 teaspoon olive oil
1 cup lettuce, chopped | 1 teaspoon salt
1 cup radish, halved | 1 tablespoon chives, chopped
1 tablespoon balsamic vinegar | 1 teaspoon lemon juice
 | 1 teaspoon sesame oil

Directions:
In the slow cooker, mix the radish with tomatoes, olive oil and balsamic vinegar and toss. Close the lid and cook the vegetables for 1 hour on High. Transfer to a salad bowl, add the rest of the ingredients, toss and serve.
Nutrition Info:calories 55, fat 5.3, fiber 0.8, carbs 2.1, protein 0.6

259. Mashed Cauliflower

Servings: 5   Cooking Time: 3 Hours
Ingredients:

3 tablespoons butter | 1 teaspoon salt
1-pound cauliflower | 1 teaspoon ground black pepper
1 tablespoons full-fat cream | 1 oz dill, chopped

Directions:
Wash the cauliflower and chop it. Place the chopped cauliflower in the slow cooker. Add butter and full-fat cream. Add salt and ground black pepper. Stir the mixture and close the lid. Cook the cauliflower for 3 hours on High. When the cauliflower is cooked, transfer it to a blender and blend until smooth. Place the smooth cauliflower in a bowl and mix with the chopped dill. Stir it well and serve!
Nutrition Info:calories 101, fat 7.4, fiber 3.2, carbs 8.3, protein 3.1

260. Butter Zucchini

Servings: 3   Cooking Time: 15 Minutes
Ingredients:

1 cup zucchinis, sliced | 1 teaspoon turmeric powder
1 teaspoon oregano, dried | 1/3 cup heavy cream
2 tablespoons butter | 1 teaspoon salt

Directions:
In the slow cooker, mix the zucchinis with the oregano and the other ingredients, toss and close the lid. Cook the green peas for 15 minutes on High.
Nutrition Info:calories 134, fat 5.9, fiber 2.6, carbs 7.6, protein 3

261. Hot Tomatoes

Servings: 4   Cooking Time: 6 Hours
Ingredients:

2 cups tomatoes, roughly cubed | 1/2 teaspoon dried basil
1 jalapeno pepper | 1/2 teaspoon dried oregano
1 teaspoon chili powder | 3/4 teaspoon ground ginger
1 teaspoon hot paprika | 1 teaspoon lemon juice
3/4 cup chicken stock |
1 teaspoon salt |

Directions:
In the slow cooker, mix the tomatoes with jalapeno pepper, chili powder and the other ingredients and toss. Close the lid and cook on Low for 6 hours. Serve warm.
Nutrition Info:calories 146, fat 1.5, fiber 0.9, carbs 2.7, protein 0.6

262. Cabbage Steaks

Servings: 4   Cooking Time: 2 Hours
Ingredients:

10 oz white cabbage | 1/2 teaspoon chili flakes
1 tablespoon butter | 4 tablespoons water
1/2 teaspoon cayenne pepper |

Directions:
Slice the cabbage into medium steaks and rub them with the cayenne pepper and chili flakes. Rub the cabbage steaks with butter on each side. Place them in the slow cooker and sprinkle with water. Close the lid and cook the cabbage steaks for 2 hours on High. When the cabbage steaks are cooked, they should be tender to the touch. Serve the cabbage steak after 10 minutes of chilling.
Nutrition Info:calories 44, fat 3, fiber 1.8, carbs 4.3, protein 1

263. Broccoli And Cauliflower Bake

Servings: 4   Cooking Time: 8 Hours
Ingredients:

2 cups broccoli florets | 4 eggs, beaten
2 cups cauliflower florets | 1/2 cup coconut milk
5 oz Cheddar cheese, shredded | 1 teaspoon turmeric powder
 | 1/2 teaspoon salt

Directions:
In the slow cooker, mix the broccoli with cauliflower and the other ingredients except the cheese and toss. Sprinkle the cheese on top. Close the lid and cook the mix for 8 hours on Low.
Nutrition Info:calories 242, fat 17.6, fiber 1.8, carbs 4.8, protein 12.4

264.	Cherry Tomatoes Sauté

Servings: 4   Cooking Time: 3 Hours

Ingredients:

- 2 cups cherry tomatoes, halved
- 1/2 cup veggie stock
- 1 teaspoon salt
- 1 teaspoon chili flakes
- 1 teaspoon dried oregano
- ¼ teaspoon ground nutmeg
- 1 tablespoon keto tomato sauce

Directions:

In the slow cooker, mix the tomatoes and the other ingredients.   Then close the slow cooker lid and cook soybeans on High for 2 hours.   Divide between plates and serve.

Nutrition Info:calories 201, fat 7, fiber 1.7, carbs 8.8, protein 7.9

265.	Tomato And Spaghetti Squash

Servings: 4   Cooking Time: 3 Hours

Ingredients:

- 10 oz spaghetti squash, halved
- 1 cup cherry tomatoes, halved
- 1 teaspoon sweet paprika
- 2 oz Parmesan
- 1 teaspoon butter
- ½ teaspoon garlic powder
- ½ teaspoon turmeric powder
- ½ cup of water

Directions:

Pour water in the slow cooker.   Add spaghetti squash and cook it on High for 3 hours.   When the squash is soft, it is cooked.   Shred the vegetable with the help of the fork.   In the shallow bowl, mix the spaghetti squash with the remaining ingredients, toss and serve.

Nutrition Info:calories 178, fat 4.4, fiber 3.1, carbs 5.8, protein 5.1

266.	Savoury Almond Bread

Servings: 8.   Cooking Time: 3 Hours On Low.

Ingredients:

- 2 cups ground almonds
- ½ cup flax seed meal
- Salt and pepper to taste
- ½ teaspoon baking soda
- 2 large eggs
- ¼ cup basil pesto sauce
- ¼ cup Parmesan
- 1 ½ Cheddar cheese, grated
- 1 cup coconut milk

Directions:

Combine dry ingredients in a bowl.   Blend wet ingredients in another bowl.   Mix the two slowly. Butter the crock-pot, pour in the batter.   Cover the crock-pot with a paper towel to absorb the water. Cover, cook on low for 3 hours.

Nutrition Info:net C 9g; P 13g; F 28g

267.	Butter Mushrooms

Servings: 2   Cooking Time: 3.5 Hours

Ingredients:

- 1 cup cremini mushrooms
- 3 tablespoons butter, melted
- 1 teaspoon black pepper
- 1 teaspoon coriander,
- 1 tablespoon turmeric ground powder
- 1 teaspoon salt

Directions:

In the slow cooker, mix the mushrooms with the other ingredients.   Cook the side dish for 3.5 hours on Low.

Nutrition Info:calories 214, fat 11.4, fiber 3.2, carbs 2.3, protein 1.1

268.	Garlic Cauliflower Steaks

Servings: 4   Cooking Time: 3 Hours

Ingredients:

- 14 oz cauliflower head
- 1 teaspoon minced garlic
- 4 tablespoons butter
- 4 tablespoons water
- 1 teaspoon paprika

Directions:

Wash the cauliflower head carefully and slice it into the medium steaks.   Mix up together the butter, minced garlic, and paprika.   Rub the cauliflower steaks with the butter mixture.   Pour the water in the slow cooker.   Add the cauliflower steaks and close the lid.   Cook the vegetables for 3 hours on High.   Transfer the cooked cauliflower steaks to a platter and serve them immediately!

Nutrition Info:calories 129, fat 11.7, fiber 2.7, carbs 5.8, protein 2.2

269.	Green Beans

Servings: 16   Cooking Time: 3 Hours

Ingredients:

- 1/2 cup of butter, melted
- 1/2 cup of packed brown swerve
- 1 1/2 teaspoons of garlic salt
- 3/4 teaspoon of soy sauce

Directions:

Start by throwing all the Ingredients: into the Crockpot.   Cover its lid and cook for 3 hours on Low setting.   Once done, remove its lid of the crockpot carefully.   Mix well and garnish as desired.   Serve warm.

Nutrition Info: Calories 237 Total Fat 22 g Saturated Fat 9 g Cholesterol 35 mg Total Carbs 5 g Sugar 1 g Fiber 2 g Sodium 118 mg Potassium 137 mg Protein 5 g

270.	Leeks And Cauliflower Mash

Servings: 2   Cooking Time: 4 Hours

Ingredients:

- 1 cup leeks, chopped
- 1 cup cauliflower florets
- 1 tablespoon coconut cream
- 1 teaspoon turmeric powder
- 1 teaspoon curry powder
- ½ teaspoon ground black pepper
- ½ teaspoon salt
- ½ cup of water

Directions:

Put leeks, cauliflower, salt and water in the slow cooker.   Close the lid and cook for 4 hours on Low. Then drain water.   Mash the mix, add the rest of the ingredients, whisk and serve.

Nutrition Info:calories 189, fat 4.3, fiber 5.4, carbs 9.5, protein 6.5

271. Parsley And Tomato Green Beans

Servings: 3   Cooking Time: 7 Hours

Ingredients:

1 ½ cup green beans, trimmed and halved	1/3 cup keto tomato sauce
2 tablespoons fresh parsley, chopped	1 teaspoon chili pepper
1 tablespoon rosemary, chopped	1 teaspoon salt
1 teaspoon butter	1 teaspoon black pepper

Directions:

In the slow cooker, mix the green beans with the parsley and the other ingredients.   Close the slow cooker lid and cook chili on Low for 7 hours. Divide between plates and serve.

Nutrition Info:calories 228, fat 12.7, fiber 5.1, carbs 11.1, protein 14.6

272.   Curled Rutabaga

Servings: 5   Cooking Time: 2 Hours

Ingredients:

1 tablespoon olive oil	13 oz rutabaga
1 teaspoon ground black pepper	1 teaspoon salt
	½ teaspoon paprika
	3 tablespoons water

Directions:

Cut the rutabaga into the long strips with the help of the scissors.   Sprinkle the rutabaga curls with the olive oil, ground black pepper, salt, and paprika. Stir gently and place in the slow cooker.   Add the water and close the lid.   Cook for 2 hours on High. Serve the side dish hot!

Nutrition Info:calories 52, fat 3, fiber 2, carbs 6.4, protein 1

273.   Cumin Green Beans

Servings: 4   Cooking Time: 10 Minutes

Ingredients:

8 oz green beans	1 oz butter
1 teaspoon cumin	1 teaspoon dried cilantro
¾ cup coconut milk, unsweetened	

Directions:

Toss the butter in the slow cooker.   Add the coconut milk, cumin and dried cilantro.   Stir the liquid with a spatula.   Add green beans and close the lid.   Cook the side dish for 6 hours on Low. Open the lid and let the beans cool for 10 minutes. Serve it!

Nutrition Info:calories 174, fat 16.7, fiber 3, carbs 6.8, protein 2.2

274.   Mint Peppers

Servings: 5   Cooking Time: 8 Hours

Ingredients:

½ cup crushed tomatoes	2 teaspoons mint, dried
2 green bell peppers, roughly chopped	1 teaspoon curry powder
2 red bell peppers, roughly chopped	1 teaspoon chili flakes
½ teaspoon turmeric	¼ cup of water

Directions:

In the slow cooker, mix the peppers with tomatoes and the other ingredients.   Close the slow cooker lid and cook for 8 hours on Low.   Divide into bowls and serve.

Nutrition Info:calories 31, fat 0.4, fiber 2.3, carbs 8.1, protein 1.7

275.   Thai Cabbage

Servings: 4   Cooking Time: 6 Hours

Ingredients:

1 tablespoon coconut oil	1 tablespoon curry paste
7 oz white cabbage, shredded	1 teaspoon salt
3 tablespoons water	3 tablespoons butter, melted

Directions:

Mix the curry paste and water.   Add salt and coconut oil and whisk.   Place the shredded cabbage in the slow cooker.   Sprinkle it with the curry paste mixture.   Add the butter and stir the vegetables gently.   Close the lid and cook the cabbage on Low for 6 hours.   When the time is done, let the cabbage rest for 10 minutes.   Serve it!

Nutrition Info:calories 143, fat 14.3, fiber 1.2, carbs 4, protein 0.9

276.	**Sardine Pate**

Servings: 6   Cooking Time: 3 Hours
Ingredients:
- ½ cup water
- 3 tablespoons butter
- 1 teaspoon onion powder
- 1 teaspoon dried parsley
- 12 oz sardine fillets, chopped

Directions:
Put the chopped sardine fillets, dried parsley, onion powder, and water in the slow cooker.   Close the lid and cook the fish for 3 hours on Low.   Strain the sardine fillet and put it in a blender.   Add butter and blend the mixture for 3 minutes on high speed.   Transfer the cooked pate into serving bowls and serve!
Nutrition Info:calories 170, fat 12.3, fiber 0, carbs 0.3, protein 14.1

277.	**Cod Fillet In Coconut Flakes**

Servings: 4   Cooking Time: 1 Hour
Ingredients:
- ¼ cup coconut flakes, unsweetened
- 1 egg, beaten
- 1 teaspoon ground black pepper
- ½ teaspoon salt
- 10 oz cod fillets
- 1 tablespoon butter
- 3 tablespoons water

Directions:
Whisk the egg, combine it with the salt, and ground black pepper.   Place the cod fillets in the egg mixture and stir well.   Coat the egged cod fillets in the coconut flakes.   Add the butter to the slow cooker.   Add water and coated cod fillets.   Close the lid and cook the fish for 1 hour on High.   Then transfer the cod fillets onto a cutting board and cut them into servings.   Enjoy the cod fillet warm!
Nutrition Info:calories 117, fat 6.3, fiber 0.6, carbs 1.2, protein 14.3

278.	**Keto Chili**

Servings: 6   Cooking Time: 3 Hours
Ingredients:
- 8 oz ground beef
- 2 cups spinach, chopped
- 1 tablespoon tomato puree
- 1 bell pepper, chopped
- ½ teaspoon ground coriander
- 1 onion, diced
- 1 teaspoon ground black pepper
- 1 teaspoon chili pepper
- ½ garlic clove, diced
- 1 cup water
- 1 teaspoon butter

Directions:
Mix the ground beef, chopped spinach, tomato puree, diced onion, ground coriander, ground black pepper, chili pepper and diced onion.   Stir the mixture until well blended and transfer it to a slow cooker.   Add water and butter.   Close the lid and cook the chili for 3 hours on High.   Cool the cooked chili slightly and serve!
Nutrition Info:calories 94, fat 3.1, fiber 1.1, carbs 4.2, protein 12.3

279.	**Duck Rolls**

Servings: 6   Cooking Time: 3 Hours
Ingredients:
- 2-pound duck fillets
- 1 teaspoon minced garlic
- 1 cup spinach, chopped
- ¼ cup water
- 1 teaspoon rosemary
- 1 tablespoon olive oil

Directions:
Beat the duck fillets gently to tenderize and flatten then sprinkle them with the minced garlic, rosemary, and olive oil.   Place the chopped spinach on each of the duck fillets and roll them up, enclosing the spinach inside the duck.   Secure the duck rolls with the toothpicks and place them in the slow cooker.   Add water and close the lid.   Cook the duck rolls for 3 hours on High.   Cool the rolls slightly and serve!
Nutrition Info:calories 210, fat 3.3, fiber 0.2, carbs 0.5, protein 44.8

280.	**Pulled Pork Salad**

Servings: 4   Cooking Time: 8 Hours
Ingredients:
- 1 avocado, chopped
- 1 cup lettuce, chopped
- 1 tablespoon olive oil
- ½ teaspoon chili flakes
- 1 tomato, chopped
- 7 oz pork loin
- 1 cup water
- 1 bay leaf
- 1 teaspoon salt
- ¼ teaspoon peppercorns

Directions:
Place the pork loin in the slow cooker.   Add the water, bay leaf, salt, and peppercorns.   Add the chili flakes and close the lid.   Cook the pork loin for 8 hours on Low.   Meanwhile, mix the chopped avocado, tomato, and lettuce in a large salad bowl. When the pork loin is cooked, remove it from the water and place it in a separate bowl.   Shred the pork loin with two forks.   Add the shredded pork loin into the salad bowl.   Stir the salad gently and sprinkle with the olive oil.   Enjoy!
Nutrition Info:calories 258, fat 20.3, fiber 3.8, carbs 5.6, protein 14.7

281.	**Chicken Liver Sauté**

Servings: 4   Cooking Time: 5 Hours
Ingredients:
- 10 oz chicken liver
- 1 onion, chopped
- 2 tablespoons full-fat cream
- 5 oz white mushrooms, chopped
- 1 cup water
- 1 tablespoon butter
- 1 teaspoon salt
- ½ teaspoon ground black pepper

Directions:
Place the chicken liver, onion, full-fat cream, mushrooms, water, butter, salt, and ground black pepper in the slow cooker and close the lid.   Cook the mixture for 5 hours on Low.   When the liver saute is cooked, let it rest for 10 minutes.   Enjoy!

282. Tuscan Chicken

Servings: 8   Cooking Time: 7 Hours

Ingredients:

1-pound chicken breast, skinless, boneless
1 tablespoon olive oil
½ cup full-fat cream
1 oz spinach, chopped
3 oz Parmesan, grated
1 teaspoon chili flakes
½ teaspoon paprika
1 teaspoon minced garlic
½ teaspoon ground black pepper

Directions:

Chop the chicken breast roughly and sprinkle it with the chili flakes, paprika, minced garlic, and ground black pepper.   Stir the chicken and transfer to the slow cooker.   Add the full-fat cream and olive oil. Add spinach and grated cheese.   Stir the chicken gently and close the lid.   Cook the chicken for 7 hours on Low.   Transfer cooked Tuscan chicken on the serving plates and serve!

Nutrition Info:calories 136, fat 7.2, fiber 0.2, carbs 1.4, protein 16

283. Chicken In Bacon

Servings: 6   Cooking Time: 3 Hours

Ingredients:

1-pound chicken thighs
7 oz bacon, sliced
1 tablespoon butter
¾ cup water
½ teaspoon ground black pepper
1 teaspoon chili flakes
1 teaspoon paprika

Directions:

Sprinkle the chicken thighs with the ground black pepper, chili flakes, and paprika.   Wrap the chicken thighs in the sliced bacon and transfer to the slow cooker.   Add the water and butter and close the lid.   Cook the chicken for 3 hours on High. Serve the cooked meal immediately!

Nutrition Info:calories 341, fat 21.4, fiber 0.2, carbs 0.8, protein 34.2

284. Spicy Bacon Strips

Servings: 4   Cooking Time: 2 Hours

Ingredients:

1 teaspoon cayenne pepper
½ teaspoon ground red pepper
1 tablespoon olive oil
¼ teaspoon ground black pepper
7 oz bacon, sliced
1 onion, sliced
1 teaspoon butter

Directions:

Cut the bacon into the strips.   Sprinkle the bacon strips with the ground red pepper, ground black pepper, and olive oil.   Place the bacon strips in the slow cooker and add sliced onion and butter. Close the lid and cook the bacon for 2 hours on High. Stir the bacon and transfer on to serving plates. Enjoy!

Nutrition Info:calories 320, fat 25.3, fiber 0.7, carbs 3.6, protein 18.8

285. Pork-jalapeno Bowl

Servings: 4   Cooking Time: 3 Hours

Ingredients:

2 jalapeno peppers, chopped
9 oz pork chops
1 onion, grated
½ cup water
1 teaspoon butter
½ teaspoon chili flakes
1 teaspoon ground black pepper

Directions:

Sprinkle the pork chops with the chili flakes and ground black pepper.   Place the pork chops in the slow cooker.   Add water, grated onion, and butter, Add the jalapeno peppers and close the lid.   Cook the meal for 3 hours on High.   Stir the cooked meal and transfer it to serving bowls.   Serve it!

Nutrition Info:calories 228, fat 17, fiber 1, carbs 3.4, protein 14.8

286. Cayenne Pepper Drumsticks

Servings: 2   Cooking Time: 5 Hours

Ingredients:

10 oz chicken drumsticks
1 teaspoon cayenne pepper
1 bell pepper, chopped
½ cup water
1 tablespoon butter
1 teaspoon thyme
1 teaspoon cumin
½ teaspoon chili pepper

Directions:

Mix the cayenne pepper, chopped bell pepper, butter, thyme, cumin, and chili pepper.   Stir the mixture until smooth,   Rub the chicken drumsticks with the spice mixture and place them in the slow cooker.   Add water and close the lid. Cook the drumsticks for 5 hours on Low.   Transfer the cooked meal onto a platter and serve!

Nutrition Info:calories 318, fat 14.4, fiber 1.4, carbs 5.9, protein 40

287. Autumn Pork Stew

Servings: 5   Cooking Time: 6 Hours

Ingredients:

1 eggplant, chopped
4 oz white mushrooms, chopped
1 white onion, chopped
2 cups water
½ teaspoon clove
½ teaspoon salt
½ teaspoon cayenne pepper
8 oz pork tenderloin

Directions:

Place the chopped eggplant, mushrooms, onion, and water in the slow cooker.   Chop the pork tenderloin roughly and sprinkle it with the cayenne pepper, salt, and clove.   Stir the meat and place it in the slow cooker too.   Close the lid and cook the stew for 6 hours on Low.   When the stew is cooked, let it rest for 20 minutes.   Enjoy!

Nutrition Info:calories 232, fat 5.1, fiber 4.1, carbs 8.4, protein 37.5

288. Rosemary Leg Of Lamb

Servings: 8   Cooking Time: 7 Hours

Ingredients:

2-pound leg of lamb
1 onion
1 garlic clove, peeled
1 tablespoon mustard
seeds

3 cups water
1 teaspoon salt
½ teaspoon turmeric
1 teaspoon ground
black pepper

Directions:
Chop the garlic clove and combine it with the mustard seeds, turmeric, black pepper and salt. Peel the onion and grate it.   Mix the grated onion and spice mixture.   Rub the leg of lamb with the grated onion mixture.   Put the leg of lamb in the slow cooker and cook it for 7 hours on Low.   Serve the cooked meal!
Nutrition Info:calories 225, fat 8.7, fiber 0.6, carbs 2.2, protein 32.4

289.   Marinated Beef Tenderloin

Servings: 6   Cooking Time: 6 Hours
Ingredients:
2 tablespoons butter
1-pound Beef
Tenderloin
1 teaspoon minced
garlic
½ teaspoon ground
nutmeg

1 teaspoon turmeric
1 teaspoon paprika
1 tablespoon apple
cider vinegar
½ teaspoon dried
oregano
1 cup water

Directions:
Melt the butter and mix it up with the minced garlic, ground nutmeg, turmeric, paprika, apple cider vinegar, and dried oregano.   Whisk the mixture. Rub the beef tenderloin with the spice mixture. Place the beef tenderloin in the slow cooker and add the remaining spice mixture.   Add water and close the lid.   Cook the beef tenderloin for 8 hours on Low.   Chop the beef tenderloin and serve it!
Nutrition Info:calories 208, fat 6, fiber .5, carbs 3, protein 24

290.   Peppered Steak

Servings: 4   Cooking Time: 4 Hours
Ingredients:
10 oz Sirloin Steak
3 cups water
1 tablespoon
peppercorns
1 teaspoon salt

½ teaspoon ground
nutmeg
2 garlic cloves, peeled
1 teaspoon olive oil

Directions:
Make the small cuts in the sirlion and chop the garlic cloves roughly.   Place the garlic cloves in the sirloin cuts.   Sprinkle the steak with the salt, ground nutmeg, and peppercorns.   Transfer the steak in the slow cooker and add water.   Close the lid and cook the steak for 4 hours on Low.   Then remove the steak from the slow cooker and slice it. Enjoy!
Nutrition Info:calories 192, fat 12, fiber 4, carbs 1, protein 12

291.   Handmade Sausage Stew

Servings: 3   Cooking Time: 3 Hours
Ingredients:
7 oz ground pork
1 egg yolk

7 oz broccoli,
chopped

½ teaspoon salt
½ teaspoon ground
black pepper

½ cup water
1 tomato, chopped
1 teaspoon butter

Directions:
Mix the ground pork and yolk. Add salt and ground black pepper.   Stir the mixture and form small sausages with your hands.   Place the sausages in the slow cooker.   Add the chopped broccoli and water.   Add chopped tomato and butter.   Close the lid and cook the stew for 3 hours on High. Place the cooked stew in bowls and enjoy!
Nutrition Info:calories 151, fat 5.4, fiber 2.1, carbs 5.6, protein 20.3

292.   Sesame Seed Shrimp

Servings: 4   Cooking Time: 30 Minutes
Ingredients:
1-pound shrimp,
peeled
2 tablespoons apple
cider vinegar
1 teaspoon paprika

1 teaspoon sesame
seeds
¼ cup water
3 tablespoons butter

Directions:
Sprinkle the shrimp with the apple cider vinegar. Add paprika and stir the shrimp.   Let the shrimp marinade for 15 minutes.   Pour water into the slow cooker.   Add the butter and marinated shrimp.   Cook the shrimp for 30 minutes on High. Transfer the shrimp to a serving bowl.   Mix together the remaining liquid and sesame seeds. Sprinkle the shrimp with the sesame mixture and enjoy!
Nutrition Info:calories 219, fat 11, fiber 0.3, carbs 2.3, protein 26.1

293.   Keto Beef Ribs

Servings: 4   Cooking Time: 5 Hours
Ingredients:
10 oz beef ribs
1 onion, grated
½ cup water
1 teaspoon ground
nutmeg
½ teaspoon chili
pepper

1 teaspoon turmeric
1 tablespoon olive oil
1 garlic clove, peeled
1 tomato, chopped

Directions:
Mix the grated onion, ground nutmeg, chili pepper, turmeric, and olive oil in a bowl.   Pour the spice mixture over the beef ribs and rub the spices into the meat.   Place the ribs in the slow cooker and add water.   Then add the chopped tomato and garlic clove.   Close the lid and cook the beef ribs for 5 hours on Low.   Cool the ribs until room temperature and serve!
Nutrition Info:calories 182, fat 8.2, fiber 1.1, carbs 4.1, protein 22.1

294.   Lamb Stew

Servings: 6   Cooking Time: 60 Minutes
Ingredients:
1 onion, chopped
5 oz broccoli,
chopped
4 oz eggplant,

1 cup water
1 zucchini, chopped
8 oz lamb fillet,
chopped

chopped
1 garlic clove, peeled

1 teaspoon cayenne pepper
1 teaspoon salt

Directions:
Place the chopped onion, broccoli, and eggplant in the slow cooker. Add water and chopped zucchini. Dice the garlic clove and add it to the slow cooker too. Add chopped lamb fillet, salt, and cayenne pepper. Stir the stew gently. Close the lid and cook the lamb stew for 7 hours on Low. Serve the lamb stew hot. Enjoy!
Nutrition Info:calories 97, fat 3, fiber 2.1, carbs 5.8, protein 12.1

295. Keto Pork Tenderloin

Servings: 2   Cooking Time: 3 Hours
Ingredients:
9 oz pork tenderloin
½ teaspoon ground black pepper
2 tablespoons butter

2 garlic clove, peeled
½ teaspoon salt
¼ cup water

Directions:
Sprinkle the pork tenderloins with the ground black pepper and salt. Place the pork tenderloin in the slow cooker. Add the peeled garlic and water. Add the butter and close the lid. Cook the pork tenderloins for 3 hours on High. When the time is done and the meat is cooked, let it cool slightly. Enjoy!
Nutrition Info:calories 290, fat 16, fiber 0.2, carbs 1.3, protein 33.8

296. Asian Chopped Beef

Servings: 4   Cooking Time: 3 Hours
Ingredients:
1-pound beef chops
2 tablespoons apple cider vinegar
1 tablespoon dried mint

1 tablespoon olive oil
1 teaspoon mustard
¼ teaspoon salt
¼ cup water

Directions:
Chop the beef roughly and sprinkle it with the apple cider vinegar, dried mint, mustard, olive oil, and salt. Stir the meat and let it sit for 20 minutes to marinate. Transfer the meat to the slow cooker and add water. Cook the beef for 3 hours on High. When the beef is cooked, let it rest for 10 minutes and serve!
Nutrition Info:calories 187, fat 8.8, fiber 0.2, carbs 2.6, protein 23.2

297. Marinated Greek Style Pork

Servings: 4   Cooking Time: 2 Hours
Ingredients:
12 oz pork chops
4 teaspoons full-fat cream
1 teaspoon ground black pepper
1 tablespoon olive oil

1 teaspoon dried oregano
1 teaspoon dried mint
½ teaspoon thyme
1 tablespoon butter
1 cup water

Directions:
Rub the pork chops with the full-fat cream, ground black pepper, olive oil, dried oregano, dried mint, and thyme. Let it sit for 20 minutes to marinate. Transfer the pork chops in the slow cooker and add

butter and water. Close the lid and cook the pork chops for 2 hours on High. Serve the cooked meat immediately!
Nutrition Info:calories 333, fat 27.8, fiber 0.4, carbs 0.8, protein 19.3

298. Corned Beef

Servings: 6   Cooking Time: 8 Hours
Ingredients:
1-pound corned beef
1 teaspoon peppercorns
1 teaspoon chili flakes
1 teaspoon mustard seeds

1 bay leaf
1 teaspoon salt
1 oz bacon fat
4 garlic cloves
1 cup water
1 tablespoon butter

Directions:
Mix the peppercorns, chili flakes, mustard seeds, and salt in the bowl. Then rub the corned beef with the spice mixture well. Peel the garlic and place it in the slow cooker. Add the corned beef. Add water, butter, and bay leaf. Add the bacon fat and close the lid. Cook the corned beef for 8 hours on Low. When the corned beef is cooked, discard the bay leaf then transfer the beef to a plate and cut into servings. Enjoy!
Nutrition Info:calories 178, fat 13.5, fiber 0.3, carbs 1.3, protein 12.2

299. Ground Pork Bowl

Servings: 4   Cooking Time: 2 Hours
Ingredients:
9 oz ground pork
2 bell peppers, chopped
1 onion, diced
1 teaspoon chili pepper

1 tablespoon butter
½ teaspoon cayenne pepper
1 teaspoon salt
¼ cup water

Directions:
Place the ground pork, chopped bell peppers, and diced onion in the slow cooker. Add butter, chili pepper, cayenne pepper, and salt. Stir the meat mixture with a spatula. Add water and close the slow cooker lid. Cook the ground pork for 2 hours on High. Transfer the cooked ground pork in the serving bowls and serve!
Nutrition Info:calories 148, fat 5.4, fiber 1.5, carbs 7.3, protein 17.7

300. Paprika Pork Sausages

Servings: 4   Cooking Time: 2 Hours
Ingredients:
10 oz ground pork
1 tablespoon paprika
2 egg yolks
1 teaspoon ground black pepper

½ teaspoon salt
½ onion, grated
1 tablespoon almond flour

Directions:
Mix the ground pork and egg yolks. Stir the ground pork with a fork until well blended. Add paprika, salt, ground black pepper, and almond flour. Stir the pork mixture and add the grated onion. Stir it well and form medium sausages using your hands. Then place the sausages in the slow cooker. Close the lid and cook for 2 hours on

High.   Then transfer the sausages to the platter and enjoy!
Nutrition Info:calories 180, fat 8.5, fiber 1.8, carbs 4.4, protein 21.9

301.   Pork Shoulder

Servings: 6   Cooking Time: 7 Hours
Ingredients:

1-pound pork shoulder	1 onion, peeled
2 cups water	1 teaspoon chili flakes
2 garlic cloves, peeled	½ teaspoon paprika
1 teaspoon peppercorns	1 teaspoon turmeric
	1 teaspoon cumin

Directions:
Sprinkle the pork shoulder with the peppercorns, chili flakes, paprika, turmeric, and cumin.   Stir it well and let it sit for 15 minutes to marinate. Transfer the pork shoulder to the slow cooker. Add water and peeled the onion.   Add garlic cloves and close the lid.   Cook the pork shoulder for 7 hours on Low.   Remove the pork shoulder from the slow cooker and serve!
Nutrition Info:calories 234, fat 16.4, fiber 0.7, carbs 2.8, protein 18

302.   Garlic Pork Belly

Servings: 8   Cooking Time: 7 Hours
Ingredients:

1-pound pork belly	2 tablespoons mustard
4 garlic cloves, peeled	
1 teaspoon peppercorns	½ teaspoon salt
	1 tablespoon butter
	1 cup water

Directions:
Dice the garlic cloves and combine them with the peppercorns and mustard.   Add the salt and butter and stir.   Rub the pork belly with the prepared mixture well.   Place the pork belly in the slow cooker.   Add the water and close the lid. Cook the pork belly for 7 hours on Low.   Slice the cooked pork belly and serve!
Nutrition Info:calories 290, fat 17.5, fiber 0.5, carbs 1.7, protein 27

303.   Prawn Stew

Servings: 4   Cooking Time: 1 Hour
Ingredients:

10 oz prawns, peeled	1 teaspoon salt
1 onion, sliced	½ cup almond milk
4 oz Parmesan, grated	1 teaspoon butter
1 garlic clove, peeled	1 teaspoon chili flakes

Directions:
Place the peeled prawns, sliced onion, garlic clove, salt, almond milk, butter, and chili flakes into the slow cooker.   Close the lid and cook the stew for 1 hour on High.   Transfer the cooked stew into serving bowls and sprinkle with the grated cheese. Serve it!
Nutrition Info:calories 265, fat 15.4, fiber 1.3, carbs 6.6, protein 26.3

304.   Delicious Turmeric Beef Stew

Servings: 4   Cooking Time: 5 Hours
Ingredients:

7 oz ground beef	1 tablespoon full-fat cream
1 tablespoon turmeric	
1 onion, diced	1 teaspoon salt
7 oz broccoli	½ teaspoon cayenne pepper
1 cup water	

Directions:
Mix the ground beef and turmeric.   Add the diced onion, salt, and cayenne pepper.   Stir the ingredients and transfer into the slow cooker. Add the broccoli and water.   Add the full-fat cream and stir the stew gently.   Close the lid and cook the stew for 5 hours on Low.   Chill the cooked stew slightly and serve!
Nutrition Info:calories 132, fat 3.9, fiber 2.3, carbs 7.3, protein 17

305.   Keto Bbq Chicken Wings

Servings: 4   Cooking Time: 2 Hours
Ingredients:

1-pound chicken wings	1 tablespoon mustard
1 teaspoon minced garlic	1 teaspoon liquid stevia
1 teaspoon cumin	1 tablespoon tomato paste
1 teaspoon ground coriander	1 teaspoon salt
1 teaspoon dried dill	1 tablespoon apple cider vinegar
1 teaspoon dried parsley	

Directions:
Mix the minced garlic, cumin, ground coriander, dried dill, dried parsley, mustard, liquid stevia, tomato paste, salt, and apple cider vinegar.   Stir the mixture until smooth.   Combine the spice mixture and chicken wings and stir well.   Transfer the chicken wings and all the remaining spice mixture into the slow cooker.   Close the lid and cook for 2 hours on High.   Cool the chicken wings slightly and serve!
Nutrition Info:calories 236, fat 9.4, fiber 0.7, carbs 2.4, protein 33.9

306.   Chicken Marsala

Servings: 4   Cooking Time: 7 Hours
Ingredients:

1-pound chicken breast, skinless, boneless	1 teaspoon garlic powder
	3 tablespoons butter
2 oz white mushrooms, chopped	1 teaspoon salt
	1 teaspoon ground black pepper
1 oz Marsala cooking wine	

Directions:
Chop the chicken breast roughly and sprinkle it with the garlic powder, salt, and ground black pepper. Stir the chicken and transfer it to the slow cooker. Add butter, Marsala cooking wine, mushrooms, and close the lid.   Cook chicken Marsala for 7 hours on Low.   Stir the cooked meal gently.   Serve it in serving bowls.   Enjoy!

Nutrition Info:calories 219, fat 11.6, fiber 0.4, carbs 2.3, protein 24.8

307.   Chicken Liver Pate

Servings: 6   Cooking Time: 2 Hours
Ingredients:
1-pound chicken liver
1 onion, chopped
2 cups water
1 teaspoon salt
¼ teaspoon ground nutmeg
2 tablespoons butter
1 bay leaf

Directions:
Place the chicken liver in the slow cooker.   Add chopped onion, water, salt, ground black pepper, and bay leaf.   Close the lid and cook the liver for 2 hours on High.   After this, strain the chicken liver, discarding the liquid, and place it in the blender. Add butter and blend the mixture until smooth (approximately for 3 minutes at maximum speed). Transfer the cooked pate into a bowl and let it cool in the freezer for 10 minutes.   Serve with keto bread!
Nutrition Info:calories 168, fat 8.8, fiber 0.5, carbs 2.5, protein 18.8

308.   Keto Adobo Chicken

Servings: 4   Cooking Time: 2 Hours
Ingredients:
1 tablespoon soy sauce
1 tablespoon olive oil
1 tablespoon apple cider vinegar
1-pound chicken breast, boneless, skinless
1 teaspoon minced garlic

Directions:
Chop the chicken breast roughly and sprinkle it with the soy sauce, olive oil, apple cider vinegar, and minced garlic.   Mix and then let sit for 20 minutes to marinate.   Transfer the chicken and all the remaining liquid into the slow cooker.   Close the lid and cook the meal for 2 hours on High.   Enjoy!
Nutrition Info:calories 163, fat 6.3, fiber 0, carbs 0.6, protein 24.3

309.   Chili Verde

Servings: 4   Cooking Time: 4 Hours
Ingredients:
1-pound pork loin
½ teaspoon cumin
½ teaspoon ground coriander
½ teaspoon chili flakes
1 garlic clove, peeled
1 cup water
½ cup Keto green chili (no sugar added)

Directions:
Chop the pork loin roughly and place it in the slow cooker.   Add cumin, ground coriander, and chili flakes.   Add the garlic clove and Keto green chili. Stir the ingredients and add water.   Close the lid and cook chili Verde for 4 hours on Low.   Serve the cooked meal immediately!
Nutrition Info:calories 287, fat 15.9, fiber 0.1, carbs 2.4, protein 31.1

310.   Keto Lasagna

Servings: 6   Cooking Time: 7 Hours
Ingredients:
10 oz ground beef
1 tablespoons tomato puree
1 zucchini
5 oz Parmesan, grated
1 tablespoon butter
½ teaspoon salt
1 teaspoon paprika
1 teaspoon chili flakes
1 tablespoon full-fat heavy cream

Directions:
Slice the zucchini lengthwise.   Mix the ground beef, salt, paprika, and chili flakes.   Then mix the full-fat cream and tomato puree.   Chop the butter and put it in the slow cooker.   Make a layer of the zucchini in the bottom of the slow cooker bowl. Put a layer of the ground beef mixture on top of the zucchini layer.   After this repeat, the same layers until you use all the ingredients.   Sprinkle the lasagna with the grated Parmesan and close the lid. Cook the lasagna for 7 hours on Low.   Chill the cooked meal little and serve!
Nutrition Info:calories 197, fat 11, fiber 0.5, carbs 2.5, protein 22.5

311. Thyme Lamb Chops

Servings: 2   Cooking Time: 7 Hours
Ingredients:
8 oz lamb chops
1 teaspoon liquid stevia
1 teaspoon thyme
1 tablespoon olive oil
¼ cup water
1 bay leaf
¾ teaspoon ground cinnamon
½ onion, chopped

Directions:
Mix the liquid stevia, thyme, olive oil, and ground cinnamon.   Rub the lamb chops with the spice mixture.   Place the lamb chops in the slow cooker and add chopped onion and water.   Add the bay leaf and close the lid.   Cook the lamb chops for 7 hours on Low.   When the meat is cooked, serve it immediately!
Nutrition Info:calories 287, fat 15.4, fiber 1.4, carbs 4, protein 32.3

312.   Duck Breast

Servings: 4   Cooking Time: 5 Hours
Ingredients:
1 teaspoon liquid stevia
1-pound duck breast, boneless, skinless
2 tablespoons butter
1 teaspoon chili pepper
½ cup water
1 bay leaf

Directions:
Rub the duck breast with the chili pepper and liquid stevia then transfer it to the slow cooker.   Add the bay leaf and water.   Add butter and close the lid. Cook the duck breast for 5 hours on Low.   Let the cooked duck breast rest for 10 minutes then remove it from the slow cooker.   Slice it into the servings. Enjoy!
Nutrition Info:calories 199 fat 10.3, fiber 0.1, carbs 0.3, protein 25.1

313.   Spare Ribs

Servings: 6   Cooking Time: 8 Hours
Ingredients:

1-pound pork loin ribs
1 teaspoon olive oil
1 teaspoon minced garlic
¼ teaspoon cumin
¼ teaspoon chili powder
1 tablespoon butter
5 tablespoons water

Directions:
Mix the olive oil, minced garlic, cumin, and chili flakes in a bowl.   Melt the butter and add to the spice mixture.   Stir it well and add water. Stir again.   Then rub the pork ribs with the spice mixture generously and place the ribs in the slow cooker.   Close the lid and cook the ribs for 8 hours on Low.   When the ribs are cooked, serve them immediately!
Nutrition Info:calories 203, fat 14.1, fiber 0.6, carbs 10, protein 9.8

---

314. Creamy Chicken Thighs

Servings: 4   Cooking Time: 6 Hours
Ingredients:
1-pound chicken thighs, skinless
¼ cup almond milk, unsweetened
1 teaspoon salt
1 tablespoon full-fat cream cheese
1 onion, diced
1 teaspoon paprika

Directions:
Mix the almond milk and full-fat cream.   Add salt, diced onion, and paprika.   Stir the mixture well. Place the chicken thighs in the slow cooker.   Add the almond milk mixture and stir it gently.   Close the slow cooker lid and cook the chicken thighs for 6 hours on High.   Transfer the cooked chicken heart in the serving bowls and serve immediately!
Nutrition Info:calories 224, fat 14.3, fiber 1.1, carbs 4.7, protein 18.9

---

315. Bacon Meatloaf

Servings: 6   Cooking Time: 3 Hours
Ingredients:
10 oz ground chicken
5 oz bacon, sliced
1 tablespoon butter
1 egg yolk
1 teaspoon salt
1 teaspoon chili pepper
½ teaspoon cayenne pepper
1 teaspoon ground black pepper
1 teaspoon olive oil
1 garlic clove, diced

Directions:
Mix the ground chicken, egg yolk, butter, chili pepper, cayenne pepper, ground black pepper, and diced garlic.   Stir the mixture and then place it in the slow cooker.   Cover the ground chicken mixture with the sliced bacon and close the lid. Cook the meatloaf for 3 hours on High.   Cool the cooked meatloaf and transfer it to a serving platter. Slice it and enjoy!
Nutrition Info:calories 253, fat 16.9, fiber 0.2, carbs 1, protein 23

---

316. Garlic Duck Breast

Servings: 6   Cooking Time: 5 Hours
Ingredients:
11 oz duck breast, boneless, skinless
4 garlic cloves, roughly diced
1 teaspoon rosemary
1 tablespoon butter
½ cup water
1 teaspoon chili flakes

Directions:
Make small cuts in the duck breast.   Sprinkle the duck breast with the rosemary and chili flakes. Fill the cuts with the diced garlic.   Place the duck breast in the slow cooker.   Add butter and water and close the lid.   Cook the duck breast for 5 hours on Low.   When the duck breast is cooked, remove it from the slow cooker and let it rest for 10 minutes. Slice the duck breast and serve!
Nutrition Info:calories 88, fat 4, fiber 0.1, carbs 0.8, protein 11.6

317. Chicken Liver With Anchovies

Servings: 2   Cooking Time: 3 Hours

Ingredients:

3/4 lb. chicken liver	1 tablespoon of
1 yellow onion,	capers, drained and
roughly diced	diced
1 bay leaf	1 tablespoon of
1/4 cup of red wine	butter, melted
1/4 cup of vegetable	Salt and black
stock	pepper- to taste
2 anchovies	

Directions:
Start by throwing all the Ingredients: into the Crockpot and mix them well.   Cover it and cook for 3 hours on Low Settings.   Garnish as desired. Serve warm.

Nutrition Info: Calories 541 Total Fat 34 g Saturated Fat 8.5 g Cholesterol 69 mg Total Carbs 3.4 g Fiber 1.2 g Sugar 1 g Sodium 547 mg Potassium 467 mg Protein 20.3 g

318. Pork Roast With Cheese

Servings: 2   Cooking Time: 6 Hours 5 Minutes

Ingredients:

1 1/2 cups of chicken	1 teaspoon of black
stock	pepper
1 cup of diced onion	For the Gravy
1/2 cup of diced	1 cup of heavy cream
mushrooms	4 oz. cream cheese,
3 4 celery stalks,	cubed
diced	1/2 stick butter
1/4 cup of parsley,	1/2 1 teaspoon of
dried	Glucomannan
1/2 stick butter	powder
2 teaspoons of salt	1 1/2 2 cups of
1 teaspoon of garlic	cooking liquid from
powder	the roast

Directions:
Start by putting all the Ingredients: except those for the gravy into your Crockpot.   Cover its lid and cook for 6 hours on high setting.   Once done, remove its lid and mix well.   Mix all the gravy Ingredients: in a saucepan and stir cook for 5 minutes.   Pour this gravy over the slow-cooked pork.   Garnish as desired.   Serve warm.

Nutrition Info: Calories 359 Total Fat 34 g Saturated Fat 10.3 g Cholesterol 112 mg Total Carbs 8.5 g Sugar 2 g Fiber 1.3 g Sodium 92 mg Protein 27.5 g

319. Pork Butt Carnitas

Servings: 8   Cooking Time: 8 Hours

Ingredients:

1/2 tablespoon of	1 tablespoon of cumin
black pepper	1 tablespoon of
1 tablespoon of chili	thyme, dried
powder	4 lb. pork butt
1 tablespoon of bacon	2 tablespoons of
grease	garlic, minced
1 small onion	1/2 cup of water

Directions:
Start by putting all the Ingredients: into your Crockpot.   Cover its lid and cook for 8 hours on High setting.   Once done, remove its lid and mix well.   Garnish as desired.   Serve warm.

Nutrition Info: Calories 329 Total Fat 34 g Saturated Fat 10.3 g Cholesterol 112 mg Total Carbs 6.5 g Sugar 2 g Fiber 1.3 g Sodium 92 mg Protein 27.5 g

320. Green Chile Chicken

Servings: 6   Cooking Time: 6 Hours

Ingredients:

1 (4 oz.) can green	optional: add in 1/2
chilis	cup of diced onions
2 teaspoons of garlic	
salt	

Directions:
Start by throwing all the Ingredients: into the Crockpot.   Cover it and cook for 6 hours on Low Settings.   Garnish as desired.   Serve warm.

Nutrition Info: Calories 248 Total Fat 2.4 g Saturated Fat 0.1 g Cholesterol 320 mg Total Carbs 2.9 g Fiber 0.7 g Sugar 0.7 g Sodium 350 mg Potassium 255 mg Protein 44.3 g

321. Pork Filled Avocado

Servings: 6   Cooking Time: 4 Hours

Ingredients:

1/2 tablespoon of	1 teaspoon of salt
cumin, ground	1/2 tablespoon of
1/2 tablespoon of chili	butter
powder	6 avocados, cut in
1/2 tablespoon of	half, pits removed
garlic powder	and scooped

Directions:
Start by putting all the Ingredients: into your Crockpot except the avocados   Cover its lid and cook for 4 hours on High setting.   Once done, remove its lid and mix well.   Shred the slow-cooked pork and return to the crockpot.   Mix well and divide this mixture into the avocados. Garnish as desired.   Serve warm.

Nutrition Info: Calories 397 Total Fat 17.1 g Saturated Fat 13.4 g Cholesterol 56 mg Sodium 146 mg Total Carbs 1.9 g Fiber 0.4 g Sugar 2.8 g Potassium 322mg Protein 41.2 g

322. Pork Tomatillo Salsa

Servings: 8   Cooking Time: 10 Hours

Ingredients:

Salt and black pepper	2 tablespoon of Olive
to taste	oil
4 teaspoon of Garlic	36 oz. Green chili
powder	tomatillo salsa

Directions:
Start by putting all the Ingredients: into your Crockpot.   Cover its lid and cook for 10 hours on medium setting.   Once done, remove its lid and mix well.   Garnish as desired.   Serve warm.

Nutrition Info: Calories 274 Total Fat 13 g Saturated Fat 7.4 g Cholesterol 132 mg Sodium 115 mg Total Carbs 8.5 g Fiber 0.9 g Sugar 1.4 g Potassium 232mg Protein 25.1 g

323. Chicken And Zucchinis

Servings: 2   Cooking Time: 2.5 Hours

Ingredients:

- 8 oz chicken fillet
- 2 zucchinis, sliced
- 2 tablespoons Dijon mustard
- 1 tablespoon butter
- 1 teaspoon chili flakes
- 1 teaspoon salt
- 1 teaspoon black pepper

Directions:

Cut the chicken fillet into 2 servings.   Combine the chicken with the zucchinis and the other ingredients in the slow cooker.   Cook the meal for 2.5 hours on High.

Nutrition Info:calories 277, fat 14.8, fiber 5.5, carbs 10.9, protein 33.3

324. Lamb And Spinach

Servings: 4   Cooking Time: 8 Hours

Ingredients:

- 1 teaspoon cumin, ground
- 1 tablespoon olive oil
- ¼ teaspoon chili powder
- ½ teaspoon black pepper
- ½ teaspoon salt
- 1-pound lamb chops
- ½ cup fresh spinach
- ¼ cup of water

Directions:

In the slow cooker, mix the lamb with cumin, oil and the other ingredients except the spinach.   Close the lid.   Cook the rack of lamb for 7 hours on Low. Add the spinach, cook on Low for 1 hour, divide into bowls and serve.

Nutrition Info:calories 328, fat 14.9, fiber 4.2, carbs 4.2, protein 23.3

325. Cheddar Chicken

Servings: 4   Cooking Time: 3 Hours

Ingredients:

- 1-pound chicken breast, skinless, boneless
- 1 teaspoon turmeric powder
- 1 teaspoon oregano, dried
- 2 oz Cheddar, grated
- 1 cup heavy cream
- 1 teaspoon ground black pepper
- 1 teaspoon almond butter

Directions:

Put the chicken breast in the slow cooker.   Add the rest of the ingredients and close the lid.   Cook chicken for 3 hours on High.

Nutrition Info:calories 324, fat 19.3, fiber 4.5, carbs 7.4, protein 30.1

326. Lamb And Leeks

Servings: 4   Cooking Time: 6 Hours

Ingredients:

- 3 oz leeks, roughly chopped
- 1-pound lamb chops
- 1 teaspoon ground paprika
- 1 garlic clove, diced
- 1 teaspoon dried basil
- 1 teaspoon Italian seasoning
- ½ teaspoon salt
- ½ teaspoon black pepper
- 2 spring onions, chopped
- ½ teaspoon chili pepper
- ¼ cup heavy cream
- 1 teaspoon olive oil

Directions:

In the slow cooker, mix the lamb with leeks, basil, seasoning and the other ingredients.   Close the lid. Cook the pot roast for 6 hours on High.

Nutrition Info:calories 296, fat 14.3, fiber 4.2, carbs 6.6, protein 17.8

327. Chicken And Hot Sauce

Servings: 6   Cooking Time: 3 Hours

Ingredients:

- 9 oz chicken breast, cooked, shredded
- 3 tablespoons hot sauce
- 1 tablespoon scallions, chopped
- 1/3 cup sour cream
- ¾ teaspoon cayenne pepper
- 1 tablespoon fresh dill, chopped

Directions:

Put the chicken and the other ingredients in the slow cooker.   Close the slow cooker lid and cook dip on Low for 3 hours.   Divide into bowls and serve

Nutrition Info:calories 218, fat 6.7, fiber 4.2, carbs 1.4, protein 12.5

328. Pumpkin Beef Chili

Servings: 6   Cooking Time: 3 Hours

Ingredients:

- 1 green bell pepper, diced
- 1 ½ lb. Beef, ground
- 6 garlic cloves, minced
- 28 oz. canned tomatoes, diced
- 1 cup of chicken stock
- 14 oz. pumpkin puree
- 2 tablespoon of Chili powder
- 1 ½ teaspoon of Cumin, ground
- 1 teaspoon of Cinnamon powder
- Salt and black pepper- to taste

Directions:

Start by putting all the Ingredients: into your Crockpot.   Cover it and cook for 4 hours on Low settings.   Once done, uncover the pot and mix well. Garnish as desired.   Serve warm.

Nutrition Info: Calories 238 Total Fat 13.8 g Saturated Fat 1.7 g Cholesterol 221 mg Sodium 120 mg Total Carbs 4.3 g Fiber 2.4 g Sugar 11.2 g Protein 34.4g

329. Chicken Fillets And Mustard Sauce

Servings: 5   Cooking Time: 7 Hours

Ingredients:

- 5 chicken fillets
- 1 tablespoon butter, softened
- 2 tablespoons mustard
- ½ cup coconut cream
- ½ teaspoon salt
- 1 teaspoon apple cider vinegar
- 4 tablespoons cream cheese

Directions:

In the slow cooker, mix the chicken with butter, mustard and the other ingredients and close the lid. Cook chicken or 7 hours on Low. Serve the cooked chicken with sauce.
Nutrition Info:calories 326, fat 15.9, fiber 4, carbs 8.2, protein 42.9

330. Chicken And Tomato Sauce

Servings: 1   Cooking Time: 3.5 Hours
Ingredients:
- 6 oz chicken fillet
- ¼ cup Cheddar, shredded
- 1 teaspoon coriander, ground
- 1 teaspoon cumin, ground
- ¼ teaspoon salt
- ½ teaspoon turmeric
- 3 tablespoons keto tomato sauce
- 1 teaspoon chives, chopped
- 1 garlic clove, diced
- 1/3 cup water

Directions:
In the slow cooker, mix the chicken with the Cheddar and the other ingredients.   Close the slow cooker lid and cook the chicken on High for 3.5 hours.   Divide into bowls and serve.
Nutrition Info:calories 341, fat 18.9, fiber 4.5, carbs 6.5, protein 51.9

331. Chicken And Walnuts

Servings: 4   Cooking Time: 6 Hours
Ingredients:
- ¼ teaspoon mustard seeds
- ½ teaspoon ground ginger
- ¾ teaspoon curry powder
- 1 teaspoon salt
- 1 teaspoon black pepper
- 1 teaspoon garam masala
- 1 tablespoon avocado oil
- ¾ cup of coconut milk
- ½ cup walnuts, chopped
- 10 oz chicken breast, skinless, boneless

Directions:
In the slow cooker, mix the chicken with walnuts and the other ingredients.   Close the slow cooker lid and cook chicken for 6 hours on Low.
Nutrition Info:calories 221, fat 16.1, fiber 7.1, carbs 6.7, protein 16.1

332. Chipotle Barbacoa Recipe

Servings: 6   Cooking Time: 10 Hours
Ingredients:
- 1/2 cup of beef broth
- 2 medium chipotle chilis in adobo
- 2 tablespoons of apple cider vinegar
- 2 tablespoons of lime juice
- 1 tablespoon of oregano, dried
- 5 cloves garlic
- 2 teaspoons of cumin
- 2 teaspoons of salt
- 1 teaspoon of black pepper
- 1/2 teaspoons of cloves, ground
- 2 whole bay leaf

Directions:
Start by putting all the Ingredients: into your Crockpot.   Cover it and cook for 10 hours on Low settings.   Once done, uncover the pot and mix well.

Shred the slow-cooked beef and return it to the pot. Serve warm.
Nutrition Info: Calories 248 Total Fat 15.7 g Saturated Fat 2.7 g Cholesterol 75 mg Sodium 94 mg Total Carbs 4.4 g Fiber 0.2 g Sugar 0.1 g Protein 43.2 g

333. Chili Chicken

Servings: 4   Cooking Time: 5 Hours
Ingredients:
- 4 chicken thighs, skinless, boneless
- 1 teaspoon coriander, ground
- 1 teaspoon chili flakes
- ½ teaspoon salt
- ½ teaspoon garlic powder
- 5 oz Pepper Jack cheese, shredded
- 4 tablespoons butter
- ¼ cup of water

Directions:
Put chicken thighs in the slow cooker.   Add the rest of the ingredients except the cheese.   Close the lid and cook chicken on High for 4 hours. Then sprinkle the chicken with shredded Pepper Jack cheese and close the lid.   Cook the chicken for 1 hour on High.
Nutrition Info:calories 336, fat 23.8, fiber 01, carbs 3.4, protein 32.3

334. Ground Pork And Veggies

Servings: 5   Cooking Time: 8 Hours
Ingredients:
- 2 cups ground pork
- 1 tablespoon minced garlic
- 1 green bell pepper, chopped
- 1 red bell pepper, chopped
- 1 zucchini, chopped
- 1 eggplant, chopped
- ½ cup cherry tomatoes, halved
- ½ cup keto tomato sauce
- 2 spring onions, chopped
- 1 teaspoon cayenne pepper
- ½ teaspoon salt
- ½ teaspoon ground coriander
- 1 tablespoon butter, softened

Directions:
In the slow cooker, mix the pork with garlic, pepper and the other ingredients, toss, close the lid and cook for 8 hours on Low.   Divide into bowls and serve.
Nutrition Info:calories 349, fat 16.3, fiber 2.3, carbs 5.5, protein 13.8

335. Chicken Ginger Curry

Servings: 4   Cooking Time: 6 Hours
Ingredients:
- 1 (13.5 oz.) can coconut milk
- 1 onion, diced
- 4 cloves garlic, minced
- 1-inch knob fresh ginger, minced
- 1 Serrano pepper, minced
- 1 tablespoon of Garam Masala
- ½ teaspoon of cayenne
- ½ teaspoon of paprika
- ½ teaspoon of turmeric

salt and pepper,
adjust to taste

Directions:
Start by throwing all the Ingredients: into the Crockpot. Cover it and cook for 6 hours on Low Settings. Garnish as desired. Serve warm.
Nutrition Info: Calories 248 Total Fat 15.7 g Saturated Fat 2.7 g Cholesterol 75 mg Total Carbs 8.4 g Fiber 0g Sugar 1.1 g Sodium 94 mg Potassium 331 mg Protein 14.1 g

336. Saucy Goose Satay

Servings: 4   Cooking Time: 6 Hours
Ingredients:

1/4 cup of sweet chili sauce	1/4 cup of extra virgin olive oil
1 sweet onion, diced	Salt and black pepper- to taste
2 teaspoons of garlic, diced	

Directions:
Start by throwing all the Ingredients: into the Crockpot and mix them well. Cover it and cook for 5-6 hours on Low Settings. Garnish as desired. Serve warm.
Nutrition Info: Calories 545 Total Fat 36.4 g Saturated Fat 10.1 g Cholesterol 200 mg Total Carbs 0.7 g Fiber 0.2 g Sugar 0 g Sodium 272 mg Potassium 433 mg Protein 42.5 g

337. Herbed Lamb Loin Chops

Servings: 1   Cooking Time: 8 Hours
Ingredients:

2 tablespoons of Butter melted	1 tablespoon of Lemon peel, grated
1 tablespoon of swerve	Salt and black pepper- to taste
¼ cup of dill, diced	1 lamb loin chop
3 green onions, diced	

Directions:
Start by putting all the Ingredients: into your Crockpot. Cover its lid and cook for 8 hours on Low setting. Once done, remove its lid and mix well. Garnish as desired. Serve warm.
Nutrition Info: Calories 298 Total Fat 14.4 g Saturated Fat 2.4 g Cholesterol 73 mg Sodium 76 mg Total Carbs 7.4 g Fiber 0.3 g Sugar 0.6 g Protein 31.4 g

338. Savoury Lamb Chili

Servings: 6   Cooking Time: 4 Hours
Ingredients:

1 green bell pepper, diced	14 oz. pumpkin puree
1 ½ lb. lamb ground	2 tablespoon of chili powder
6 garlic cloves, minced	1 ½ teaspoon of cumin, ground
28 oz. canned tomatoes, diced	1 teaspoon of cinnamon powder
1 cup of chicken stock	Salt and black pepper- to taste

Directions:
Start by putting all the Ingredients: into your Crockpot. Cover it and cook for 5 hours on Low settings. Once done, uncover the pot and mix well. Garnish as desired. Serve warm.
Nutrition Info: Calories 238 Total Fat 13.8 g Saturated Fat 1.7 g Cholesterol 221 mg Sodium 120 mg Total Carbs 4.3 g Fiber 2.4 g Sugar 11.2 g Protein 34.4g

339. Thai Chicken Curry

Servings: 2   Cooking Time: 2.5 Hours
Ingredients:

1/2 cup of chicken stock	1 lb. boneless, skinless chicken thighs, diced
1 2 tablespoons of red curry paste	Salt and black pepper-to taste
1 tablespoon of coconut aminos	red pepper flakes as desired
1 tablespoon of fish sauce	1 bag frozen mixed veggies
2 3 garlic cloves, minced	

Directions:
Start by throwing all the Ingredients: except vegetables into the Crockpot. Cover it and cook for 2 hours on Low Settings. Remove its lid and thawed veggies. Cover the crockpot again then continue cooking for another 30 minutes on Low settings. Garnish as desired. Serve warm.
Nutrition Info: Calories 327 Total Fat 3.5 g Saturated Fat 0.5 g Cholesterol 162 mg Total Carbs 56g Fiber 0.4 g Sugar 0.5 g Sodium 142 mg Potassium 558 mg Protein 21.5 g

340. Duck And Vegetable Stew

Servings: 4   Cooking Time: 5 Hours
Ingredients:

1 tablespoon of wine	1-inch ginger pieces, diced
2 carrots, diced	
2 cups of water	Salt and black pepper- to taste
1 cucumber, diced	

Directions:
Start by throwing all the Ingredients: except into the Crockpot and mix them well. Cover it and cook for 5 hours on Low Settings. Garnish with cucumber. Serve warm.
Nutrition Info: Calories 449 Total Fat 23.4 g Saturated Fat 1.5 g Cholesterol 210 mg Total Carbs 0.4 g Fiber 1.3 g Sugar 22g Sodium 838 mg Potassium 331 mg Protein 28.5g

341. Wine Dipped Pork Ribs

Servings: 4   Cooking Time: 8.5 Hours
Ingredients:

¾ teaspoon of erythritol	¼ teaspoon of coriander powder
½ teaspoon of garlic powder	¼ cup of tomato ketchup
½ teaspoon of allspice	¾ tablespoon of red wine vinegar
½ teaspoon of salt	
¼ teaspoon of black pepper	½ teaspoon of ground mustard
½ teaspoon of onion powder	¼ teaspoon of liquid smoke

Directions:
Start by putting all the Ingredients: into your Crockpot. Cover its lid and cook for 8 hours on Low setting. Once done, remove its lid and mix well. Transfer the ribs to the serving plate. Cook the remaining sauce in the crockpot for 30 minutes on high heat. Pour this sauce over the ribs on the plate. Garnish as desired. Serve warm.
Nutrition Info: Calories 244 Total Fat 17.4 g Saturated Fat 14.8 g Cholesterol 44 mg Sodium 164 mg Total Carbs 4.5 g Fiber 2.4 g Sugar 0.1 g Potassium 222mg Protein 31.2 g

342. Mushroom Cream Goose Curry

Servings: 6   Cooking Time: 6.5 Hours
Ingredients:
- 1 goose breast, fat: trimmed off and cut into pieces
- 1 goose leg, skinless
- 1 yellow onion, diced
- 3 ½ cups of water
- 2 teaspoons of garlic, minced
- 1 goose thigh, skinless
- Salt and black pepper- to taste

Directions:
Start by throwing all the Ingredients: into the Crockpot except cream and mix them well. Cover it and cook for 6 hours on Low Settings. Stir in mushroom cream and cook for another 30 minutes on low heat. Give it a stir and garnish as desired. Serve warm.
Nutrition Info: Calories 288 Total Fat 5.7g Saturated Fat 1.8 g Cholesterol 60 mg Total Carbs 2.9 g Fiber 0.2 g Sugar 0.1 g Sodium 554 mg Potassium 431 mg Protein 25.6g

343. Fennel Chicken Mix

Servings: 7   Cooking Time: 5 Hours
Ingredients:
- 3-pound chicken drumsticks
- 1 fennel, chopped
- ½ teaspoon fennel seeds
- ½ teaspoon salt
- ½ teaspoon cayenne pepper
- ½ teaspoon garlic powder
- ½ teaspoon coriander, ground
- ½ teaspoon saffron
- ¼ teaspoon ground nutmeg
- ½ teaspoon turmeric
- 2 tablespoons butter
- 1/3 cup almond milk
- ¼ cup fresh cilantro, chopped

Directions:
In the slow cooker, mix the chicken with fennel and the other ingredients. Close the lid and cook chicken for 5 hours on High. Divide between plates and serve.
Nutrition Info:calories 388, fat 17.2, fiber 0.6, carbs 1.5, protein 53.9

344. Chicken And Spring Onions

Servings: 6   Cooking Time: 3 Hours
Ingredients:
- 2 tablespoons sweet paprika
- 1 cup spring onions, chopped
- 1 tablespoon olive oil
- ½ teaspoon minced garlic
- 1 teaspoon paprika
- ½ teaspoon salt
- 1 tablespoon olive oil
- 2-pound chicken fillet

Directions:
In the slow cooker mix the chicken and the other ingredients and close the lid. Cook it on High for 3 hours.
Nutrition Info:calories 286, fat 16.9, fiber 6.7, carbs 6.6, protein 24.7

345. Ground Beef And Broccoli

Servings: 4   Cooking Time: 2 Hours
Ingredients:
- 3 oz. butter
- ½ cup of beef stock
- 9 oz. broccoli, trimmed and diced
- Salt and black pepper-to taste
- ½ cup of mayonnaise or crème Fraiche

Directions:
Start by putting all the Ingredients: into your Crockpot. Cover it and cook for 2 hours on Low settings. Once done, uncover the pot and mix well. Garnish as desired. Serve warm.
Nutrition Info: Calories 272 Total Fat 18 g Saturated Fat 5 g Cholesterol 6.1 mg Sodium 3 mg Total Carbs 4 g Fiber 3 g Sugar 4 g Protein 19.4 g

346. Lamb Curry

Servings: 6 – 8   Cooking Time: Approximately 8 Hours
Ingredients:
- 2 ½ lb boneless lamb (shoulder is a good cut to choose for this dish), cubed
- 2 onions, roughly chopped
- 5 garlic cloves, finely chopped
- 4 tbsp curry paste
- 1 lamb stock cube
- 2 ½ full-fat coconut milk
- 2 tomatoes, chopped
- Fresh coriander, roughly chopped
- Full-fat Greek yogurt, to serve

Directions:
Heat some oil in skillet or pan. Add the lamb to the hot pan and seal on all sides, about 3 minutes. Drizzle some olive oil into the Crock Pot. Add the lamb, onions, garlic, curry paste, salt, and pepper to the pot. Stir to coat the lamb in curry paste. Add the coconut milk, stock cube, chopped tomatoes, and 1 cup of water to the pot. Place the lid onto the pot and set the temperature to LOW. Cook for 8 hours. Serve with a dollop of Greek yoghurt and fresh coriander.

347. Stuffed Chicken Breasts

Servings: 4 – 6   Cooking Time: Approximately 4 Hours
Ingredients:
- 4 large chicken breasts, skin off
- 4 garlic cloves, finely chopped
- ½ pound mozzarella cheese, sliced
- 1 cup baby spinach, roughly chopped
- 12 black olives, pit removed, chopped into chunks
- 2 tomatoes, chopped
- ½ tsp dried mixed herbs

½ cup grated mozzarella cheese

Directions:
Slice the chicken breasts lengthways, so that a cavity opens (don't slice them into two pieces). Rub the chicken breasts with olive oil and sprinkle with salt and pepper. Stuff each breast with the garlic, mozzarella, olive, and spinach. Place the chicken breasts into the Slow Cookerand pour the tinned tomatoes over the top, sprinkle the mixed herbs over the top. Set the temperature to HIGH. Place the lid onto the pot and cook for 4 hours. Sprinkle the extra mozzarella over the top and place the lid back onto the pot, cook until the cheese has melted. Serve while hot!

348. Beef Stuffed Mushrooms

Servings: 4   Cooking Time: 3 Hours
Ingredients:

1 cup cremini mushroom caps	½ cup ground beef
1 tablespoon butter, soft	1 teaspoon sweet paprika
1 teaspoon coriander, ground	1 teaspoon dried dill
	1 oz Parmesan, grated
	¾ cup of water

Directions:
In a bowl, mix ground beef, butter, coriander, dill and paprika. Fill every mushroom cap with the meat mixture and arrange them in the slow cooker. Add water. Top every mushroom cap with Parmesan and close the lid. Cook the mushroom caps for 3 hours on High.
Nutrition Info:calories 260, fat 5.8, fiber 4.4, carbs 8.6, protein 7.4

349. Southwest Jalapeno Beef

Servings: 4   Cooking Time: 6 Hours
Ingredients:

1 red onion, diced	3 cup of chicken stock
½ green pepper, diced	3 tablespoons of chili powder
2 oz. olive oil	1 tablespoon of salt
10 oz. diced tomatoes	1 tablespoon of pepper
1 cup of carrots, diced	2 oz. diced cilantro
3 diced jalapeños	
3 cup of cauliflower rice	

Directions:
Start by putting all the Ingredients: into your Crockpot. Cover it and cook for 6 hours on Low settings. Once done, uncover the pot and mix well. Garnish as desired. Serve warm.
Nutrition Info: Calories 391 Total Fat 21.8 g Saturated Fat 12.6 g Cholesterol 16 mg Sodium 162 mg Total Carbs 1.5 g Fiber 9.2 g Sugar 4.5 g Protein 11.6 g

350. Lemon Beef

Servings: 4   Cooking Time: 5 Hours
Ingredients:

1-pound beef sirloin, chopped	1 teaspoon lemon zest, grated
3 tablespoons lemon	1 tablespoon keto

juice
1 teaspoon curry powder
1 teaspoon chili flakes
½ teaspoon salt

tomato sauce
1 teaspoon butter
½ cup of water
½ teaspoon cayenne pepper

Directions:
In the slow cooker, mix the beef with lemon juice and zest and the other ingredients and toss. Close the lid and cook beef sirloin for 5 hours on High. Divide between plates and serve.
Nutrition Info:calories 229, fat 8.7, fiber 0.2, carbs 1.2, protein 34.5

351. Chicken With Nuts

Servings: 4   Cooking Time: 4.5 Hours
Ingredients:

1-pound chicken fillet	1 cup coconut cream
1 tablespoon butter, softened	1 tablespoon almonds, chopped
1 tablespoon walnuts, chopped	1 teaspoon salt
1 tablespoon pecans, chopped	¼ cup heavy cream
	1 teaspoon oregano, dried

Directions:
In the slow cooker, mix the chicken with the cream and the other ingredients and close the lid. Cook the chicken for 4.5 hours on High. Divide between plates and serve.
Nutrition Info:calories 281, fat 15.3, fiber 4.3, carbs 7.8, protein 33.7

352. Caraway Ribs

Servings: 4   Cooking Time: 4.5 Hours
Ingredients:

1 ½ teaspoons caraway seeds	15 oz pork spare ribs
½ teaspoon cumin, ground	½ teaspoon dried oregano
½ teaspoon sweet paprika	½ teaspoon dried basil
½ teaspoon garam masala	1 tablespoon olive oil
	1/3 cup water

Directions:
In your slow cooker, mix the ribs with caraway seeds and the other ingredients. Close the lid. Cook the spare ribs for 4.5 hours on High.
Nutrition Info:calories 311 fat 15, fiber 3.2, carbs 7.3, protein 20.1

353. Dinner Lamb Shanks

Servings: 3   Cooking Time: 8 Hours
Ingredients:

1 tablespoon of olive oil	3/4 cup of bone broth
½ teaspoon of rosemary, dried, crushed	Salt and black pepper, to taste
1 tablespoon of melted butter	3/4 tablespoon of Sugar-free tomato paste
3 whole garlic cloves, peeled	1 ¼ tablespoon of fresh lemon juice

Directions:

Start by putting all the Ingredients: into your Crockpot. Cover its lid and cook for 8 hours on Low settings. Once done, remove its lid and mix well. Garnish as desired. Serve warm.
Nutrition Info: Calories 188 Total Fat 12.5 g Saturated Fat 4.4 g Cholesterol 53 mg Sodium 1098 mg Total Carbs 4.9 g Sugar 0.3 g Fiber 2 g Potassium 332mg Protein 14.6 g

354. Chicken With Lemon Parsley Butter

Servings: 10   Cooking Time: 3 Hours
Ingredients:
1 cup of water
1/2 teaspoon of kosher salt
1/4 teaspoon of black pepper
1 whole lemon, sliced
4 tablespoons of butter
2 tablespoons of fresh parsley, chopped

Directions:
Start by seasoning the chicken with all the herbs and spices. Place this chicken in the Crockpot. Cover it and cook for 3 hours on High Settings. Meanwhile, melt butter with lemon slices and parsley in a saucepan. Drizzle the butter over the Crockpot chicken. Serve warm.
Nutrition Info: Calories 379 Total Fat 29.7 g Saturated Fat 18.6 g Cholesterol 141 mg Total Carbs 9.7g Fiber 0.9 g Sugar 1.3 g Sodium 193 mg Potassium 131 mg Protein 25.2 g

355. Mint Lamb Roast

Servings: 4   Cooking Time: 3.5 Hours
Ingredients:
1-pound rack of lamb, chopped
1 tablespoon minced garlic
½ teaspoon black pepper
1 teaspoon mint, dried
½ teaspoon salt
½ cup sour cream
1 tablespoon balsamic vinegar
2 tablespoons olive oil
½ teaspoon fresh rosemary, chopped

Directions:
In the slow cooker, mix the lamb with garlic, salt, pepper and the other ingredients, Close the lid and cook lamb for 3.5 hours on High.
Nutrition Info:calories 370, fat 26.6, fiber 4.1, carbs 6.3, protein 29.5

356. Pork Roast With Cabbage Stir Fry

Servings: 2   Cooking Time: 4 Hours 5minutes
Ingredients:
1 Pork tenderloin
¼ cup of Tomato passata
¼ cup of beef stock
1 Red cabbage head, shredded
Cabbage Stir fry
4 Green onions diced
2 tablespoons of Balsamic vinegar
1 Jalapeno diced

Directions:
Start by putting all the Ingredients: into your Crockpot. Cover its lid and cook for 4 hours on High setting. Once done, remove its lid and mix well. Now prepare the cabbage stir fry by sautéing all its Ingredients: for 5 minutes. Garnish the pork with cabbage stir fry. Serve warm.
Nutrition Info: Calories 338 Total Fat 9.5 g Saturated Fat 2.7 g Cholesterol 103 mg Sodium 403 mg Total Carbs 1.8 g Sugar 0 g Fiber 0 g Potassium 342mg Protein 34.2 g

357. Pork Shoulder And Zucchinis

Servings: 7   Cooking Time: 11 Hours
Ingredients:
2.5-pound pork shoulder, boneless
1 teaspoon salt
1 teaspoon black pepper
1 cup zucchinis, cubed
1 teaspoon sweet paprika
1 teaspoon chili flakes
1 tablespoon olive oil
1 ½ cup water

Directions:
In the slow cooker, mix the pork with salt, pepper and the other ingredients. Close the lid and cook the meat for 11 hours.
Nutrition Info:calories 368, fat 26.3, fiber 0.1, carbs 7.2, protein 17.8

358. Chicken And Okra

Servings: 2   Cooking Time: 4.5 Hours
Ingredients:
8 oz chicken breast, skinless, boneless
1 tablespoon keto tomato sauce
1 cup okra, sliced
1 teaspoon sweet paprika
¼ cup of water
½ teaspoon chili powder
½ teaspoon salt
½ teaspoon dried oregano

Directions:
In the slow cooker, mix the chicken with the tomato sauce and the other ingredients. Close the lid. Cook pulled chicken for 4 hours and 30 minutes.
Nutrition Info:calories 213, fat 7.5, fiber 5.2, carbs 8.9, protein 25.9

359. Chili Lamb

Servings: 4   Cooking Time: 10 Hours
Ingredients:
1 teaspoon stevia
½ teaspoon cayenne pepper
1 teaspoon cumin, ground
1 teaspoon green chili, minced
1 teaspoon minced garlic
1 teaspoon keto tomato sauce
1 tablespoon mustard
1-pound lamb shoulder, boneless
½ cup of water
1 tablespoon olive oil
½ teaspoon chili powder
¾ teaspoon garam masala

Directions:
In your slow cooker, mix the lamb with the stevia, cayenne and the other ingredients. Close the lid and cook the pork for 10 hours on Low. Divide between plates and serve.

Nutrition Info:calories 309, fat 18.6, fiber 3.8, carbs 8.4, protein 27.3

360. Indian Lamb Stew

Servings: 8   Cooking Time: 10 Hours 15 Minutes

Ingredients:

- 1 ½ teaspoons of cayenne pepper
- 1 cup of Greek yogurt
- ¼ cup of vegetable oil
- 4 lbs. boneless lamb shoulder
- 1 ½ teaspoons of ground ginger
- 1 ½ teaspoon of ground coriander
- ½ teaspoon of ground turmeric
- ¼ teaspoon of cloves, ground
- 2 small cinnamon sticks
- 8 cardamom pods
- 1 medium tomato, diced
- Black pepper
- 1 tablespoon of xanthan gum
- 2 tablespoons of water

Directions:

Start by throwing all the Ingredients: except the butter and flour into your Crockpot.   Cover its lid and cook for 10 hours on Low settings.   Once done, remove its lid and mix well.   Mix corn starch and water in a small bowl then pour into the crockpot. Continue cooking the remaining sauce for 15 minutes on high heat until it thickens.   Garnish as desired.   Serve warm.

Nutrition Info: Calories 265 Total Fat 26.1 g Saturated Fat 7.8 g Cholesterol 143 mg Sodium 65 mg Total Carbs 5.9 g Fiber 3.2 g Sugar 1.3 g Protein 6.1 g

361. Debdoozie's Beef Chili

Servings: 6   Cooking Time: 4 Hours

Ingredients:

- 1 teaspoon of black pepper
- ½ teaspoon of garlic salt
- 2 ½ cups of sugar-free tomato sauce
- ½ onion, diced
- 1 (8 oz.) jar salsa
- 4 tablespoons of chili seasoning mix
- ½ cup of green bell pepper, diced

Directions:

Start by putting all the Ingredients: into your Crockpot.   Cover it and cook for 4 hours on Low settings.   Once done, uncover the pot and mix well. Garnish as desired.   Serve warm.

Nutrition Info: Calories 416 Total Fat 24.5 g Saturated Fat 10 g Cholesterol 32 mg Sodium 123 mg Total Carbs 0.8 g Fiber 3.6 g Sugar 5.5 g Protein 14.3 g

362. Mozzarella Chicken

Servings: 4   Cooking Time: 9 Hours

Ingredients:

- 1 cup Mozzarella cheese, shredded
- ½ teaspoon cayenne pepper
- ½ teaspoon coriander, ground
- 1 teaspoon basil, dried
- 1-pound chicken breast, skinless, boneless and cubed
- 3 spring onions, chopped
- 1 cup heavy cream
- Cooking spray

Directions:

Spray the slow cooker bottom with cooking spray. Chop the keto tortillas and chicken breast. Combine the chicken with the cheese and the other ingredients, and close the slow cooker lid.   Cook the chicken for 9 hours on Low.

Nutrition Info:calories 269, fat 17.2, fiber 2.4, carbs 7, protein 30.6

363. Paprika Drumsticks

Servings: Makes 10 Drumsticks   Cooking Time: Approximately 4 Hours

Ingredients:

- 10 chicken drumsticks
- 2 eggs, lightly beaten
- 2 tsp smoky paprika
- ¼ cup ground almond

Directions:

Mix together the paprika, ground almond, salt, and pepper and spread onto a plate   Prepare the chicken drumsticks by dipping them in the beaten egg, then rolling them in the paprika/almond mixture   Drizzle some olive oil into the Slow Cooker   Place the chicken drumsticks into the pot and set the temperature to HIGH   Cook for 4 hours   Serve hot or cold, with a few fresh salads!

364. Beef And Asparagus

Servings: 5   Cooking Time: 11 Hours

Ingredients:

- 1-pound beef steak
- 1 cup asparagus, trimmed and halved
- 3 scallions, chopped
- 1 teaspoon sweet paprika
- 1 teaspoon coriander, ground
- 1 teaspoon butter
- ½ teaspoon dried dill
- 1/3 cup water

Directions:

In the slow cooker, mix the beef with scallions and the other ingredients except the asparagus and close the lid.   Cook the beef roll for 10 hours on Low. Add the asparagus, close the lid, cook on Low for 1 more hour and serve.

Nutrition Info:calories 301, fat 11.2, fiber 3.2, carbs 6.1, protein 32.1

365. Butter Turkey And Olives

Servings: 3   Cooking Time: 5.5 Hours

Ingredients:

- 1-pound turkey breast, skinless, boneless and cut into strips
- 1 cup kalamata olives, pitted and halved
- 3 spring onions, chopped
- ½ teaspoon salt
- ½ teaspoon cayenne pepper
- ½ teaspoon ground black pepper
- ½ tablespoon apple cider vinegar
- 2 tablespoons butter

Directions:

Grease the slow cooker with the butter, add the turkey and the other ingredients inside and toss. Close the lid and cook for 5.5 hours on Low.

Nutrition Info:calories 364, fat 10.1, fiber 3.2, carbs 5.7, protein 49.4

366. Vegetable Beef Stew

Servings: 2   Cooking Time: 8 Hours

Ingredients:

½ yellow onion, diced
3 oz. tomato paste
1 garlic clove, minced
½ tablespoon of thyme, diced
1.5 celery stalks, diced
1 carrot, diced
1 tablespoon of parsley, chopped
1 tablespoon of white vinegar
salt and black pepper to taste

Directions:

Start by putting all the Ingredients: into your Crockpot.   Cover it and cook for 8 hours on Low settings.   Once done, uncover the pot and mix well. Garnish as desired.   Serve warm.

Nutrition Info: Calories 311 Total Fat 25.5 g Saturated Fat 12.4 g Cholesterol 69 mg Sodium 58 mg Total Carbs 1.4 g Fiber 0.7 g Sugar 7.3 g Protein 3.4 g Protein 17.5 g

367. Crockpot Chicken Adobo

Servings: 6   Cooking Time: 8 Hours

Ingredients:

1 onion, diced into slices
2 tablespoons of olive oil
10 cloves garlic, smashed
12 chicken drumsticks
1 cup of gluten-free tamari
1/4 cup of diced green onion

Directions:

Place the drumsticks in the Crockpot and then add the remaining Ingredients: on top.   Cover it and cook for 8 hours on Low Settings.   Mix gently, then serve warm.

Nutrition Info: Calories 249 Total Fat 11.9 g Saturated Fat 1.7 g Cholesterol 78 mg Total Carbs 1.8 g Fiber 1.1 g Sugar 0.3 g Sodium 79 mg Potassium 131 mg Protein 25 g

368. Chicken With Celery Stick

Servings: 4   Cooking Time: 6 Hours

Ingredients:

4 carrots, diced
1 yellow onion, diced
1/2 teaspoon of thyme, dried
1 tablespoon of chives
3 celery stalks, diced
3/4 cup of chicken stock
Salt and black pepper- to taste

Directions:

Start by throwing all the Ingredients: into the Crockpot except chives and mix them well.   Cover it and cook for 5 6 hours on Low Settings.   Garnish with chives.   Serve warm.

Nutrition Info: Calories 188 Total Fat 6 g Saturated Fat 1 g Cholesterol 72 mg Total Carbs 5 g Fiber 1.6 g Sugar 2.3 g Sodium 472 mg Potassium 271 mg Protein 25 g

369. Parmesan Pork Schnitzel

Servings: 4   Cooking Time: 8 Hours

Ingredients:

¼ cup of parmesan cheese, grated
½ cup of water
1 teaspoon of salt

½ teaspoon of garlic powder
1 teaspoon of black pepper

Directions:

Start by putting all the Ingredients: into your Crockpot except the cheese.   Cover its lid and cook for 8 hours on Low setting.   Once done, remove its lid and mix well.   Garnish with cheese on top. Serve warm.

Nutrition Info: Calories 248 Total Fat 15.7 g Saturated Fat 2.7 g Cholesterol 75 mg Sodium 94 mg Total Carbs 0.4 g Fiber 0g Sugar 0 g Potassium 122mg Protein 12.9 g

370. Passata Mixed Pulled Pork

Servings: 2   Cooking Time: 10 Hours

Ingredients:

2 tablespoon of chili powder
½ cup of tomato passata
2 tablespoons of mustard
2 tablespoon of olive oil
2 tablespoons of balsamic vinegar
Salt and black pepper- to taste

Directions:

Start by putting all the Ingredients: into your Crockpot.   Cover its lid and cook for 10 hours on Low setting.   Once done, remove its lid and mix well.   Shred the slow-cooked pork and return the pot.   Mix well and garnish as desired.   Serve warm.

Nutrition Info: Calories 487 Total Fat 37.4 g Saturated Fat 8.8 g Cholesterol 71 mg Sodium 501 mg Total Carbs 12.6 g Sugar 1.2 g Fiber 9.2 g Potassium 411mg Protein 28.1 g

371. Lamb Chops With Dill Butter

Servings: 3   Cooking Time: 6 Hours

Ingredients:

1-pound lamb chops
3 tablespoons butter, softened
1/3 cup fresh dill, chopped
¼ teaspoon turmeric powder
½ teaspoon garam masala
½ teaspoon salt
½ teaspoon ground black pepper
1 teaspoon olive oil

Directions:

In the slow cooker, mix the lamb with the butter, dill and the other ingredients and close the lid.   Cook the mix for 6 hours on Low. Divide between plates and serve.

Nutrition Info:calories 375, fat 6.5, fiber 3.8, carbs 3.4, protein 22.2

372. Rosemary Rainbow Pork Sautee

Servings: 2   Cooking Time: 9 Hours

Ingredients:

Salt and black pepper- to taste
1 and ½ teaspoon of rosemary, diced
1 tablespoon of olive oil
3 garlic cloves, minced
1 red bell pepper, cut into strips
1 yellow bell pepper, cut into strips
2 teaspoons of balsamic vinegar

¼ cup of vegetable stock

Directions:
Start by putting all the Ingredients: into your Crockpot. Cover its lid and cook for 9 hours on Low setting. Once done, remove its lid and mix well. Garnish as desired. Serve warm.
Nutrition Info: Calories 238 Total Fat 23.2 g Saturated Fat 13 g Cholesterol 61 mg Sodium 115 mg Total Carbs 6.8 g Sugar 0 g Fiber 0.9 g Potassium 157mg Protein 22.3 g

373. Steak And Dill Sauce

Servings: 4   Cooking Time: 5 Hours
Ingredients:
- 14 oz flank steak
- 1 teaspoon minced garlic
- 2 tablespoons fresh dill, chopped
- ½ teaspoon turmeric powder
- 1 teaspoon curry powder
- ½ cup of coconut milk
- 1 teaspoon oregano, dried
- ½ teaspoon salt
- 1 teaspoon almond butter
- 1 teaspoon chili powder

Directions:
In the cockpit, mix the steaks with the garlic and the other ingredients. Close the lid, and cook on High for 5 hours. Serve the flank steak hot.
Nutrition Info:calories 405, fat 21.6, fiber 5.1, carbs 4.7, protein 31.3

374. Lamb, Celery And Tomatoes

Servings: 4   Cooking Time: 5 Hours
Ingredients:
- 1 cup cherry tomatoes, halved
- 1 garlic clove, diced
- 3 oz celery stalk, chopped
- ½ teaspoon black pepper
- 1 tablespoon olive oil
- ½ teaspoon salt
- 1-pound lamb shank
- 1 cup chicken stock
- ½ teaspoon ground black pepper
- 1 teaspoon chili powder
- ½ teaspoon dried cilantro

Directions:
In the slow cooker, mix the lamb with tomatoes and the other ingredients and toss. Close the lid and cook the meat for 5 hours on High.
Nutrition Info:calories 307, fat 14.6, fiber 4.3, carbs 4.9, protein 22.4

375. Garlic Creamy Beef Steak

Servings: 2   Cooking Time: 4 Hours
Ingredients:
- 2 garlic cloves, minced
- ¾ cup of cream
- ¼ cup of butter
- Salt and black pepper, to taste

Directions:
Start by putting all the Ingredients: into your Crockpot. Cover it and cook for 4 hours on High settings. Once done, uncover the pot and mix well. Garnish as desired. Serve warm.

Nutrition Info: Calories 287 Total Fat 17.5 g Saturated Fat 4.8 g Cholesterol 283 mg Sodium 1212 mg Total Carbs 2.4 g Fiber 1.8 g Sugar 0.8 g Protein 17.4 g

376. Mustard Rubbed Lamb Chops

Servings: 4   Cooking Time: 6 Hours
Ingredients:
- 1 tablespoon of olive oil
- ½ cup of vegetable broth
- ¼ cup of apricot preserves
- 3 tablespoons of mustard
- Salt and black pepper- to taste

Directions:
Start by putting all the Ingredients: into your Crockpot. Cover its lid and cook for 6 hours on High setting. Once done, remove its lid and mix well. Garnish as desired. Serve warm.
Nutrition Info: Calories 324 Total Fat 20.7 g Saturated Fat 6.7 g Cholesterol 45 mg Sodium 241 mg Total Carbs 8.6 g Sugar 1.4 g Fiber 0.5 g Protein 35.3 g

377. Sweet Passata Dipped Steaks

Servings: 4   Cooking Time: 2 Hours
Ingredients:
- 1 teaspoon of Ginger, grated
- 1 tablespoon of Mustard
- 1 Garlic clove, minced
- 1 teaspoon of Garlic, minced
- 1 tablespoon of Stevia
- 1 tablespoon of Olive oil
- 1 and ½ lbs. Beef steaks

Directions:
Start by putting all the Ingredients: into your Crockpot. Cover it and cook for 2 hours on High settings. Once done, uncover the pot and mix well. Garnish as desired. Serve warm.
Nutrition Info: Calories 371 Total Fat 17.2 g Saturated Fat 9.4 g Cholesterol 141 mg Sodium 153 mg Total Carbs 6 g Fiber 0.9 g Sugar 1.4 g Protein 32 g

378. Lamb Pepper Stew

Servings: 12   Cooking Time: 12 Hours
Ingredients:
- 4 garlic cloves sliced thin
- 2 teaspoons of salt
- 2 teaspoons of garlic powder
- 2 teaspoons of oregano
- 2 tablespoons of cumin
- 4 teaspoons of ground coriander
- 4 teaspoons of chili powder
- 1/2 teaspoon of black pepper
- 1/2 teaspoon of onion powder
- 1 tablespoon of olive oil
- 4 tablespoons of apple cider vinegar
- 2 cups of peppers sliced
- 1 onion sliced
- 1 7 oz. can of chipotle peppers
- 1 14.5 oz. can tomato, diced
- 1 4 oz. can of green chilis

Directions:

Start by putting all the Ingredients: into your Crockpot. Cover its lid and cook for 12 hours on medium setting. Once done, remove its lid and mix well. Garnish as desired. Serve warm.
Nutrition Info: Calories 449 Total Fat 28.7 g Saturated Fat 14.9 g Cholesterol 163 mg Sodium 844 mg Total Carbs 8.4 g Sugar 2.6 g Fiber 1.9 g Potassium 236 mg Protein 39.3 g

379. Pork Tenderloin With Swiss Chard

Servings: 4   Cooking Time: 10 Hours
Ingredients:

2 lemons, sliced	2 garlic cloves, minced
4 teaspoon of olive oil	2 bunches swiss chard, diced
Salt and black pepper- to taste	½ cup of beef stock

Directions:
Start by putting all the Ingredients: into your Crockpot. Cover its lid and cook for 10 hours on Low setting. Once done, remove its lid and mix well. Garnish as desired. Serve warm.
Nutrition Info: Calories 434 Total Fat 36.4 g Saturated Fat 17.1 g Cholesterol 257 mg Sodium 1038 mg Total Carbs 2.5 g Sugar 0.9 g Fiber 0.2 g Potassium 312mg Protein 24.2 g

380. Cajun Lamb

Servings: 4   Cooking Time: 5.5 Hours
Ingredients:

13 oz lamb chops	1 teaspoon oregano, dried
1 tablespoon Cajun seasonings	1 tablespoon butter
1 teaspoon curry powder	½ teaspoon dried rosemary
1 teaspoon coriander, ground	1 teaspoon salt
	1/3 cup heavy cream

Directions:
In the slow cooker, mix the lamb with Cajun seasoning and the other ingredients. Close the lid. Cook meat for 5.5 hours on High.
Nutrition Info:calories 312, fat 12.3, fiber 4.1, carbs 4.4, protein 28.2

381. Chunky Chicken Salsa

Servings: 2   Cooking Time: 6 Hours
Ingredients:

1 cup of chunky salsa	Salt and black pepper- to taste
3/4 teaspoon of cumin	
A pinch oregano	

Directions:
Start by throwing all the Ingredients: into the Crockpot and mix them well. Cover it and cook for 6 hours on Low Settings. Garnish as desired. Serve warm.
Nutrition Info: Calories 541 Total Fat 34 g Saturated Fat 8.5 g Cholesterol 69 mg Total Carbs 3.4 g Fiber 1.2 g Sugar 1 g Sodium 547 mg Potassium 467 mg Protein 20.3 g

382. Lamb Tomato Stew

Servings: 2   Cooking Time: 10 Hours
Ingredients:

1 (½ -1 ¾) lb. lamb stew meat	2 teaspoons of cinnamon
2 onions, diced	1 teaspoon of chili flakes
8 garlic cloves, diced	4 tablespoons of tomato paste
2 teaspoons of salt	½ cup of apple cider vinegar
2 teaspoons of pepper	4 tablespoons of swerve
2 teaspoons of cumin	2 ½ cups of chicken broth
2 teaspoons of coriander	
2 teaspoons of turmeric,	

Directions:
Start by throwing all the Ingredients: except the cilantro into your Crockpot. Cover its lid and cook for 10 hours on Low settings. Once done, remove its lid and mix well. Garnish as desired. Serve warm.
Nutrition Info: Calories 347 Total Fat 11.6 g Saturated Fat 2.3 g Cholesterol 421 mg Sodium 54 mg Total Carbs 6.3 g Fiber 0.6 g Sugar 1.1 g Protein 2.4 g

383. Coconut Milk Turkey Breast

Servings: 5   Cooking Time: 4.5 Hours
Ingredients:

1 cup of coconut milk	9 oz turkey breast, boneless
1 teaspoon onion powder	½ teaspoon dried oregano
¾ teaspoon garlic powder	3 oz leek, chopped
1 teaspoon butter	

Directions:
Pour coconut milk in the slow cooker and add onion powder, garlic powder, dried oregano, and leek. Then add butter. Chop the turkey breast roughly and transfer it in the slow cooker. Close the lid and cook the meal for 5 hours on High. Serve the turkey breast with coconut milk-leek gravy.
Nutrition Info:calories 184, fat 13.1, fiber 1.8, carbs 8, protein 10.2

384. Chicken And Cabbage

Servings: 4   Cooking Time: 2 Hours
Ingredients:

1-pound chicken wings	1 tablespoon paprika
1 tablespoon chili powder	½ teaspoon turmeric
1 and ½ cups red cabbage, shredded	½ teaspoon onion powder
¼ cup chicken stock	1 teaspoon olive oil

Directions:
In the slow cooker, mix the chicken with cabbage and the other ingredients. Close the lid and cook the chicken wings for 2 hours on High.
Nutrition Info:calories 240, fat 10.5, fiber 1, carbs 1.9, protein 33.2

| **385.** | **Pork Roast With Cinnamon** |

Servings: 2   Cooking Time: 4 Hours
Ingredients:

1 ½ teaspoon of red pepper, crushed
2 tablespoon of olive oil
2 yellow onions, cut into wedges
2 tablespoons of butter, melted
3-star anise
¼ cup of apple vinegar
2 teaspoons of cinnamon powder
5 garlic slices, diced
1 tablespoon of parsley, chopped

Directions:
Start by putting all the Ingredients: into your Crockpot.   Cover its lid and cook for 4 hours on High setting.   Once done, remove its lid and mix well.   Garnish as desired.   Serve warm.
Nutrition Info: Calories 369 Total Fat 24.9 g Saturated Fat 8.5 g Cholesterol 112 mg Sodium 537 mg Total Carbs 3.8 g Sugar 1.4 g Fiber 3.4 g Potassium 252mg Protein 31.5 g

| **386.** | **Chicken And Tomatoes** |

Servings: 4   Cooking Time: 5.5 Hours
Ingredients:

3 spring onions, chopped
1 tablespoon keto tomato sauce
¼ cup crushed tomatoes
½ teaspoon ground black pepper
1 ½-pound chicken breast, skinless, boneless
1/3 teaspoon salt
1 teaspoon balsamic vinegar
1 tablespoon olive oil
1 tablespoon basil, chopped
½ teaspoon garlic powder
½ cup of chicken stock

Directions:
Heat up a pan with the oil over medium-high heat, add the chicken, brown for 5 minutes and transfer to the slow cooker.   Add the rest of the ingredients and close the lid.   Cook cacciatore for 5.5 hours on Low.
Nutrition Info:calories 283, fat 8.7, fiber 1.1, carbs 6.4, protein 37

| **387.** | **Beef With Bok Choy** |

Servings: 2   Cooking Time: 5.5 Hours
Ingredients:

7 oz beef loin, cubed
3 spring onions, chopped
1 cup bok choy, chopped
1 teaspoon salt
1 teaspoon coconut oil
¼ teaspoon sweet paprika
1 cup of water

Directions:
Place coconut oil in the skillet and melt it.   Add the meat, brown for 5 minutes and transfer to the slow cooker.   Add the rest of the ingredients and toss. Close the lid.   Cook the mix for 5.5 hours on High.
Nutrition Info:calories 362, fat 12.5, fiber 3.1, carbs 8.4, protein 27.8

| **388.** | **Butter And Lemon Lamb** |

Servings: 7   Cooking Time: 4.5 Hours
Ingredients:

1-pound lamb chops
2 tablespoons stevia
4 tablespoons lemon juice
2 tablespoons lemon zest, grated
3 tablespoons butter
1 teaspoon turmeric powder
1 teaspoon coriander, ground

Directions:
In the slow cooker, mix the lamb with stevia, butter and the other ingredients.   Close the lid and cook on High for 4.5 hours.
Nutrition Info:calories 234, fat 11.8, fiber 4.1, carbs 7.5, protein 13.2

| **389.** | **Chicken And Creamy Onions And Peppers** |

Servings: 5   Cooking Time: 9 Hours
Ingredients:

1 tablespoon olive oil
1 teaspoon salt
1 teaspoon black pepper
15 oz chicken fillet, chopped
1 teaspoon curry powder
½ cup of coconut milk
¼ cup heavy cream
2 spring onions, chopped
1 red bell pepper, sliced
1 green bell pepper, sliced
½ cup of water
½ teaspoon minced ginger
1 teaspoon apple cider vinegar

Directions:
In the slow cooker, mix the chicken with the oil, salt, pepper and the other ingredients..   Close the slow cooker lid and cook the mix overnight (for 9 hours). Divide into bowls and serve.
Nutrition Info:calories 314, fat 15.9, fiber 5.5, carbs 6.1, protein 26.6

| **390.** | **Basil Chicken** |

Servings: 2   Cooking Time: 2 Hours
Ingredients:

9 oz chicken breast, skinless, boneless
¼ cup fresh basil, chopped
1 tablespoon olive oil
1 teaspoon coriander, ground
1 teaspoon chili powder
1 tomato, chopped
½ teaspoon cayenne pepper
½ teaspoon salt
½ teaspoon paprika
1 tablespoon olive oil
¼ cup of chicken stock

Directions:
In the slow cooker, mix the chicken with the basil and the other ingredients, close the lid and cook on High for 2 hours.
Nutrition Info:calories 287, fat 18, fiber 4.8, carbs 8.1, protein 28.9

| **391.** | **Green Chile Shredded Beef Cabbage Bowl** |

Servings: 4   Cooking Time: 4 Hours

Ingredients:

2 lb. beef chuck roast, well-trimmed and cut into thick strips
1 tablespoon of Kalyn's taco seasoning 2 3 teaspoons of olive oil
2 cans (4 oz. can) diced chilis with juice
For Cabbage Slaw and Dressing:
1 small head green cabbage
1/2 small head red cabbage
1/2 cup of sliced green onion
6 tablespoons of mayo or light mayo
4 teaspoons of fresh-squeezed lime juice
2 teaspoons of green tabasco sauce

Directions:
Start by putting all the Ingredients: for beef into your Crockpot. Cover it and cook for 4 hours on High settings. Once done, uncover the pot and mix well. Now toss all the coleslaw Ingredients: in a salad bowl. Serve the beef with coleslaw.
Nutrition Info: Calories 429 Total Fat 11.9 g Saturated Fat 1.7 g Cholesterol 78 mg Sodium 79 mg Total Carbs 1.8 g Fiber 1.1 g Sugar 0.3 g Protein 35 g

392. Beef And Cauliflower

Servings: 4   Cooking Time: 5 Hours
Ingredients:

2 cups cauliflower florets
1-pound beef stew meat, cubed
½ cup chicken stock
1 tablespoon chives, chopped
½ teaspoon salt
1 teaspoon black pepper

Directions:
In the slow cooker, mix the cauliflower with the beef and the other ingredients. Close the lid and cook on High for 5 hours.
Nutrition Info:calories 216, fat 12.2, fiber 4.3, carbs 4.2, protein 10.9

393. Cumin Chicken

Servings: 5   Cooking Time: 5.5 Hours
Ingredients:

1-pound chicken thighs, skinless, boneless
1 teaspoon oregano, dried
¼ teaspoon basil, chopped
½ teaspoon salt
1 teaspoon olive oil
1/3 cup chicken stock
½ teaspoon garlic powder
½ teaspoon chili powder
½ teaspoon ground cumin

Directions:
In the slow cooker, mix the chicken with the oregano and the other ingredients. Close the lid and cook the mix for 5.5 hours on Low.
Nutrition Info:calories 394, fat 7.8, fiber 4.3, carbs 7.8, protein 27

394. Chicken Cubes And Pesto

Servings: 4   Cooking Time: 3.5 Hours
Ingredients:

2 teaspoons hot paprika
½ teaspoon minced garlic
3 tablespoons basil pesto
1-pound chicken breast, skinless, boneless, chopped
1 teaspoon salt
2 spring onions, chopped
½ teaspoon cayenne pepper
½ cup chicken stock

Directions:
In the slow cooker, mix the chicken with paprika, pesto and the other ingredients, and close the lid. Cook the chicken for 3.5 hours on High.
Nutrition Info:calories 320, fat 8.3, fiber 0.9, carbs 3.2, protein 26.3

395. Coconut Lamb Stew

Servings: 2   Cooking Time: 10 Hours.
Ingredients:

1 tablespoon of curry powder, divided
¼ cup of unsweetened coconut milk
2 tablespoons of coconut cream
1 tablespoon of coconut oil
1 medium yellow onion, diced
½ cup of chicken broth
1 tablespoon of fresh lemon juice
Salt and black pepper, to taste
2 tablespoons of fresh basil, diced

Directions:
Start by putting all the Ingredients: into your Crockpot except basil. Cover its lid and cook for 10 hours on Low settings. Once done, remove its lid and mix well. Garnish with basil Serve warm.
Nutrition Info: Calories 141 Total Fat 11.3 g Saturated Fat 3.8 g Cholesterol 181 mg Sodium 334 mg Total Carbs 0.6 g Sugar 0.5 g Fiber 0 g Potassium 332 mg Protein 8.9 g

396. Irish Chop Stew

Servings: 8   Cooking Time: 10 Hours.
Ingredients:

8 large onions, sliced into thin rounds
4 cups of water
4 tablespoons of olive oil
9 large carrots, chunked
4 sprigs thyme
2 teaspoons of salt
2 teaspoons of black pepper

Directions:
Start by putting all the Ingredients: into your Crockpot. Cover its lid and cook for 10 hours on Low settings. Once done, remove its lid and mix well. Garnish as desired. Serve warm.
Nutrition Info: Calories 280 Total Fat 23 g Saturated Fat 13.8 g Cholesterol 82 mg Sodium 28 mg Total Carbs 3.1 g Fiber 2.5 g Sugar 0.5 g Protein 3.9 g

397. Chives Chicken Teriyaki

Servings: 3   Cooking Time: 4.5 Hours
Ingredients:

1 teaspoon apple cider vinegar
1 teaspoon soy sauce
1 teaspoon turmeric
1 tablespoon Erythritol
½ teaspoon salt

powder
1 teaspoon oregano, dried
2 tablespoons chives, chopped
1 teaspoon olive oil

½ teaspoon ground ginger
8 oz chicken fillet, chopped
1 tablespoon almond butter

Directions:
Put the chicken fillet in the slow cooker.   Add the rest of the ingredients and toss.   Close the lid and cook chicken for 4.5 hours on Low.   Divide between plates and serve.
Nutrition Info:calories 201, fat 10.8, fiber 1, carbs 7.1, protein 23.4

398.	Lamb Leg With Thyme

Servings: 4   Cooking Time: 10 Hours.
Ingredients:

1 teaspoon of fine salt
2 ½ tablespoons of olive oil
6 sprigs thyme
6 garlic cloves, minced

1 ½ cup of bone broth
1 ½ teaspoon of black pepper
1 ½ small onion
3/4 cup of vegetable stock

Directions:
Start by putting all the Ingredients: into your Crockpot.   Cover its lid and cook for 10 hours on Low settings.   Once done, remove its lid and mix well.   Garnish as desired.   Serve warm.
Nutrition Info: Calories 112 Total Fat 4.9 g Saturated Fat 1.9 g Cholesterol 10 mg Sodium 355 mg Total Carbs 1.9 g Sugar 0.8 g Fiber 0.4 g Protein 3 g

---

399.	Pork Brisket Bo Kho

Servings: 2   Cooking Time: 4 Hours
Ingredients:

1 tablespoon of oil
½ small onion, diced
1 tablespoon of fresh ginger, grated
1 tablespoon of red boat fish sauce
½ large stalk lemongrass, cut into 3-inch lengths
½ cup of diced tomatoes

½ bay leaf
½ lb carrots, peeled and diced
1 teaspoon of Madras curry powder
1 tablespoon of sugar free applesauce
1 whole star anises
½ cup of bone broth
Salt to taste

Directions:
Start by putting all the Ingredients: into your Crockpot.   Cover its lid and cook for 4 hours on High setting.   Once done, remove its lid and mix well.   Garnish as desired.   Serve warm.
Nutrition Info: Calories 303 Total Fat 11.9 g Saturated Fat 1.7 g Cholesterol 78 mg Sodium 79 mg Total Carbs 7.8 g Fiber 1.1 g Sugar 0.3 g Potassium 211 mg Protein 20 g

---

400.	Chicken And Eggplant

Servings: 6   Cooking Time: 7 Hours
Ingredients:

2 spring onions, chopped
1 big eggplant, cubed
2 pounds chicken breast, skinless, boneless and sliced
1 tablespoon capers
1 teaspoon ground black pepper
1 teaspoon salt

2 garlic cloves, chopped
1 teaspoon chili flakes
1 tablespoon keto tomato sauce
1 cup of water
1 teaspoon avocado oil

Directions:
Pour the oil in the skillet and bring it to boil.   Place the chicken breast in the skillet and cook it on high heat for 4 minutes from each side.   Then transfer the chicken breast in the slow cooker.   Add the rest of the ingredients and toss.   Close the lid. Cook for 7 hours on Low.
Nutrition Info:calories 230, fat 4.9, fiber 1, carbs 3.3, protein 40.6

401.	Chili Lamb Skewers

Servings: 2   Cooking Time: 3.5 Hours
Ingredients:

7 oz lamb stew meat, cubed
½ cup cremini mushroom caps
1 tablespoon avocado oil
1 teaspoon curry powder

1 teaspoon cumin, ground
½ teaspoon salt
1 teaspoon chili powder
1 tablespoon apple cider vinegar

Directions:
In a bowl, mix the lamb with mushroom and the other ingredients and toss.   Then string the lamb and mushroom caps one-by-one on the skewers. Place the skewers in the slow cooker and close the lid.   Cook the meal for 3.5 hours on High.
Nutrition Info:calories 326, fat 36.2, fiber 0.4, carbs 5.1, protein 14.8

402.	Lamb Shanks And Olives

Servings: 2   Cooking Time: 7.hours
Ingredients:

8 oz lamb shank, boneless
½ cup black olives, pitted and halved
1 teaspoon curry powder

1 tablespoon thyme
1/3 teaspoon ground black pepper
½ teaspoon salt
1 cup of coconut milk

Directions:
Pour coconut milk in the slow cooker.   Add the lamb, curry powder and the other ingredients, close the lid and cook for 7 hours on Low.
Nutrition Info:calories 392, fat 22.7, fiber 4.2, carbs 7.7, protein 34.8

403.	Beef Lasagna

Servings: 6 – 8   Cooking Time: Approximately 8 Hours
Ingredients:

2 lb minced beef
1 onion, finely chopped
5 garlic cloves, finely

2 large zucchinis, cut into slices lengthways
2 cups baby spinach
4 tomatoes, chopped

chopped
2 tsp dried mixed
herbs – oregano,
rosemary, thyme
1 large eggplant, cut
into slices width ways
(rounds)

2 cups grated
cheddar cheese
1 cup grated
mozzarella cheese
1 cup ricotta cheese

Directions:
Heat some olive oil in a deep-sided frying pan. Add the onions and garlic to the pan and sauté until soft.   Add the minced beef to the pan and cook for about 3 minutes to brown.   Add the tomatoes and mixed herbs to the beef and sprinkle with salt and pepper, cook for about 5 minutes.   Drizzle some olive oil into the Crock Pot.   Spread a layer of beef mixture into the pot.   Place a layer of eggplant over the beef.   Add another thin layer of beef mixture over the eggplant.   Place a layer of zucchini over the beef.   Add another layer of beef over the zucchini.   Place the spinach leaves over the beef.   Add the remaining beef mixture over the spinach.   In a large bowl, mix together the cheddar cheese, mozzarella, ricotta cheese, salt, and pepper.   Spread the cheese mixture over the lasagna.   Place the lid onto the pot and set the temperature to HIGH.   Cook for 4 hours.   Serve while hot!

---

404.   Ground Duck Chili

Servings: 8   Cooking Time: 6 Hours
Ingredients:

1 garlic heat, top
trimmed off
2 cloves
1 bay leaf
6 cups of water
Salt- to taste
15 oz. Canned
tomatoes and their
juices, diced
4 oz. Canned green
chilies and their juice

For the duck:
1 lb. Duck, ground
1 teaspoon of Swerve
1 tablespoon of
Vegetable oil
1 yellow onion,
minced
2 carrots, diced
Salt and black
pepper- to taste
Handful cilantro,
diced

Directions:
Start by throwing all other Ingredients: into the Crockpot and mix them well.   Cover it and cook for 6 hours on Low Settings.   Garnish as desired. Serve warm.
Nutrition Info: Calories 548 Total Fat 22.9 g Saturated Fat 9 g Cholesterol 105 mg Total Carbs 7.5 g Sugar 10.9 g Fiber 6.3 g Sodium 350 mg Potassium 433 mg Protein 40.1 g

---

405.   Lemongrass Pork Meatballs

Servings: 2   Cooking Time: 8 Hours
Ingredients:

3 garlic cloves,
minced
1 shallot, diced
1 lemongrass stalk,
diced
1 lb. pork, ground
1 teaspoon of tomato
passata

½ teaspoon of chili
pepper
1 tablespoon of
cilantro, diced
2 tablespoon of olive
oil
1/2 cup of beef stock

Directions:

Thoroughly mix garlic, mint, lemongrass, pork, shallots, chili, cilantro, and tomato passata in a bowl. Make small meatballs out of this mixture and keep them aside.   Now start by putting all the Ingredients:, including the meatballs into your Crockpot.   Cover its lid and cook for 8 hours on Low setting.   Once done, remove its lid and mix well.   Garnish as desired.   Serve warm.
Nutrition Info: Calories 455 Total Fat 34.4 g Saturated Fat 3.4 g Cholesterol 64 mg Sodium 58 mg Total Carbs 10.8 g Sugar 1.7 g Fiber 5.2 g Potassium 43mg Protein 29.6 g

---

406.   Blue Cheese Casserole

Servings: 4   Cooking Time: 10 Hours
Ingredients:

1 lb. ground beef
1 yellow onion, diced
7 oz. fresh green
beans, trimmed and
diced
5 oz. blue cheese
1 cup of heavy
whipping cream

4 oz. shredded
cheddar cheese
salt and pepper
Scrving
5 oz. leafy greens
4 tablespoons of olive
oil

Directions:
Start by putting all the Ingredients: into your Crockpot except blue cheese.   Mix well and spread evenly then drizzle the cheese on top.   Cover it and cook for 10 hours on Low settings.   Once done, uncover the pot and mix well.   Garnish as desired. Serve warm.
Nutrition Info: Calories 301 Total Fat 12.2 g Saturated Fat 2.4 g Cholesterol 110 mg Sodium 276 mg Total Carbs 2.4 g Fiber 0.9 g Sugar 1.4 g Protein 28.8 g

---

407.   Lime Chicken Drumsticks

Servings: 4   Cooking Time: 4.5 Hours
Ingredients:

½ jalapeno pepper,
chopped
2 spring onions,
chopped
1 red bell pepper,
chopped
Juice of 1 lime
Zest of 1 lime, grated

1-pound chicken
drumsticks
1 cup of water
1 teaspoon salt
½ teaspoon chili
flakes
2 tablespoons tahini
paste

Directions:
In the slow cooker, mix the chicken with lime juice and the other ingredients.   Close the lid and cook chicken for 4.5 hours on High.
Nutrition Info:calories 301, fat 10.6, fiber 5.6, carbs 6.7, protein 33.1

---

408.   Paprika Chicken

Servings: 8   Cooking Time: 8 Hours
Ingredients:

1 tablespoon of olive
oil
1 tablespoon of dried
paprika
1 teaspoon of salt

1 tablespoon of curry
powder
1 teaspoon of dried
turmeric

Directions:

Start by mixing all the spices and oil in a bowl except chicken. Now season the chicken with these spices liberally. Add the chicken and spices to your Crockpot. Cover the lid of the crockpot and cook for 8 hours on Low. Serve warm.

Nutrition Info: Calories 313 Total Fat 134g Saturated Fat 78 g Cholesterol 861 mg Total Carbs 6.3 g Fiber 0.7 g Sugar 19 g Sodium 62 mg Potassium 211 mg Protein 24.6 g

409. Nutmeg Chicken

Servings: 8   Cooking Time: 5.5 Hours

Ingredients:

2 teaspoons ground nutmeg	3-pound whole chicken
1 teaspoon ground paprika	½ teaspoon salt
1 teaspoon ground black pepper	½ teaspoon chili flakes
	1 tablespoon Erythritol

Directions:
Line the slow cooker bottom with foil. Combine the chicken with nutmeg and the other ingredients inside. Close the lid and cook chicken for 5.5 hours on High. For the crunchy crust, bake the chicken for 20 minutes at the preheated to the 360F oven.

Nutrition Info:calories 347, fat 12.7, fiber 3.2, carbs 2.6, protein 29.4

410. Chicken Stew

Servings: 4   Cooking Time: 10 Hours

Ingredients:

8 oz. Bacon, diced	A drizzle of olive oil for serving
1 cup of Yellow onion, diced	2 Bay leaves
8 oz. wild rice	1-quart Chicken stock
2 Carrots, diced	2 teaspoon of Sherry vinegar
12 Parsley springs, diced	Salt and black pepper- to taste
2 tablespoon of Extra virgin olive oil	

Directions:
Start by throwing all the Ingredients: into the Crockpot and mix them well. Cover it and cook for 10 hours on Low Settings. Remove the cooked chicken and shred its meat. Return the chicken meat to the stew and mix well. Garnish as desired. Serve warm.

Nutrition Info: Calories 201 Total Fat 8.9 g Saturated Fat 4.5 g Cholesterol 57 mg Total Carbs 4.7 g Fiber 1.2 g Sugar 1.3 g Sodium 340 mg Potassium 315 mg Protein 15.3g

411. Lamb Mushroom Curry

Servings: 4   Cooking Time: 9 Hours

Ingredients:

1 (1-ounce) packet onion soup mix	1/2 cup of dry red wine
1 (10 3/4-ounce) can golden mushroom soup	1 (4-ounce) can mushrooms

Directions:

Start by putting all the Ingredients: into your Crockpot. Cover it and cook for 9 hours on Low settings. Once done, uncover the pot and mix well. Garnish as desired. Serve warm.

Nutrition Info: Calories 233 Total Fat 20.2 g Saturated Fat 4.4 g Cholesterol 120 mg Sodium 76 mg Total Carbs 4.5 g Fiber 0.9 g Sugar 1.4 g Protein 41.9 g

412. Stevia Pork Mix

Servings: 2   Cooking Time: 3 Hours

Ingredients:

10 oz pork tenderloins	1 teaspoon cayenne pepper
1 tablespoon avocado oil	½ teaspoon apple cider vinegar
1 and ½ teaspoon stevia	¾ teaspoon ground nutmeg
½ teaspoon salt	

Directions:
In the slow cooker, mix the pork with the oil, stevia and the other ingredients. Close the lid and cook meat on High for 3 hours.

Nutrition Info:calories 322, fat 18.8, fiber 3.5, carbs 5.1, protein 42.5

413. Tangy Lamb Meat Balls

Servings: 6   Cooking Time: 9 Hours

Ingredients:

Salt and black pepper, to taste	¼ teaspoon of red pepper flakes, crushed
2 small tomatoes, diced roughly	5 mini bell peppers, seeded and halved
½ small yellow onion, diced roughly	½ tablespoon of olive oil
½ cup of sugar-free tomato sauce	1 teaspoon of adobo seasoning
2 garlic cloves, peeled	

Directions:
Mix lamb meat, adobo seasoning, black pepper, and salt in a suitable bowl. Now use this lamb mixture to make small meatballs of 1-inch diameter. Start putting all the Ingredients:, including the meatballs into your Crockpot. Cover its lid and cook for 9 hours on Low settings. Once done, remove its lid and mix well. Garnish as desired. Serve warm.

Nutrition Info: Calories 345 Total Fat 27.2 g Saturated Fat 15.2 g Cholesterol 53 mg Sodium 65 mg Total Carbs 3.9 g Fiber 1.2 g Sugar 0.9 g Protein 6.4 g

414. Jalapeno Pork Tenderloin Soup

Servings: 2   Cooking Time: 8 Hours

Ingredients:

cooking spray	2 teaspoon of chili powder
2/3 cup of green bell pepper, diced	1 teaspoon of cumin, ground
1 tablespoon of garlic, minced	Salt and black pepper -to taste
1 jalapeno pepper, diced	14 oz. canned tomatoes, diced
1 lb. pork tenderloin,	

cubed
2 cups of chicken stock

2 tablespoons of Cilantro, diced

Directions:
Start by putting all the Ingredients: into your Crockpot. Cover its lid and cook for 8 hours on Low setting. Once done, remove its lid and mix well. Garnish as desired. Serve warm.
Nutrition Info: Calories 392 Total Fat 40.4 g Saturated Fat 6 g Cholesterol 20 mg Sodium 423 mg Total Carbs 7.2 g Sugar 3 g Fiber 4.2 g Potassium 422mg Protein 21 g

415.	**Char Siu Glazed Pork**

Servings: 4   Cooking Time: 4 Hours
Ingredients:

4 tablespoons of Char Siu sauce
2 tablespoons of soy sauce
2 tablespoons of dry sherry
1 teaspoon of peanut oil

2 lbs pork belly
2 tablespoons of sugar-free ketchup
2 teaspoons of sesame oil
¼ cup of vegetable stock

Directions:
Start by putting all the Ingredients: into your Crockpot. Cover its lid and cook for 4 hours on High setting. Once done, remove its lid and mix well. Garnish as desired. Serve warm.
Nutrition Info: Calories 257 Total Fat 7.5 g Saturated Fat 1.1 g Cholesterol 20 mg Sodium 97 mg Total Carbs 7.4 g Fiber 0 g Sugar 0 g Potassium 382 mg Protein 20.1g

416.	**Pork Tenderloin And Kale**

Servings: 4   Cooking Time: 8 Hours
Ingredients:

1 tablespoon chives, chopped
1 cup kale, chopped
10 oz pork tenderloin, sliced
1 cup heavy cream
1 teaspoon curry powder

½ teaspoon salt
½ teaspoon black pepper
1 teaspoon lemongrass, crushed
½ teaspoon garlic powder

Directions:
In the slow cooker, mix the pork with kale, chives and the other ingredients, Close the lid and cook for 8 hours on Low. Divide between plate sand serve.
Nutrition Info:calories 262, fat 13.7, fiber 4.3, carbs 6.8, protein 19.3

417.	**Herbed Lamb Stew**

Servings: 2   Cooking Time: 9 Hours.
Ingredients:

3/4 tablespoon of olive oil
1 celery stalk, diced
1 cup of tomatoes, diced
1 ½ tablespoon of fresh lemon juice
½ teaspoon of salt

½ large red bell pepper, cut into 8 slices
½ cup of bone broth
½ small onion, diced
½ tablespoon of

½ teaspoon of black pepper
½ large green bell pepper, cut into 8 slices

garlic, minced
½ teaspoon of oregano, dried, crushed
½ teaspoon of dried basil, crushed

Directions:
Start by putting all the Ingredients: into your Crockpot. Cover its lid and cook for 9 hours on Low settings. Once done, remove its lid and mix well. Garnish as desired. Serve warm.
Nutrition Info: Calories 260 Total Fat 22.9 g Saturated Fat 7.3 g Cholesterol 0 mg Sodium 9 mg Total Carbs 47 g Sugar 1.8 g Fiber 1.4 g Protein 5.6 g

418.	**Pork Carne Asada**

Servings: 4   Cooking Time: 8 Hours
Ingredients:

¾ tablespoon of chili powder
1½ tablespoons of olive oil
½ cup of beef bone broth

Salt to taste
½ large onion, sliced
¾ tablespoon of cumin
1 tablespoon of lemon juice
1½ oz tomato paste

Directions:
Start by putting all the Ingredients: into your Crockpot. Cover its lid and cook for 8 hours on Low setting. Once done, remove its lid and mix well. Garnish as desired. Serve warm.
Nutrition Info: Calories 272 Total Fat 11.1 g Saturated Fat 5.8 g Cholesterol 610 mg Sodium 749 mg Total Carbs 10.9 g Fiber 0.2 g Sugar 0.2 g Potassium 152mg Protein 23.5 g

419.	**Pork Roast**

Servings: 5   Cooking Time: 4 Hours
Ingredients:

5 slices thick-cut bacon

1.5 cups of BBQ sauce

Directions:
Start by putting all the Ingredients: into your Crockpot. Cover its lid and cook for 4 hours on Low setting. Once done, remove its lid and mix well. Garnish as desired. Serve warm.
Nutrition Info: Calories 254 Total Fat 15 g Saturated Fat 7 g Cholesterol 79 mg Total Carbs 17 g Sugar 3 g Fiber 1 g Sodium 812 mg Protein 21 g

420.	**Chicken Dipped In Tomatillo Sauce**

Servings: 4   Cooking Time: 6 Hours
Ingredients:

2 tablespoon of extra virgin olive oil
1 yellow onion, sliced
1 garlic clove, crushed
4 oz. canned green chilies, diced
1 handful cilantro,

15 oz. cauliflower rice, already cooked
15 oz. cheddar cheese, grated
4 oz. black olives, pitted and diced
Salt and black pepper- to taste

diced
5 oz. tomatoes, diced

15 oz canned
tomatillos, diced

Directions:
Start by throwing all the Ingredients: into the Crockpot and mix them well. Cover it and cook for 5 6 hours on Low Settings. Shred the slow-cooked chicken and return to the pot. Mix well and garnish as desired. Serve warm.
Nutrition Info: Calories 427 Total Fat 31.1 g Saturated Fat 4.2 g Cholesterol 0 mg Total Carbs 9 g Sugar 12.4 g Fiber 19.8 g Sodium 86 mg Potassium 100 mg Protein 23.5 g

421.	Dill Turkey

Servings: 3   Cooking Time: 3.5 Hours
Ingredients:

2 pounds turkey breast, skinless and sliced

½ teaspoon turmeric powder

¼ cup fresh dill, chopped

½ teaspoon salt

½ cup of water

1 teaspoon olive oil

Directions:
In the slow cooker, mix the turkey with dill and the other ingredients. Close the slow cooker lid and cook for 3.5 hours on High.
Nutrition Info:calories 236, fat 5, fiber 4.6, carbs 17.5, protein 25.4

422.	Meatballs With Saucy Mushrooms

Servings: 4   Cooking Time: 6 Hours
Ingredients:

1 yellow onion, minced

4 garlic cloves, minced

¼ cup of parsley, chopped

salt, and black pepper to taste

1 teaspoon of oregano, dried

1 egg whisked

¼ cup of almond milk

2 teaspoon of coconut aminos

12 mushrooms, diced

1 cup of chicken stock

2 tablespoon of olive oil

2 tablespoons of butter

Directions:
Thoroughly mix beef meat with garlic, onion, parsley, pepper, salt, egg, aminos, and oregano in a bowl. Make 1-inch small meatballs out of this mixture. Now start by putting all the Ingredients: into your Crockpot including the meatballs Cover it and cook for 6 hours on medium settings. Once done, uncover the pot and mix well. Serve warm.
Nutrition Info: Calories 231 Total Fat 17.8 g Saturated Fat 10.3 g Cholesterol 112 mg Total Carbs 1.2 g Sugar 0.2 g Fiber 0 g Sodium 92 mg Protein 16.4 g

423.	Thyme And Coriander Brisket

Servings: 6   Cooking Time: 12 Hours
Ingredients:

1 cup water

½ cup chicken stock

1 teaspoon ground coriander

½ teaspoon basil, dried

½ teaspoon chili

1 teaspoon ground thyme

½ teaspoon salt

1 teaspoon cumin, ground

½ teaspoon ground black pepper

powder

½ teaspoon paprika

1 tablespoon olive oil

1 tablespoon balsamic vinegar

2-pound beef brisket

Directions:
In a bowl, mix the beef with coriander, thyme and the other ingredients except the water and stock and leave aside for 20 minutes. Transfer the mix to the slow cooker, add the remaining ingredients and toss. Close the lid and cook the meat for 12 hours on Low.
Nutrition Info:calories 376, fat 12, fiber 4.4, carbs 4.8, protein 46

424.	Tarragon Lamb Chops

Servings: 4   Cooking Time: 10 Hours
Ingredients:

2 tablespoons of tarragon, diced

Salt and black pepper- to taste

1 lb. Asparagus, trimmed and halved

2 tablespoon of Olive oil

1 bunch green onions, diced

½ cup of vegetable broth

1 tablespoon of Mustard

Directions:
Start by putting all the Ingredients: into your Crockpot and mix them well. Cover its lid and cook for 10 hours on Low setting. Once done, remove its lid and mix well. Garnish as desired. Serve warm.
Nutrition Info: Calories 355 Total Fat 15 g Saturated Fat 1.4 g Cholesterol 128 mg Sodium 1271 mg Total Carbs 11.8 g Sugar 2.5 g Fiber 2.7 g Potassium 232mg Protein 44.2 g

425.	Lamb Chops Curry

Servings: 2   Cooking Time: 6 Hours
Ingredients:

1 garlic clove, crushed

3/4 teaspoon of rosemary, dried, crushed

1 tablespoon of xanthan gum

1 ½ tablespoons of butter

½ cup of bone broth

½ small onion, sliced

3/4 cup of Sugar-free diced tomatoes

1 cup of carrots, peeled and sliced

Salt and black pepper

½ tablespoon of cold water

Directions:
Start by putting all the Ingredients: into your Crockpot. Cover its lid and cook for 6 hours on Low settings. Once done, remove its lid and mix well. Garnish as desired. Serve warm.
Nutrition Info: Calories 184 Total Fat 12.7 g Saturated Fat 7.3 g Cholesterol 35 mg Sodium 222 mg Total Carbs 6.3 g Sugar 2.7 g Fiber 1.6 g Potassium 342mg Protein 12.2 g

426.	Pomegranate Lamb

Servings: 4   Cooking Time: 10 Hours 15 Minutes

Ingredients:

- 1 cup of pomegranate juice
- 1 cup of white wine
- 1 cup of chicken stock
- ½ cup of pomegranate seeds
- 4 mint leaves
- 4 cloves garlic, peeled and minced
- 1 teaspoon of black pepper, ground
- 1 teaspoon of salt
- 3 tablespoons of olive oil

Directions:
Start by throwing all the Ingredients: except the pomegranate seeds, butter, and flour into your Crockpot. Cover its lid and cook for 10 hours on Low settings. Once done, remove its lid and mix well. Slice the slow-cooked lamb then transfer to a plate Mix flour with butter in a small bowl then pour into the crockpot. Continue cooking the remaining sauce for 15 minutes on high heat. Pour this sauce around the slices lamb. Garnish with pomegranate seeds. Serve warm.

Nutrition Info: Calories 225 Total Fat 20.4 g Saturated Fat 8.7 g Cholesterol 30 mg Sodium 135 mg Total Carbs 7.7 g Fiber 4.3 g Sugar 2.2 g Protein 5.2 g

427. Pork Mushroom Stew

Servings: 3   Cooking Time: 8 Hours

Ingredients:

- ½ garlic clove, minced
- 1 lb. pork loin, cubed
- Salt and black pepper to taste
- 1 tablespoon of oregano, dried
- ¼ teaspoon of nutmeg, ground
- 1 lb. mushrooms, sliced
- 1 tablespoon of white vinegar
- 2/3 cups of vegetable broth
- 1/8 cup of coconut milk

Directions:
Start by putting all the Ingredients: into your Crockpot. Cover its lid and cook for 8 hours on Low setting. Once done, remove its lid and mix well. Garnish as desired. Serve warm.

Nutrition Info: Calories 213 Total Fat 23.4 g Saturated Fat 6.1 g Cholesterol 102 mg Sodium 86 mg Total Carbs 4.5 g Sugar 2.1 g Fiber 1.5 g Potassium 362mg Protein 33.2 g

428. Beef And Broccoli

Servings: 4   Cooking Time: 4 Hours

Ingredients:

- 1 cup broccoli florets
- 1-pound beef sirloin, sliced
- 1 teaspoon ground coriander
- 1 teaspoon cumin, ground
- 1 teaspoon sweet paprika
- ½ teaspoon salt
- 1 teaspoon olive oil
- 3 spring onions, chopped
- ½ teaspoon ground black pepper
- 1 tablespoon butter
- 1/3 cup water
- 1 tablespoon chives, chopped

Directions:
In the slow cooker, mix the broccoli with the beef and the other ingredients. Close the lid and cook on High for 4 hours. Divide into bowls and serve.

Nutrition Info: calories 308, fat 8.3, fiber 4.1, carbs 3.8, protein 7.5

429. Chicken With Romano Cheese

Servings: 6   Cooking Time: 6 Hours

Ingredients:

- 1 teaspoon of chicken bouillon granules
- 1 cup of Romano cheese, grated
- 1 yellow onion, diced
- 4 oz. mushrooms, sliced
- 1 teaspoon of garlic, minced
- 1/2 cup of white almond flour
- 2 tablespoon of vegetable oil
- 10 oz. sugar-free tomato sauce
- 1 teaspoon of basil, dried
- 1 teaspoon of white wine vinegar
- 1 tablespoon of swerve
- 1 tablespoon of oregano, dried
- Salt and black pepper- to taste

Directions:
Start by throwing all the Ingredients: into the Crockpot except cheese and mix them well. Cover it and cook for 6 hours on Low Settings. Garnish with cheese. Serve warm.

Nutrition Info: Calories 361 Total Fat 16.3 g Saturated Fat 4.9 g Cholesterol 114 mg Total Carbs 9.3 g Fiber 0.1 g Sugar 18.2 g Sodium 515 mg Potassium 343 mg Protein 33.3 g

430. Pork With Green Onion Sauce

Servings: 2   Cooking Time: 8 Hours

Ingredients:

- 1/3 cup of chicken stock
- 2 tablespoon of coconut aminos
- 1 teaspoon of garlic sauce
- Salt and black pepper- to taste
- cooking spray
- 1 and ½ teaspoon of olive oil
- ¼ cup of water
- 2 teaspoons of ginger, grated
- ¼ cup of green onions, diced

Directions:
Start by putting all the Ingredients: into your Crockpot. Cover its lid and cook for 8 hours on Low setting. Once done, remove its lid and mix well. Garnish as desired. Serve warm.

Nutrition Info: Calories 474 Total Fat 40.8 g Saturated Fat 25.5 g Cholesterol 105 mg Sodium 345 mg Total Carbs 3.9 g Sugar 1.8 g Fiber 0.8 g Potassium 341mg Protein 24.5 g

431. Slow CookerWhole Chicken

Servings: Makes 1 Whole Chicken   Cooking Time: Approximately 6 Hours

Ingredients:

- 1 medium-sized chicken
- 1 tsp fresh dried herbs
- 1 lemon
- 6 garlic cloves, skin kept on
- 2 onions, cut into rough chunks
- 3 celery sticks, cut into rough chunks
- ¾ cup chicken stock
- 3 tbsp butter

Directions:

Drizzle some olive oil into the Crock Pot. Prepare the chicken by rubbing with olive oil and sprinkling with dried herbs, salt, and pepper. Stuff the lemon into the chicken cavity. Add the onion chunks, celery chunks, and garlic cloves to the pot, pour the stock over the vegetables. Lay the chicken on top of the vegetables. Place a knob of butter on top of the chicken and press into the skin. Place the lid onto the pot and set the temperature to HIGH. Cook for 6 hours. Remove the lid, take the chicken out of the pot and leave to rest on a board to cool slightly before serving! Use the remaining liquid and vegetables from the pot to make a gravy by reducing in a pan and adding more liquid or thickeners if need be.

432. Creamy Chicken

Servings: 2   Cooking Time: 3 Hours
Ingredients:

8 oz chicken fillet, boneless and cut into cubes	1 teaspoon sweet chili pepper, minced
½ teaspoon salt	½ teaspoon chili powder
1 teaspoon turmeric powder	1 tablespoon butter
	¾ cup coconut cream

Directions:
In the slow cooker, mix the chicken with the salt, turmeric and the other ingredients. Close the lid and cook the chicken for 3 hours on High.
Nutrition Info:calories 295, fat 20.6, fiber 5.2, carbs 10.3, protein 19

433. Barbecue Beef Short Ribs

Servings: 6   Cooking Time: 6 Hours
Ingredients:

1 1/2 teaspoons of kosher salt	1 cup of barbecue sauce
1/2 teaspoon of black pepper	1 teaspoon of Worcestershire sauce
2 tablespoons of olive oil	1/2 teaspoon of onion powder
1/3 cup of beef stock	1/2 teaspoon of chili powder
1/4 cup of red wine	1/2 teaspoon of garlic powder
1/2 cup of water	
1/2 teaspoon of liquid smoke	

Directions:
Start by putting all the Ingredients: into your Crockpot. Cover it and cook for 6 hours on Low settings. Once done, uncover the pot and mix well. Garnish as desired. Serve warm.
Nutrition Info: Calories 314 Total Fat 18.2 g Saturated Fat 2.4 g Cholesterol 110 mg Sodium 231 mg Total Carbs 4.7 g Fiber 0.9 g Sugar 1.4 g Protein 26.3 g

434. Spicy Mexican Luncheon

Servings: 4   Cooking Time: 8 Hours
Ingredients:

6 tomatoes, diced	2 red onion, diced
10 oz. canned green chilies, diced	2 teaspoons of oregano, dried
4 teaspoon of chili powder	4 cups of vegetable broth
2 teaspoon of cumin powder	salt and black pepper to taste

Directions:
Start by putting all the Ingredients: into your Crockpot. Cover it and cook for 8 hours on Low settings. Once done, uncover the pot and mix well. Garnish as desired. Serve warm.
Nutrition Info: Calories 338 Total Fat 34 g Saturated Fat 8.5 g Cholesterol 69 mg Sodium 217 mg Total Carbs 5.1 g Fiber 1.2 g Sugar 12 g Protein 30.3 g

435. Mustard Beef

Servings: 4   Cooking Time: 8 Hours
Ingredients:

1 teaspoon garam masala	½ teaspoon salt
½ cup of water	1 tablespoon olive oil
1-pound beef chuck roast	¼ teaspoon cayenne pepper
1 tablespoon mustard	½ teaspoon mayonnaise

Directions:
In the slow cooker, mix the beef with mustard, masala and the other ingredients. Close the lid. Cook harissa braised beef for 8 hours on Low.
Nutrition Info:calorie 327, fat 22.6, fiber 4.3, carbs 4.1, protein 30

436. Full Meal Turmeric Lamb

Servings: 2   Cooking Time: 6 Hours.
Ingredients:

½ cup of onion diced	¼ teaspoon of ground coriander
½ tablespoon of garlic	½ teaspoon of salt
½ tablespoon of minced ginger	¼ teaspoon of cumin
¼ teaspoon of turmeric	¼ teaspoon of cayenne pepper

Directions:
Start by putting all the Ingredients: into your Crockpot. Cover its lid and cook for 6 hours on Low settings. Once done, remove its lid and mix well. Garnish as desired. Serve warm.
Nutrition Info: Calories 132 Total Fat 10.9 g Saturated Fat 2.7 g Cholesterol 164 mg Sodium 65 mg Total Carbs 3.3 g Sugar 0.5 g Fiber 2.3 g Protein 6.3 g

437. Slow CookerBeef Shank

Servings: 6   Cooking Time: Approximately 8 Hours
Ingredients:

2 lb beef shanks	2 cups red wine
1 onion, finely chopped	3 cups beef stock
5 garlic cloves, finely chopped	Sprig of fresh rosemary

Directions:
Heat some olive oil in a skillet or fry pan and brown the beef shanks until sealed on all sides. Remove

the beef shanks and set aside.   Pour the wine into the skillet and simmer to reduce.   Drizzle some olive oil into the Crock Pot.   Add the beef shanks, onion, garlic, reduced wine, stock, rosemary, salt, and pepper.   Secure the lid onto the pot and set the temperature to LOW.   Cook for 8 hours, the meat should be very tender.   Serve while hot, with a side of vegetables.

438.   Vegetable Lamb Stew

Servings: 2   Cooking Time: 10.5 Hours.
Ingredients:

- 1 tablespoon of fresh ginger, grated
- ½ teaspoon of lime juice
- ¼ teaspoon of black pepper
- 3/4 cup of diced tomatoes
- ½ teaspoon of turmeric powder
- ½ cup of coconut milk
- 1 ½ medium carrots, sliced
- 2 garlic cloves, minced
- ¼ teaspoon of salt
- 1 tablespoon of olive oil
- ½ medium onion, diced
- ½ medium zucchini, diced

Directions:
Start by putting all the Ingredients: into your Crockpot except zucchini.   Cover its lid and cook for 10 hours on Low settings.   Once done, remove its lid and mix well.   Stir in zucchini and continue cooking for 30 minutes on high heat.   Garnish as desired.   Serve warm.
Nutrition Info: Calories 108 Total Fat 9 g Saturated Fat 4.3 g Cholesterol 180 mg Sodium 146 mg Total Carbs 1.1 g Sugar 0.5 g Fiber 0.1 g Protein 6 g

439.   Pozole Blanco

Servings: 4   Cooking Time: 3.5 Hours
Ingredients:

- 3 tablespoons almond butter
- 2 spring onions, chopped
- ½ teaspoon minced garlic
- ½ jalapeno pepper, chopped
- 1 teaspoon dried oregano
- 11 oz chicken breast, skinless, boneless, chopped
- 1 tablespoon lime juice
- ¾ teaspoon lime zest, grated
- ½ cup of water
- ¼ cup fresh cilantro, chopped

Directions:
Put chopped chicken breast and 1 tablespoon of almond butter in the skillet.   Roast the poultry for 5 minutes over the medium heat.   Then transfer the chicken breast in the slow cooker, add remaining almond butter, diced onion, minced garlic, chopped jalapeno pepper, dried oregano, lime juice, and lime zest.   Mix up the ingredients and pour water. Close the lid and cook the meal for 3.5 hours on High. When Pozole Blanco is cooked, transfer it in the serving plates and garnish with chopped fresh cilantro.
Nutrition Info:calories 176, fat 8.8, fiber 2.1, carbs 5.4, protein 19.5

440.   Dijon Chicken

Servings: 4   Cooking Time: 6 Hours
Ingredients:

- 3/4 cup of chicken stock
- 1/4 cup of lemon juice
- 2 tablespoon of extra virgin olive oil
- 3 tablespoon of Dijon mustard
- 2 tablespoons of Italian seasoning
- Salt and black pepper- to taste

Directions:
Start by throwing all the Ingredients: into the Crockpot and mix them well.   Cover it and cook for 6 hours on Low Settings.   Garnish as desired. Serve warm.
Nutrition Info: Calories 398 Total Fat 13.8 g Saturated Fat 5.1 g Cholesterol 200 mg Total Carbs 3.6 g Fiber 1 g Sugar 1.3 g Sodium 272 mg Potassium 531 mg Protein 51.8 g

441.   Garlic Sirloin

Servings: 12   Cooking Time: 12 Hours
Ingredients:

- 4 teaspoons of garlic powder
- 8 cloves garlic, minced
- 1 cup of butter
- Salt and pepper, to taste
- ½ cup of beef stock

Directions:
Start by putting all the Ingredients: into your Crockpot.   Cover it and cook for 12 hours on Low settings.   Once done, uncover the pot and mix well. Garnish as desired.   Serve warm.
Nutrition Info: Calories 335 Total Fat 10.7 g Saturated Fat 2.7 g Cholesterol 168 mg Sodium 121 mg Total Carbs 1.9 g Fiber 3.5 g Sugar 2.3 g Protein 19.7 g

442.   Thyme Sea Bass

Servings: 4   Cooking Time: 4 Hours
Ingredients:
11 oz sea bass, trimmed
2 tablespoons coconut cream
3 oz spring onions, chopped
1 teaspoon fennel seeds
½ teaspoon dried thyme
1 teaspoon olive oil
1/3 cup water
1 teaspoon apple cider vinegar
½ teaspoon salt
Directions:
In the slow cooker, mix the sea bass with the cream and the other ingredients.   Close the lid and cook sea bass for 4 hours on Low.
Nutrition Info:calories 304, fat 11.4, fiber 0.9, carbs 6.2, protein 0.7

443.   Butter-dipped Lobsters

Servings: 8   Cooking Time: 1 Hour
Ingredients:
4 tablespoons of unsalted butter, melted
Salt to taste
4 lbs. lobster tails, cut in half
Black pepper to taste
Directions:
Start by throwing all the Ingredients: into your Crockpot.   Cover its lid and cook for 1 hour on Low setting.   Once done, remove its lid and give it a stir. Serve warm.
Nutrition Info: Calories 324 Total Fat 20.7 g Saturated Fat 6.7 g Cholesterol 45 mg Sodium 241 mg Total Carbs 8.6 g Sugar 1.4 g Fiber 0.5 g Protein 15.3 g

444.   Creamy Vanilla Custard

Servings: 8   Cooking Time: Approximately 3 Hours
Ingredients:
3 cups full-fat cream
4 egg yolks, lightly beaten
2 tsp vanilla extract
Few drops of stevia
Directions:
In a medium-sized bowl, whisk together the cream, egg yolks, vanilla extract, and stevia.   Pour the mixture into a heat-proof dish (one that fits into the Crock Pot!).   Place the dish into the Crock Pot. Pour enough hot water into the pot, around the dish, so that it reaches half way up the sides of the dish. Place the lid onto the pot and set the temperature to HIGH.   Cook for 3 hours.   Serve hot or cold!

445.   Fish And Salsa Bowl

Servings: 5   Cooking Time: 2 Hours
Ingredients:
1-pound white fish fillets, boneless and cubed
½ teaspoon Italian seasoning
1 cup keto salsa
½ teaspoon paprika
2 tablespoons olive oil
½ cup red cabbage, shredded
1 tablespoon chives, chopped
Directions:
In the slow cooker, mix the fish with the salsa and the other ingredients.   Close the lid and cook on High for 2 hours.   Divide into bowls and serve.
Nutrition Info:calories 238, fat 16.3, fiber 1.9, carbs 5.8, protein 11.8

446.   Butter Glazed Mussels

Servings: 6   Cooking Time: 2 Hours
Ingredients:
A splash of lemon juice
2 garlic cloves, peeled and minced
2 lb. mussels, debearded and scrubbed
Directions:
Start by throwing all the Ingredients: into your Crockpot.   Cover its lid and cook for 2 hours on High setting.   Once done, remove its lid and give it a stir.   Serve warm.
Nutrition Info: Calories 266 Total Fat 26.4 g Saturated Fat 4 g Cholesterol 13 mg Sodium 455 mg Total Carbs 5.4 g Sugar 2 g Fiber 1.6 g Protein 20.6 g

447.   Calamari Rings And Broccoli

Servings: 6   Cooking Time: 4.5 Hours
Ingredients:
1 1/2-pound calamari rings
1 cup broccoli florets
1 jalapeno pepper, minced
1 tablespoon keto tomato sauce
1/3 cup heavy cream
½ teaspoon salt
½ teaspoon chili powder
1 teaspoon cumin, ground
2 garlic cloves, diced
1 tablespoon butter
Directions:
In the slow cooker, mix the calamari with broccoli and the other ingredients, toss and close the lid. Cook the meal on Low for 4.5 hours.
Nutrition Info:calories 210, fat 6.1, fiber 2.2, carbs 4.7, protein 18.1

448.   Citrus Enriched Salmon

Servings: 6   Cooking Time: 2 Hours
Ingredients:
1 ½ teaspoon of fresh ginger, minced
1 ½ tablespoon of olive oil
1 ½ cup of white wine
4 tablespoons of fresh lemon juice
2 ½ teaspoons of fresh orange zest, grated finely
Black pepper, to taste
Fresh herbs (garnish)
Directions:
Start by throwing all the Ingredients: into your Crockpot.   Cover its lid and cook for 2 hours on Low setting.   Once done, remove its lid and give it a stir.   Garnish with cilantro.   Serve warm.
Nutrition Info: Calories 487 Total Fat 37.4 g Saturated Fat 8.8 g Cholesterol 71 mg Sodium 501

mg Total Carbs 10.6 g Sugar 1.2 g Fiber 9.2 g
Protein 28.1 g

449.   Shrimp Mushroom Alfredo

Servings: 4   Cooking Time: 4 Hours
Ingredients:

- 2 tablespoon of olive oil
- 1 onion, peeled and diced
- 8 oz. mushrooms, diced
- 1 asparagus bunch, cut into pieces
- 1 lb. shrimp, peeled and deveined
- 1 cup of heavy cream
- Salt and black pepper ground, to taste
- 2 teaspoons of Italian seasoning
- 1 teaspoon of red pepper flakes
- 1 cup of Parmesan cheese, shredded
- 2 garlic cloves, peeled and minced

Directions:
Start by throwing all the Ingredients: into your Crockpot except shrimp.   Cover its lid and cook for 4 hours on High setting.   Once done, remove its lid and give it a stir.   Stir in shrimp and continue cooking for 1 hour on low heat.   Serve warm.
Nutrition Info: Calories 213 Total Fat 23.4 g Saturated Fat 6.1 g Cholesterol 102 mg Sodium 86 mg Total Carbs 4.5 g Sugar 2.1 g Fiber 1.5 g Protein 33.2 g

450.   Cod Soup

Servings: 4   Cooking Time: 2 Hours
Ingredients:

- ½ cup cream
- 12 oz cod, boneless and cubed
- 1 cup cherry tomatoes, halved
- 1 oz bacon, chopped, roasted
- 2 cups of water
- 1 teaspoon salt
- 1 teaspoon ground black pepper
- 1/3 cup fresh cilantro, chopped

Directions:
In the slow cooker, mix the cod with the cream and the other ingredients, close the lid and cook on High for 2 hours.   Divide into bowls and serve.
Nutrition Info:calories 342, fat 5.6, fiber 4.3, carbs 3.8, protein 19.7

451.   Herbed Shrimp

Servings: 4   Cooking Time: 1.5 Hours
Ingredients:

- 1-pound shrimp, peeled and deveined
- 1 tablespoon oregano, chopped
- ½ teaspoon dried basil
- ½ teaspoon nutmeg, ground
- 1 tablespoon chives, chopped
- 1 tablespoon sage, chopped
- 1 tablespoon cilantro, chopped
- 1 teaspoon curry powder
- ½ teaspoon paprika
- 1 cup organic almond milk

Directions:
In the slow cooker, mix the shrimp with the oregano, basil and the other ingredients.   Close the lid and cook curry shrimps on High for 1.5 hours.

Nutrition Info:calories 212, fat 3.9, fiber 2.8, carbs 4.6, protein 20.4

452.   Warming Mussels Tomato Soup

Servings: 4   Cooking Time: 3 Hours
Ingredients:

- 1 tablespoon of olive oil
- 2 cups of chicken stock
- 1 onion, peeled and diced
- 1 teaspoon of red pepper flakes
- 1 (28 oz.) can diced tomatoes
- 3 garlic cloves, peeled and minced
- ½ cup of fresh parsley, diced
- 1 (28 oz.) can crushed tomatoes
- Salt and black pepper ground, to taste

Directions:
Start by throwing all the Ingredients: into your Crockpot.   Cover its lid and cook for 3 hours on Low setting.   Once done, remove its lid and give it a stir.   Serve warm.
Nutrition Info: Calories 321 Total Fat 9 g Saturated Fat 4.9 g Cholesterol 108 mg Sodium 184 mg Total Carbs 10.8 g Sugar 8.2 g Fiber 3.2 g Protein 24.3 g

453.   Shrimp Curry

Servings: 4   Cooking Time: 1.5 Hours
Ingredients:

- 1-pound shrimp, peeled and deveined
- 1 tablespoon red curry paste
- 1 teaspoon curry powder
- 1 tablespoon curry paste
- 1 cup of coconut milk
- 1/3 jalapeno pepper, chopped
- ½ teaspoon garlic powder
- 1 teaspoon olive oil
- ½ cup spring onions, chopped

Directions:
In the slow cooker, mix the shrimp with curry paste and the other ingredients.   Close the lid and cook the curry for 1.5 hours on High.
Nutrition Info:calories 261, fat 13.8, fiber 1.7, carbs 6, protein 21

454.   Salmon With Leeks And Cream

Servings: 4   Cooking Time: Approximately 4 Hours
Ingredients:

- 4 fresh salmon fillets
- 1 cup heavy cream
- One leek, finely sliced
- ½ cup white wine

Directions:
Pour the cream and wine into a pot, bring to a simmer and reduce until slightly thickened.   Rub the salmon fillets with olive oil, and sprinkle with salt and pepper.   Drizzle some olive oil into the Crock Pot.   Add the leeks to the pot and sprinkle with salt and pepper.   Place the salmon fillets on top of the leeks.   Pour the reduced cream and wine mixture into the pot.   Place the lid onto the pot and set the temperature to LOW.   Cook for 4

hours. Serve the salmon with a generous serving of leeks and creamy sauce! Desserts

455. Shrimp Tomato Medley

Servings: 8   Cooking Time: 1 Hour
Ingredients:
- 1½ tablespoon of coconut oil
- 1 small ginger root, diced
- 8 cups of chicken stock
- ¼ cup of coconut aminos
- ¼ teaspoon of fish sauce
- 4 scallions, diced
- 1 lb. shrimp, peeled and deveined
- ½ lb. tomatoes
- Black pepper ground, to taste
- 1 tablespoon of sesame oil
- 1 (5 oz.) can bamboo shoots, sliced

Directions:
Start by throwing all the Ingredients: into your Crockpot. Cover its lid and cook for 1 hour on Low setting. Once done, remove its lid and give it a stir. Serve warm.
Nutrition Info: Calories 371 Total Fat 3.7 g Saturated Fat 2.7 g Cholesterol 168 mg Sodium 121 mg Total Carbs 4 g Fiber 1.5 g Sugar 0.3 g Protein 26.5 g

456. Fish And Tomato Stew

Servings: 4   Cooking Time: Approximately 4 Hours
Ingredients:
- 4 tomatoes, chopped
- 2 cups fish stock
- 5 garlic cloves, finely chopped
- 1 tsp ground cumin
- 1 tsp ground coriander
- 1 tsp ground chili
- 3 large white fish fillets, cut into chunks
- Handful of fresh parsley, chopped

Directions:
Drizzle some olive oil into the Crock Pot. Add the tinned tomatoes, fish stock, garlic, cumin, chili, coriander, fish, salt, and pepper, stir to combine. Place the lid onto the pot and set the temperature to HIGH. Cook for 4 hours. Serve the stew while hot, with a generous sprinkling of fresh parsley!

457. Shrimp And Zucchini

Servings: 6   Cooking Time: 2 Hours
Ingredients:
- 1-pound shrimp, peeled and deveined
- 2 zucchinis, roughly cubed
- 1 cup cherry tomatoes, halved
- ½ cup Mozzarella cheese, shredded
- 4 tablespoons cream cheese
- 1 tablespoon butter, melted
- 1 teaspoon salt
- 1 tablespoon keto tomato sauce
- ¾ cup of water

Directions:
In the slow cooker, mix the shrimp with zucchinis and the other ingredients except the cheese and toss. Sprinkle the cheese on top, close the lid and cook on High for 2 hours.
Nutrition Info:calories 223, fat 8.9, fiber 0.8, carbs 3.2, protein 19.3

458. Coffee Creams With Toasted Seed Crumble Topping

Servings: Makes 6 Ramekins   Cooking Time: Approximately 4 Hours
Ingredients:
- 2 cups heavy cream
- 3 egg yolks, lightly beaten
- 3 tbsp strong espresso coffee (or 3tsp instant coffee dissolved in 3tbsp boiling water)
- 1 tsp vanilla extract
- ½ cup mixed seeds – sesame seeds, pumpkin seeds, chia seeds, sunflower seeds,
- 1 tsp cinnamon
- 1 tbsp coconut oil

Directions:
Heat the coconut oil in a small fry pan until melted. Add the mixed seeds, cinnamon, and a pinch of salt, toss in the oil and heat until toasted and golden, place into a small bowl and set aside. In a medium-sized bowl, whisk together the cream, egg yolks, vanilla, and coffee. Pour the cream/coffee mixture into the ramekins. Place the ramekins into the Crock Pot. Pour enough hot water into the pot to reach half way up the ramekins. Place the lid onto the pot and set the temperature to LOW. Cook for 4 hours. Remove the ramekins from the Slow Cookerand leave to cool slightly on the bench. Sprinkle the seed mixture over the top of each custard before serving.

459. Cod & Peas With Sour Cream

Servings: 2   Cooking Time: 1 Hour
Ingredients:
- 1 tablespoon of fresh parsley
- 1 garlic clove, diced
- ½ lb. frozen peas
- ½ teaspoon of paprika
- 1 cup of sour cream
- ½ cup of white wine

Directions:
Start by throwing all the Ingredients: into your Crockpot except sour cream. Cover its lid and cook for 1 hour on High setting. Once done, remove its lid and give it a stir. Stir in sour cream and mix it gently Serve warm.
Nutrition Info: Calories 349 Total Fat 31.9 g Saturated Fat 15 g Cholesterol 46 mg Sodium 237 mg Total Carbs 6.6 g Sugar 1.4 g Fiber 3.4 g Protein 11 g

460. Slow CookerTuna Steaks

Servings: 4   Cooking Time: Approximately 3 Hours
Ingredients:
- 4 tuna steaks
- 3 garlic cloves, crushed
- 1 lemon, sliced into 8 slices
- ½ cup white wine

Directions:
Reduce the white wine in a pot by simmering until the strong alcoholic smell is cooked off. Rub the tuna steaks with olive oil, and sprinkle with salt and pepper. Place the tuna steaks into the Crock Pot. Sprinkle the crushed garlic on top of the tuna steaks. Place 2 lemon slices on top of each tuna steak. Pour the reduced wine into the pot. Secure the lid

onto the pot and set the temperature to HIGH. Cook for 3 hours.   Serve with a drizzle of leftover liquid from the pot, and a side of crispy greens!

461.   Tilapia And Radish Bites

Servings: 2   Cooking Time: 2.5 Hours
Ingredients:
1 ½ cups radishes, halved
1 teaspoon sweet paprika
½ teaspoon dried rosemary
½ teaspoon salt
¼ teaspoon ground black pepper
9 oz tilapia fillet, boneless and cubed
2 oz Cheddar cheese, sliced
¼ cup veggie stock

Directions:
In the slow cooker, mix the radishes with the fish and the other ingredients and toss.   Close the lid and cook the fish for 5 hours on High.
Nutrition Info:calories 251, fat 8.4, fiber 0.2, carbs 1.3, protein 6.6

462.   Shrimp & Pepper Stew

Servings: 4   Cooking Time: 2 Hours
Ingredients:
14 oz. canned diced tomatoes
¼ cup of yellow onion, peeled and diced
2 tablespoon of lime juice
¼ cup of olive oil
1½ lbs. shrimp, peeled and deveined
¼ cup of red pepper, roasted and diced
1 garlic clove, peeled and diced
1 cup of coconut milk
¼ cup of fresh cilantro, diced
Salt and black pepper ground, to taste

Directions:
Start by throwing all the Ingredients: into your Crockpot except shrimp.   Cover its lid and cook for 2 hours on Low setting.   Once done, remove its lid and give it a stir.   Stir in shrimp and continue cooking for 1 hour on low heat.   Serve warm.
Nutrition Info: Calories 392 Total Fat 40.4 g Saturated Fat 6 g Cholesterol 20 mg Sodium 423 mg Total Carbs 7.2 g Sugar 3 g Fiber 4.2 g Protein 21 g

463.   Chili Squid

Servings: 4   Cooking Time: 2.5 Hours
Ingredients:
16 oz squid tubes, trimmed (4 squid tubes)
1 cup spring onions, chopped
1 teaspoon salt
½ teaspoon chili powder
½ teaspoon hot paprika
1 tablespoon butter
1/3 cup heavy cream
1 teaspoon ground black pepper
1 tablespoon dried dill

Directions:
In the slow cooker, mix the squid with spring onions and the other ingredients.   Close the slow cooker lid and cook for 5 hours on High.
Nutrition Info:calories 244, fat 8.2, fiber 3.8, carbs 7.1, protein 13.2

464.   Creamy Seafood Chowder

Servings: 6   Cooking Time: Approximately 5 Hours
Ingredients:
5 garlic cloves, crushed
1 small onion, finely chopped
1 cup prawns, (frozen is fine, thaw first)
1 cup shrimp, (frozen is fine, thaw first)
1 cup white fish, chopped into small chunks
2 cups full-fat cream
1 cup dry white wine
Handful of fresh parsley, finely chopped

Directions:
Drizzle some olive oil into the Crock Pot.   Add the garlic, onion, prawns, shrimp, white fish, cream, wine, salt, and pepper into the Crock Pot, stir to combine.   Place the lid onto the pot and set the temperature to LOW.   Cook for 5 hours.   Serve while hot, with a sprinkling of fresh parsley!

465.   Luscious Herbed Clams

Servings: 12   Cooking Time: 2 Hours
Ingredients:
½ cup of butter
2 cups of white wine
1 teaspoon of fresh parsley, roughly diced
1 teaspoon of red pepper flakes
36 clams, scrubbed
5 garlic cloves, peeled and minced

Directions:
Start by throwing all the Ingredients: into your Crockpot.   Cover its lid and cook for 2 hours on Low setting.   Once done, remove its lid and give it a stir.   Serve warm.
Nutrition Info: Calories 455 Total Fat 34.4 g Saturated Fat 3.4 g Cholesterol 64 mg Sodium 58 mg Total Carbs 10.8 g Sugar 1.7 g Fiber 5.2 g Protein 29.6 g

466.   Dinner Mussels

Servings: 8   Cooking Time: 3 Hours
Ingredients:
2 medium yellow onions, diced
1 teaspoon of rosemary, dried, crushed
4 lbs. mussels, cleaned and de-bearded
2 garlic cloves, minced
2 cups of chicken broth
¼cup of fresh lemon juice
Salt and black pepper, to taste

Directions:
Start by throwing all the Ingredients: into your Crockpot.   Cover its lid and cook for 3 hours on Low setting.   Once done, remove its lid and give it a stir.   Serve warm.
Nutrition Info: Calories 238 Total Fat 9.5 g Saturated Fat 2.7 g Cholesterol 103 mg Sodium 403 mg Total Carbs 1.8 g Sugar 0.2 g Fiber 0.2 g Protein 34.2 g

467.   Salmon Casserole

Servings: 6   Cooking Time: 8 Hours
Ingredients:

8 oz. cream of mushroom soup
1 cup of mushrooms, diced
3 tablespoons of almond flour
1 (16oz.) can salmon (drained and flaked)
¼ cup of water
½ cup of diced scallion
¼ teaspoon of ground nutmeg
Salt and black pepper, to taste

Directions:
Start by throwing all the Ingredients: into your Crockpot. Cover its lid and cook for 8 hours on medium setting. Once done, remove its lid and give it a stir. Serve warm.
Nutrition Info: Calories 211 Total Fat 18.5 g Saturated Fat 11.5 g Cholesterol 173 mg Sodium 280 mg Total Carbs 0.5 g Sugar 0.3 g Fiber 0.2 g Protein 11.5 g

468. Creamy Tuna

Servings: 6   Cooking Time: 4 Hours
Ingredients:
1-pound tuna fillet, boneless and cubed
1 red chili pepper, minced
1 tablespoon butter
2 shallots, chopped
½ cup heavy cream
1 cup Mozzarella cheese, shredded
1 teaspoon salt
1 teaspoon paprika
1 teaspoon basil, dried

Directions:
Put butter in the bottom of slow cooker. Add the tuna and the other ingredients and toss. Close the lid and cook for 4 hours on High.
Nutrition Info:calories 205, fat 12.7, fiber 3.7, carbs 9.7, protein 21.9

469. Cinnamon Mackerel

Servings: 4   Cooking Time: 3 Hours
Ingredients:
1 ½ pound mackerel, trimmed
1 tablespoon avocado oil
1 teaspoon garlic powder
1/3 cup coconut milk
½ teaspoon salt
½ teaspoon basil, dried
1 teaspoon cumin, ground
¾ teaspoon ground cinnamon

Directions:
In the slow cooker, mix the mackerel with the oil and the other ingredients and close the lid. Cook the fish for 3 hours on High. Divide between plates and serve.
Nutrition Info:calories 228, fat 8.8, fiber 0.9, carbs 2.2, protein 11.2

470. Lime Cod And Shrimps

Servings: 4   Cooking Time: 3 Hours
Ingredients:
1-pound cod fillet, boneless and cubed
½ pound shrimp, peeled and deveined
1 teaspoon Italian seasoning
Juice of 1 lime
1/3 teaspoon cayenne pepper
½ teaspoon ginger
¾ teaspoon ground

1 teaspoon dried rosemary
cinnamon
1 tablespoon butter
Directions:
In the slow cooker, mix the cod with shrimp, lime juice and the other ingredients, toss and close the lid. Cook fish for 3 hours on High. Divide into bowls and serve.
Nutrition Info:calories 220, fat 6, fiber 3.4, carbs 4.8, protein 20.4

471.Cheesy Tuna

Servings: 4   Cooking Time: 9 Hours
Ingredients:
1 cup coconut cream
1 tablespoon Ricotta cheese
½ teaspoon white pepper
10 ounces tuna fillet, boneless and cubed
1 teaspoon salt
1 teaspoon olive oil
1 garlic clove, crushed
1 teaspoon fennel seeds
1/2 cup Cheddar, shredded

Directions:
In the slow cooker, mix the tuna with the cream and the other ingredients. Close the lid and cook snapper for 9 hours on Low.
Nutrition Info:calories 211, fat 4.3, fiber 3.3, carbs 7.8, protein 21

472. Salty-sweet Almond Butter And Chocolate Sauce

Servings: Makes 1 Jar Of Sauce   Cooking Time: Approximately 4 Hours
Ingredients:
2 ounces salted butter
1 ounce dark chocolate
1 cup almond butter
½ tsp sea salt
Few drops of stevia

Directions:
Place the almond butter, butter, dark chocolate, sea salt, and stevia to the Crock Pot. Place the lid onto the pot and set the temperature to LOW. Cook for 4 hours, stirring every 30 minutes to combine the butter and chocolate as they melt. Pour into a jar and leave to cool before storing in the fridge.

473. Fish And Bacon Soup

Servings: 6   Cooking Time: Approximately 4 Hours
Ingredients:
5 slices streaky bacon, chopped
4 fillets of fresh white fish, chopped into chunks
5 garlic cloves, crushed
4 cups fish stock
1 cup crème fraiche

Directions:
Drizzle some olive oil into the Crock Pot. Add the bacon, fish, garlic, stock, salt, and pepper to the pot, stir to combine. Place the lid onto the pot and set the temperature to HIGH. Cook for 4 hours. Remove the lid and stir the crème fraiche into the soup. Serve with an extra dollop of crème fraiche and some freshly chopped herbs!

474. Nutritious Salmon Dinner

Servings: 2   Cooking Time: 3 Hours

Ingredients:
- 1 garlic clove, minced
- 1 teaspoon of powdered stevia
- 1 tablespoon of red chili powder
- 1 teaspoon of cumin, ground
- Salt and Black pepper
- ½ cup of red wine
- ½ cup of broth

Directions:
Start by throwing all the Ingredients: into your Crockpot. Cover its lid and cook for 3 hours on Low setting. Once done, remove its lid and give it a stir. Serve warm.
Nutrition Info: Calories 238 Total Fat 23.2 g Saturated Fat 13 g Cholesterol 61 mg Sodium 115 mg Total Carbs 6.8 g Sugar 0.2 g Fiber 0.9 g Protein 22.3 g

475.	Coconut Squares With Blueberry Glaze

Servings: About 20 Small Squares   Cooking Time: Approximately 3 Hours
Ingredients:
- 2 cups desiccated coconut
- 1 ounce butter, melted
- 3 ounces cream cheese
- 1 egg, lightly beaten
- ½ tsp baking powder
- 2 tsp vanilla extract
- 1 cup frozen berries

Directions:
In a large bowl, place the coconut, butter, cream cheese, egg, baking powder, and vanilla extract, beat with a wooden spoon until combined and smooth. Grease a heat-proof dish (make sure it fits inside the Crock Pot) with butter. Spread the coconut mixture into the dish. Place the blueberries into a small bowl and defrost in the microwave until they resemble a thick sauce. Spread the blueberries over the coconut mixture. Place the dish into the Slow Cookerand pour enough hot water into the pot so that it reaches half way up the dish. Place the lid onto the pot and set the temperature to HIGH. Cook for 3 hours. Remove the dish from the pot and leave to cool on the bench before slicing into small squares.

476.	Balsamic Mussels

Servings: 4   Cooking Time: 2 Hours
Ingredients:
- 1-pound mussels
- 1 tablespoon Balsamic vinegar
- ½ teaspoon stevia extract
- 1 teaspoon lemon juice
- 1 teaspoon lemon zest
- 2 tablespoon sesame oil
- ¼ cup butter
- 4 tablespoons coconut cream

Directions:
In the slow cooker, mix the mussels with vinegar, stevia and the other ingredients. Close the slow cooker lid and cook the catfish for 2 hours on High. Divide into bowls and serve,
Nutrition Info:calories 279, fat 20.1, fiber 4.5, carbs 5.2, protein 6.1

477.	Maple Glazed Salmon Fillet

Servings: 1   Cooking Time: 2 Hours
Ingredients:
- 2 tablespoons of mustard
- 1 tablespoon of maple syrup (sugar-free)
- 1 salmon fillet
- Salt and black pepper ground, to taste

Directions:
Start by throwing all the Ingredients: into your Crockpot. Cover its lid and cook for 2 hours on High setting. Once done, remove its lid and give it a stir. Serve warm.
Nutrition Info: Calories 434 Total Fat 36.4 g Saturated Fat 17.1 g Cholesterol 257 mg Sodium 1038 mg Total Carbs 2.5 g Sugar 0.9 g Fiber 0.2 g Protein 24.2 g

478.	Cider Soaked Pancetta Clams

Servings: 6   Cooking Time: 2 Hours
Ingredients:
- 2 lbs. clams, scrubbed
- 1 tablespoon of olive oil
- Juice from ½ lemon
- 1 bottle infused cider
- 3 tablespoons of butter
- Salt and black pepper ground, to taste
- 2 garlic cloves, peeled and diced
- 2 thyme sprigs, diced

Directions:
Start by throwing all the Ingredients: into your Crockpot. Cover its lid and cook for 2 hours on Low setting. Once done, remove its lid and give it a stir. Serve warm.
Nutrition Info: Calories 355 Total Fat 15 g Saturated Fat 1.4 g Cholesterol 128 mg Sodium 1271 mg Total Carbs 11.8 g Sugar 2.5 g Fiber 2.7 g Protein 44.2 g

479.	Cod Platter

Servings: 6   Cooking Time: 4 Hours
Ingredients:
- 2 ½ tablespoons of fresh rosemary, diced
- 6 (4-oz.) cod fillets
- 3 garlic cloves, minced
- 2 tablespoon of olive oil
- Salt and black pepper, to taste

Directions:
Start by throwing all the Ingredients: into your Crockpot. Cover its lid and cook for 4 hours on Low setting. Once done, remove its lid and give it a stir. Serve warm.
Nutrition Info: Calories 335 Total Fat 5.4 g Saturated Fat 3.3 g Cholesterol 16 mg Sodium 708 mg Total Carbs 2.1 g Sugar 0.7 g Fiber 0.4 g Protein 18.5 g

480.	Tuna And Cabbage Mix

Servings: 4   Cooking Time: 3 Hours
Ingredients:
- 2 oz cabbage, shredded
- 11 oz tuna, drained, chopped
- 2 tablespoons keto tomato sauce
- 1/3 cup water
- 1 teaspoon salt
- 1 tablespoon butter
- 1 teaspoon turmeric powder

Directions:
In the slow cooker, mix the cabbage with the tuna and the other ingredients, and close the lid.   Cook cabbage for 3 hours on High.   Divide into bowls and serve.
Nutrition Info:calories 227, fat 8.3, fiber 0.8, carbs 3.2, protein 15.9

481.   Seafood Stew

Servings: 6   Cooking Time: 2.5 Hours
Ingredients:

1 tablespoon of tomato paste	1/2 teaspoon of celery salt
4 cups of vegetable broth	1/4 teaspoon of crushed red pepper flakes
3 garlic cloves, minced	1/8 teaspoon of cayenne pepper
1/2 cup of diced white onion	Salt and pepper to taste
1 teaspoon of thyme, dried	1 lb. large shrimp
1 teaspoon of dried basil	1 lb. scallops
1 teaspoon of oregano, dried	A handful of fresh parsley, chopped

Directions:
Start by throwing all the Ingredients: into your Crockpot except seafood.   Cover its lid and cook for 2 hours on Low setting.   Once done, remove its lid and give it a stir.   Stir in seafood and continue cooking for 30 minutes on low heat.   Serve warm.
Nutrition Info: Calories 335 Total Fat 5.4 g Saturated Fat 3.3 g Cholesterol 16 mg Sodium 708 mg Total Carbs 2.1 g Sugar 0.7 g Fiber 0.4 g Protein 18.5 g

482.   Salmon And Garlic Greens

Servings: 4   Cooking Time: Approximately 3 Hours
Ingredients:

4 salmon fillets, skin on	1/2 a head of broccoli, cut into florets
4 garlic cloves, crushed	2 cups frozen green beans

Directions:
Drizzle some olive oil into the Crock Pot.   Place the salmon fillets, (skin-side down) into the pot and sprinkle them with salt and pepper.   Place the broccoli, beans, and garlic on top of the salmon, sprinkle the veggies with salt and pepper.   Drizzle some more olive oil over top of the veggies and fish. Place the lid onto the pot and set the temperature to HIGH.   Cook for 3 hours.   Serve immediately!

483.   Jalapeno Cheese Oysters

Servings: 9   Cooking Time: 2 Hours
Ingredients:

2 tomatoes, cored and diced	18 oysters, scrubbed
2 limes, cut into wedges	1/2 cup of Monterey Jack cheese, shredded
1/2 cup of fresh cilantro, diced	1/4 cup of onion, diced

Salt and black pepper ground, to taste	1/2 cup of vegetable stock
	Juice from 1 lime

Directions:
Start by throwing all the Ingredients: into your Crockpot.   Cover its lid and cook for 2 hours on Low setting.   Once done, remove its lid and give it a stir.   Serve warm.
Nutrition Info: Calories 487 Total Fat 37.4 g Saturated Fat 8.8 g Cholesterol 71 mg Sodium 501 mg Total Carbs 10.6 g Sugar 1.2 g Fiber 9.2 g Protein 28.1 g

484.   Chocolate And Blackberry Cheesecake Sauce

Servings: Makes 1 Jar Of Sauce   Cooking Time: Approximately 6 Hours
Ingredients:

3/4 lb cream cheese	1 1/2 ounces butter
1/2 cup heavy cream	1 tsp vanilla extract
3 ounces dark chocolate	Few drops of stevia (optional, depending on how sweet you prefer your sauce)
1/2 cup fresh blackberries, chopped	

Directions:
Place the cream cheese, cream, butter, dark chocolate, blackberries, vanilla, and stevia into the Crock Pot.   Place the lid onto the pot and set the temperature to LOW.   Cook for 6 hours, stirring every 30 minutes to combine the butter and chocolate as it melts.   Pour into a jar and leave to cool before storing in the fridge.   Have a spoonful here and there to curb your sweet cravings! Or pour over Keto desserts or berries!

485.   Sage Halibut

Servings: 5   Cooking Time: 4.5 Hours
Ingredients:

5 halibut fillets, boneless	1 teaspoon turmeric powder
1/4 cup coconut cream	1 teaspoon salt
1/2 teaspoon black pepper	1/2 teaspoon sage
	1/3 cup butter

Directions:
In the slow cooker, mix the fish with coconut cream and the other ingredients.   Close the lid and cook the fish on Low for 4.5 hours.
Nutrition Info:calories 278, fat 19, fiber 4.1, carbs 6.2, protein 20.7

486.   Cajun Shrimp

Servings: 4   Cooking Time: 3 Hours
Ingredients:

1-pound shrimps, peeled	1 teaspoon basil, dried
1 tomato, chopped	1 teaspoon oregano, dried
1 tablespoon keto tomato sauce	1 teaspoon salt
2 green bell peppers, chopped	1/2 teaspoon ground black pepper
1/3 teaspoon Cajun seasoning	1/2 cup of water

Directions:

Pour water in the slow cooker.   Add shrimp and the other ingredients.   Close the lid and cook liquid for 2 hours on High.   Divide into bowls and serve.
Nutrition Info:calories 150, fat 2.1, fiber 1.2, carbs 5.1, protein 26.5

487.   Salmon And Spinach Bake

Servings: 2   Cooking Time: 6 Hours
Ingredients:

- 1-pound salmon fillet, chopped
- 1/3 cup spinach, chopped
- ½ cup Cheddar cheese, shredded
- 1 teaspoon butter
- ¾ cup organic coconut milk
- ½ teaspoon ground thyme
- ½ teaspoon salt
- 1/3 cup of water

Directions:
In the slow cooker mix the salmon with spinach and the other ingredients, toss and close the lid.   Cook the salmon bake for 6 hours on Low.
Nutrition Info:calories 423, fat 16.1, fiber 1.9, carbs 3.8, protein 17.4

488.   Peanut Butter, Chocolate And Pecan Cupcakes

Servings: Makes 14 Chocolate Cups   Cooking Time: Approximately 4 Hours
Ingredients:

- 14 paper cupcake cases
- 1 cup smooth peanut butter
- 2 ounces butter
- 2 tsp vanilla extract
- 5 ounces dark chocolate
- 2 tbsp coconut oil
- 2 eggs, lightly beaten
- 1 cup ground almonds
- 1 tsp baking powder
- 1 tsp cinnamon
- 10 pecan nuts, toasted and finely chopped

Directions:
Melt together the dark chocolate and coconut oil in the microwave, stir to combine and set aside. Place the peanut butter and butter into a medium-sized bowl, microwave for 30 seconds at a time until the butter has just melted.   Stir together the peanut butter and butter until combined and smooth.   Stir the vanilla extract into the peanut butter mixture.   In a small bowl, mix together the ground almonds, eggs, baking powder, and cinnamon.   Pour the melted chocolate and coconut oil evenly into the 14 paper cases.   Spoon half of the almond/egg mixture evenly into the cases, on top of the chocolate and press down slightly. Spoon the peanut butter mixture into the cases, on top of the almond/egg mixture.   Spoon the remaining almond/egg mixture into the cases. Sprinkle the chopped pecans on top of each cupcake. Very carefully place the filled cases into the Crock Pot, if they don't all fit, use a rack (so there are 2 levels of cakes).   Place the lid onto the pot and set the temperature to HIGH.   Cook for 4 hours. Remove the cakes from the pot and leave to cool. Serve warm, with a dollop of whipped cream!

489.   Salmon Cake

Servings: 4 – 6   Cooking Time: Approximately 4 Hours
Ingredients:

- 3 tbsp heavy cream
- 2 ounces smoked salmon strips, or 1 large fillet of hot smoked salmon, roughly chopped or flaked
- 4 eggs, lightly beaten
- 1 cup baby spinach, roughly chopped
- Handful of fresh coriander, roughly chopped

Directions:
Drizzle some olive oil into the Crock Pot.   Place the beaten egg, cream, spinach, salmon, salt, and pepper into the pot and gently stir to combine. Place the lid onto the pot and set the temperature to LOW.   Cook for 4 hours.   Serve with a generous sprinkling of fresh coriander!

490.   Tangy Pepper Oysters

Servings: 6   Cooking Time: 1 Hour
Ingredients:

- 1 Serrano chili pepper, diced
- 12 oysters, shucked
- Juice from 1 lime
- ½ teaspoon of fresh ginger, shredded
- ¼ teaspoon of garlic, minced
- Juice of 2 lemons
- Zest from 2 limes
- ¼ cup of scallions, diced
- 1 cup of tomato juice
- Salt, to taste
- ¼ cup of fresh cilantro, diced

Directions:
Start by throwing all the Ingredients: into your Crockpot.   Cover its lid and cook for 1 hour on High setting.   Once done, remove its lid and give it a stir.   Serve warm.
Nutrition Info: Calories 449 Total Fat 28.7 g Saturated Fat 14.9 g Cholesterol 163 mg Sodium 744 mg Total Carbs 8.4 g Sugar 2.6 g Fiber 1.9 g Protein 39.3 g

491.   Shrimp Bake

Servings: 2   Cooking Time: 2 Hours
Ingredients:

- 1-pound shrimp, peeled and deveined
- 2 tablespoons lime juice
- 1 teaspoon apple cider vinegar
- 1 teaspoon salt
- 1 tablespoon butter
- ¾ cup heavy cream
- 2 oz Provolone cheese, shredded

Directions:
In the slow cooker, mix the shrimp with the lime juice and the other ingredients except the cheese. Toss, sprinkle the cheese on top and cook on High for 2 hours.
Nutrition Info:calories 290, fat 5.2, fiber 0.2, carbs 2.5, protein 18.8

492.   Spiced Shrimp

Servings: 2   Cooking Time: 1 Hour
Ingredients:

- 8 oz shrimp, peeled and deveined
- 1 teaspoon chili
- ½ teaspoon minced garlic

powder
1 teaspoon nutmeg,
ground
1 teaspoon coriander,
ground

1 tablespoon olive oil
2 tablespoon coconut
cream
½ teaspoon salt
2 tablespoons water

Directions:
In the slow cooker, mix the shrimp with chili powder, nutmeg and the other ingredients.   Close the lid. Cook for 1 hour on High.
Nutrition Info:calories 200, fat 11.7, fiber 4.9, carbs 4.7, protein 9.6

493.   Fish Curry Delight

Servings: 6   Cooking Time: 4 Hours
Ingredients:

2 tablespoons of olive oil
4 curry leaves
4 medium onions, diced
2 tablespoons of fresh ginger, grated finely
4 garlic cloves, minced
4 tablespoons of curry powder
4 teaspoons of cumin, ground

4 teaspoons of ground coriander
2 teaspoons of red chili powder
1 teaspoon of ground turmeric
4 cups of unsweetened coconut milk
2 ½ cups of tomatoes, diced
2 Serrano peppers, seeded and diced
2 tablespoons of fresh lemon juice

Directions:
Start by throwing all the Ingredients: into your Crockpot.   Cover its lid and cook for 4 hours on Low setting.   Once done, remove its lid and give it a stir.   Garnish with cilantro.   Serve warm.
Nutrition Info: Calories 231 Total Fat 17.6 g Saturated Fat 7.6 g Cholesterol 383 mg Sodium 244 mg Total Carbs 3.1 g Sugar 1.3 g Fiber 0.8 g Protein 15.7 g

494.   Shrimp And Salmon Skewers

Servings: 4   Cooking Time: 1.5 Hour
Ingredients:

9 ounces salmon fillets, boneless and cubed
1 teaspoon garlic powder
1 teaspoon ginger powder
1 tablespoon lime juice

9 oz shrimps, peeled
1/3 teaspoon oregano, dried
1 tablespoon sesame oil
1 teaspoon heavy cream
¾ cup of water

Directions:
String the shrimps and salmon into the skewers one-by-one.   After this, pour water in the slow cooker. Arrange the shrimp and salmon skewers in the slow cooker, and add the rest of the ingredients as well. Close the lid and cook shrimps for 1.5 hours on High. Then transfer the cooked shrimp skewers on the plates and sprinkle with slow cooker gravy.
Nutrition Info:calories 185, fat 5, fiber 3.3, carbs 5.4, protein 14.7

495.   Coconut Catfish

Servings: 6   Cooking Time: 6.5 Hours
Ingredients:

13 oz catfish, chopped
½ cup of coconut milk
1 tablespoon Cajun seasoning
1 teaspoon curry powder
1 teaspoon salt

½ teaspoon chili flakes
1 bay leaf
1 garlic clove, peeled
1/3 teaspoon coriander, ground

Directions:
In the slow cooker, mix the catfish with coconut milk, seasoning and the other ingredients.   Close the lid and cook the stew for 6.5 hours on Low.   Transfer in the serving bowls and enjoy.
Nutrition Info:calories 299, fat 13.4, fiber 4.5, carbs 7.9, protein 12

496.   Balsamic Salmon

Servings: 3   Cooking Time: 1 Hour
Ingredients:

1-pound salmon fillet, sliced
½ teaspoon garlic powder
¼ teaspoon cayenne pepper

½ teaspoon salt
3 tablespoons balsamic vinegar
1/3 cup water
½ teaspoon olive oil

Directions:
In the slow cooker, mix the salmon with garlic powder, salt and the other ingredients and toss gently.   Close the lid and cook salmon for 1 hour on High.   Serve the salmon with the balsamic sauce.
Nutrition Info:calories 226, fat 10.1, fiber 4.1, carbs 8.6, protein 20.5

497.   Ambrosia

Servings: 8 – 10   Cooking Time: Approximately 4 Hours
Ingredients:

1 cup unsweetened shredded coconut
¾ cup slivered almonds
3 ounces dark chocolate (high cocoa percentage), roughly chopped
1/3 cup pumpkin seeds

2 ounces salted butter
1 tsp cinnamon
2 cups heavy cream
2 cups full-fat Greek yogurt
1 cup fresh berries – strawberries and raspberries are best

Directions:
Place the shredded coconut, slivered almonds, dark chocolate, pumpkin seeds, butter, and cinnamon into the Crock Pot.   Place the lid onto the pot and set the temperature to HIGH.   Cook for 3 hours, stirring every 45 minutes to combine the chocolate and butter as it melts.   Remove the mixture from the Crock Pot, place in a bowl, and leave to cool. In a large bowl, whip the cream until softly whipped. Stir the yoghurt through the cream.   Chop the strawberries into small pieces and add to the cream mixture, along with the other berries you are using, fold through.   Sprinkle the cooled coconut

mixture over the cream mixture.   Serve in bowls with an extra grating of dark chocolate on top!

498.   Shrimp Creole

Servings: 4   Cooking Time: 1 Hour
Ingredients:

- 1 tablespoon of olive oil
- 1 (28 oz.) can crush whole tomatoes
- 1 cup of celery stalk, sliced
- ¾ cup of diced white onion
- 1 (8oz.) can sugar-free tomato sauce
- 1/2 cup of green bell pepper, diced
- 1/2 teaspoon of minced garlic
- ¼ teaspoon of black pepper
- 1 tablespoon of Worcestershire sauce
- 4 drops hot pepper sauce
- Salt, to taste

Directions:
Start by throwing all the Ingredients: into your Crockpot.   Cover its lid and cook for 1 hour on High setting.   Once done, remove its lid and give it a stir.   Serve warm.
Nutrition Info: Calories 139 Total Fat 10.1 g Saturated Fat 5 g Cholesterol 216 mg Sodium 238 mg Total Carbs 2.3 g Sugar 1.5 g Fiber 0.2 g Protein 10.1 g

499.   Balsamic Scallops

Servings: 4   Cooking Time: 2 Hours
Ingredients:

- 8 scallops
- 1 tablespoon balsamic vinegar
- 1 teaspoon hot paprika
- ½ teaspoon salt
- 2 tablespoons olive oil
- ½ teaspoon dried rosemary

Directions:
In the slow cooker, mix the scallops with the vinegar and the other ingredients, toss and close the lid. Cook bacon scallops for 2 hours on High.
Nutrition Info:calories 215, fat 6.2, fiber 0.1, carbs 1.8, protein 7.1

500.   Oregano Crab

Servings: 4   Cooking Time: 40 Minutes
Ingredients:

- 1 tablespoon dried oregano
- 2 cups crab meat
- ½ cup spring onions, chopped
- ¾ teaspoon minced garlic
- 1 tablespoon lemon juice
- ½ cup of coconut milk

Directions:
In the slow cooker, mix the crab with oregano and the other ingredients and close the lid   Cook for 40 minutes on High, divide into bowls and serve.
Nutrition Info:calories 151, fat 3.4, fiber 1, carbs 6.8, protein 5.2

501.   Creamy Lobster

Servings: 8   Cooking Time: 1 Hour
Ingredients:

- 4 lbs. fresh lobster tails
- 2 teaspoons of old bay seasoning
- 1 cup of mayonnaise
- 2 scallions, diced
- ¼ cup of unsalted butter, melted
- 4 tablespoons of fresh lemon juice

Directions:
Start by throwing all the Ingredients: into your Crockpot except mayonnaise.   Cover its lid and cook for 1 hour on Low setting.   Once done, remove its lid and give it a stir.   Peel the slow-cooked lobster tail and transfer the meat to a bowl. Mix the meat with mayonnaise in that bowl. Garnish as desired.   Serve warm.
Nutrition Info: Calories 349 Total Fat 31.9 g Saturated Fat 15 g Cholesterol 46 mg Sodium 237 mg Total Carbs 6.6 g Sugar 1.4 g Fiber 3.4 g Protein 11 g

502.   Prawn And Sausage Slow CookerCasserole

Servings: 6   Cooking Time: Approximately 6 Hours
Ingredients:

- 1 ½ cups frozen prawns, (thawed)
- 3 sausages, chopped into chunks
- 5 garlic cloves, crushed
- 1 small onion, finely chopped
- 4 tomatoes, chopped
- 1 tsp mixed dried herbs
- 2 tsp mixed dried spices – coriander, cumin, chili (choose your favorites)

Directions:
Drizzle some olive oil into the Crock Pot.   Place the prawns, sausages, garlic, onion, tinned tomatoes, herbs, spices, salt, and pepper into the pot and stir to combine.   Place the lid onto the pot and set the temperature to LOW.   Cook for 6 hours.   Serve while hot, with a sprinkling of fresh herbs such as coriander and parsley!

503.   Herbed Swordfish Delight

Servings: 4   Cooking Time: 2 Hours
Ingredients:

- 4 swordfish steaks
- 1 tablespoon of fresh parsley, diced
- 3 tablespoon of olive oil
- 1 lemon, cut into wedges
- 3 garlic cloves, peeled and minced
- ½ teaspoon of dried marjoram
- ½ teaspoon of rosemary, dried
- ⅓ cup of chicken stock
- Salt and black pepper ground, to taste
- ¼ cup of lemon juice

Directions:
Start by throwing all the Ingredients: into your Crockpot.   Cover its lid and cook for 2 hours on High setting.   Once done, remove its lid and give it a stir.   Serve warm.
Nutrition Info: Calories 311 Total Fat 8.3 g Saturated Fat 4.9 g Cholesterol 69 mg Sodium 896 mg Total Carbs 1.9 g Sugar 0.8 g Fiber 0.6 g Protein 17.4 g

504. Sea Bass And Celery

Servings: 2   Cooking Time: 3.5 Hours

Ingredients:

- 2 sea bass fillets, boneless
- 1 cup celery stalks, peeled and cubed
- ½ teaspoon black pepper
- 1 teaspoon salt
- 1 tablespoon paprika
- ¼ teaspoon chili powder
- 1/3 cup sour cream

Directions:

In the slow cooker, mix the sea bass with the celery and the other ingredients and close the lid.   Cook the cod on High for 3.5 hours.

Nutrition Info: calories 263, fat 9.5, fiber 4.4, carbs 7.7, protein 21.8

505. Shrimp And Fennel Soup

Servings: 6   Cooking Time: 2 Hours

Ingredients:

- ½ cup fennel, shredded
- 12 oz shrimps, peeled
- ½ teaspoon sweet paprika
- 1 teaspoon turmeric powder
- ½ teaspoon salt
- ½ teaspoon cayenne pepper
- 1 teaspoon coriander seeds
- 2 cups of water
- 2 cups of coconut milk
- 1 teaspoon chili powder
- 1 cup spinach, chopped

Directions:

In the slow cooker, mix the shrimp with fennel and the other ingredients and toss.   Divide into bowls and serve.

Nutrition Info: calories 275, fat 20.3, fiber 3.4, carbs 5.3, protein 16

506. Slow Cooked Coconut Lime Mussels

Servings: 4   Cooking Time: Approximately 2 ½ Hours

Ingredients:

- 16 fresh mussels
- 1 ½ cup full-fat coconut milk
- ½ red chili, finely chopped
- 4 garlic cloves
- 1 lime
- ½ cup fish stock
- Handful of fresh coriander, chopped

Directions:

Drizzle some olive oil into the Crock Pot.   Add the garlic, coconut milk, chili, fish stock, salt, pepper, and juice of one lime to the pot, stir to combine. Place the lid onto the pot and set the temperature to HIGH.   Cook for 2 hours.   Remove the lid, place the mussels into the liquid and place the lid back onto the pot.   Cook for about 20 minutes, or until the mussels open.   Serve while hot, with a generous serving of coconut and lime sauce over the top, and a big handful of fresh coriander!

507. Seafood Jambalaya

Servings: 4-6   Cooking Time: 1 Hour

Ingredients:

- 4 oz. shrimp, peeled and deveined
- 2 bacon strips, diced
- 1 cup of uncooked

1 tablespoon of olive oil
1 1/5 cups of vegetable broth
¾ cup of sliced celery stalk
1/4 teaspoon of minced garlic
1/2 cup of diced onion
1 cup of canned diced tomatoes
cauliflower rice
1/2 tablespoon of Cajun seasoning
1/4 teaspoon of thyme, dried
1/4 teaspoon of cayenne pepper
1/2 teaspoon of oregano, dried
Salt and black pepper, to taste

Directions:

Start by throwing all the Ingredients: into your Crockpot.   Cover its lid and cook for 1 hour on High setting.   Once done, remove its lid and give it a stir.   Serve warm.

Nutrition Info: Calories 231 Total Fat 17.6 g Saturated Fat 7.6 g Cholesterol 383 mg Sodium 244 mg Total Carbs 3.1 g Sugar 1.3 g Fiber 0.8 g Protein 15.7 g

508. Cod Patties

Servings: 3   Cooking Time: 1 Hour

Ingredients:

- 8 oz cod fillets, boneless, finely chopped
- 1 teaspoon cilantro, dried
- 1 teaspoon Italian seasoning
- ¼ cup fresh basil, blended
- 1 egg, beaten
- ½ teaspoon salt
- ¼ teaspoon chili powder
- 1/3 cup coconut milk
- 1 tablespoon butter
- 1 tablespoon almond flour

Directions:

In the mixing bowl, mix up together the cod with cilantro, seasoning, flour, basil, salt and chili powder, stir and shape medium patties out of this mix. Toss the butter in the skillet and bring it to boil. Add the patties and cook for 1 minute over medium high heat.   Transfer the patties in the slow cooker and add coconut milk.   Close the lid and cook patties for 1 hour on High.

Nutrition Info: calories 301, fat 21, fiber 4.7, carbs 5.8, protein 19.3

509. Lobster Dinner

Servings: 4   Cooking Time: 1 Hour

Ingredients:

- 2 tablespoons of unsalted butter, melted
- Pinch of salt
- 2 oz. white wine
- 4 oz. water

Directions:

Start by throwing all the Ingredients: into your Crockpot.   Cover its lid and cook for 1 hour on Low setting.   Once done, remove its lid and give it a stir. Serve warm.

Nutrition Info: Calories 324 Total Fat 20.7 g Saturated Fat 6.7 g Cholesterol 45 mg Sodium 241 mg Total Carbs 8.6 g Sugar 1.4 g Fiber 0.5 g Protein 15.3 g

510. Parsley Salmon

Servings: 4   Cooking Time: 2 Hours

Ingredients:

10 oz salmon fillet
2 tablespoons parsley, chopped
½ cup coconut cream
½ teaspoon chili flakes
½ teaspoon salt
1 teaspoon turmeric powder
2 oz Parmesan, grated
3 tablespoons coconut oil

Directions:
In the slow cooker, mix the salmon with the parsley and the other ingredients.   Close the lid and cook the meal for 2 hours on High.
Nutrition Info:calories 283, fat 22.2, fiber 0.8, carbs 2.3, protein 21.2

511. Curried Shrimp

Servings: 4   Cooking Time: 2.5 Hours
Ingredients:

1 medium onion, diced
½ teaspoon of cumin, ground
1½ teaspoons of red chili powder
1 teaspoon of ground turmeric
2 medium tomatoes, diced
Pinch of salt
¼ cup of water
1¾ lbs. medium shrimp, peeled and deveined
1 tablespoon of fresh lemon juice
¼ cup of fresh cilantro, diced

Directions:
Start by throwing all the Ingredients: into your Crockpot except shrimp.   Cover its lid and cook for 2 hours on Low setting.   Once done, remove its lid and give it a stir.   Add shrimp and continue cooking for 30 minutes on low heat.   Serve warm.
Nutrition Info: Calories 287 Total Fat 29.5 g Saturated Fat 3 g Cholesterol 743 mg Sodium 388 mg Total Carbs 5.9 g Sugar 1.4g Fiber 4.3 g Protein 4.2 g

512.   Salmon With Juicy Shallots

Servings: 2   Cooking Time: 2 Hours
Ingredients:

1 shallot, peeled and diced
2 medium salmon fillets
¼ cup of and 1 tablespoon of olive oil
Salt and black pepper ground, to taste
1 lemon, cut into thin wedges
2 tablespoons of fresh parsley, diced

Directions:
Start by throwing all the Ingredients: into your Crockpot.   Cover its lid and cook for 2 hours on High setting.   Once done, remove its lid and give it a stir.   Serve warm.
Nutrition Info: Calories 207 Total Fat 15 g Saturated Fat 5.2 g Cholesterol 64 mg Sodium 252 mg Total Carbs 5.4 g Sugar 0.2 g Fiber 1.8 g Protein 11.1 g

513.   Oregano Salmon

Servings: 2   Cooking Time: 1.5 Hours
Ingredients:

2 salmon steaks (2 fillets 6 oz each)
2 tablespoons olive oil
1 tablespoon oregano, dried
1 teaspoon smoked paprika
6 tablespoons water
½ teaspoon salt
½ teaspoon balsamic vinegar

Directions:
In the slow cooker, mix the salmon with the oregano and the other ingredients.   Close the lid and cook salmon for 1.5 hours on High.
Nutrition Info:calories 222, fat 12.1, fiber 0.7, carbs 1.5, protein 14.7

514.   Lemon-butter Fish

Servings: 6   Cooking Time: Approximately 5 Hours
Ingredients:

6 fillets of fresh white fish
2 ounces butter, soft but not melted
1 lemon
2 garlic cloves, crushed
Handful of fresh parsley, finely chopped

Directions:
In a small bowl, combine the butter, garlic, zest of one lemon, chopped parsley, salt and pepper. Drizzle some olive oil into the Crock Pot.   Place the fish fillets into the Slow Cookerand sprinkle with salt and pepper.   Place a dollop of lemon butter onto each fish fillet and gently spread it out.   Place the lid onto the Slow Cookerand set the temperature to LOW.   Cook for 5 hours.   Serve each fish fillet with a generous spoonful of melted lemon butter from the bottom of the Crock Pot, and a small squeeze of lemon juice over the top!

515. Caraway Cod

Servings: 2   Cooking Time: 5 Hours
Ingredients:

8 oz cod fillet
1 teaspoon caraway seeds
½ teaspoon cayenne pepper
1 teaspoon coriander, ground
½ teaspoon salt
1 tablespoon lime juice
1 tablespoon coconut cream
3 tablespoons avocado oil

Directions:
In the slow cooker, mix the cod with caraway seeds, salt, pepper and the other ingredients.   Close the lid and cook cod for 5 hours on Low.
Nutrition Info:calories 290, fat 23.4, fiber 4.7, carbs 11.7, protein 20.7

516.   Coconut, Chocolate, And Almond Truffle Bake

Servings: 6 – 8   Cooking Time: Approximately 4 Hours
Ingredients:

3 ounces butter, melted
3 ounces dark chocolate, melted
1 cup desiccated coconut
3 tbsp unsweetened cocoa powder
1 cup ground almonds
2 tsp vanilla extract
1 cup heavy cream
A few extra squares of dark chocolate, grated

¼ cup toasted almonds, chopped

Directions:
In a large bowl, mix together the melted butter, chocolate, ground almonds, coconut, cocoa powder, and vanilla extract. Roll the mixture into balls. Grease a heat-proof dish (make sure it fits in the Crock Pot). Place the balls into the dish. Place the lid onto the pot and set the temperature to LOW. Cook for 4 hours. Leave the truffle dish to cool until warm. Whip the cream until it is soft and pillowy. Spread the cream over the truffle dish and sprinkle the grated chocolate and chopped toasted almonds over the top. Serve immediately!

517. Saffron Tilapia

Servings: 4   Cooking Time: 2 Hours
Ingredients:
15 oz tilapia fillet
1 cup coconut cream
1 teaspoon coconut oil
¼ teaspoon cumin
¼ teaspoon turmeric
¼ teaspoon ginger
¼ teaspoon paprika
¼ teaspoon saffron
¾ teaspoon ground black pepper
1 teaspoon salt

Directions:
In the slow cooker, mix the tilapia with cream and the other ingredients and toss gently. Close the lid and cook fish for 2 hours on High.
Nutrition Info:calories 274, fat 13.3, fiber 4.3, carbs 7.5, protein 20.5

518. Salmon Curry

Servings: 6   Cooking Time: 4 Hours
Ingredients:
2 tablespoons of olive oil
2 Serrano peppers, diced
1 teaspoon of ground turmeric
4 tablespoons of curry powder
4 teaspoons of cumin, ground
4 teaspoons of ground coriander
2 small yellow onion, diced
4 curry leaves
2 teaspoons of red chili powder
4 garlic cloves, minced
4 cups of unsweetened coconut milk
2 ½ cups of tomatoes, diced
2 tablespoons of fresh lemon juice
Fresh cilantro leaves (Garnish)

Directions:
Start by throwing all the Ingredients: into your Crockpot. Cover its lid and cook for 4 hours on Low setting. Once done, remove its lid and give it a stir. Garnish with cilantro. Serve warm.
Nutrition Info: Calories 335 Total Fat 5.4 g Saturated Fat 3.3 g Cholesterol 16 mg Sodium 708 mg Total Carbs 2.1 g Sugar 0.7 g Fiber 0.4 g Protein 18.5 g

519. Mouth-watering Casserole

Servings: 4   Cooking Time: 4 Hours
Ingredients:

2 teaspoons of olive oil
12 oz. water-packed tuna
15 oz. cream of mushroom soup
8 oz. egg noodles, cooked and drained
8 oz. thawed frozen mixed vegetables
2 tablespoons of parsley, dried
Salt and black pepper, to taste
1/4 cup of toasted almonds, sliced

Directions:
Start by throwing all the Ingredients: into your Crockpot. Cover its lid and cook for 4 hours on High setting. Once done, remove its lid and give it a stir. Serve warm.
Nutrition Info: Calories 489 Total Fat 43.3 g Saturated Fat 15.2 g Cholesterol 128 mg Sodium 662 mg Total Carbs 5 g Sugar 0.1 g Fiber 2 g Protein 22.2 g

520. Tilapia And Tomatoes

Servings: 2   Cooking Time: 2 Hours
Ingredients:
8 oz tilapia fillet (2 servings)
1 and ½ cups cherry tomatoes, halved
1 tablespoon keto tomato sauce
½ teaspoon lemongrass
1 tablespoon butter, melted
3 tablespoons coconut cream
½ teaspoon salt
¼ teaspoon chili flakes

Directions:
In the slow cooker, mix the tilapia with tomatoes and the other ingredients. Close the slow cooker lid and cook tilapia for 2 hours on High.
Nutrition Info:calories 308, fat 12.2, fiber 0.5, carbs 1.9, protein 32.3

521. Tomato Shrimps

Servings: 2   Cooking Time: 1 Hour
Ingredients:
8 oz king shrimps, peeled
1/4 cup keto tomato sauce
1 tablespoon sweet paprika
1 green chili pepper, chopped
2 tablespoons butter
¼ cup of water
½ teaspoon chili powder

Directions:
Pour water in the slow cooker. Add the shrimp and the other ingredients, stir and close the lid. Cook for 1 hour on High and serve.
Nutrition Info:calories 174, fat 12.7, fiber 0.8, carbs 2.6, protein 12.7

522. Lemon Crab Legs

Servings: 4   Cooking Time: 3 Hours
Ingredients:
12 oz King crab legs
1/3 cup butter
Zest of 1 lemon, grated
1 tablespoon yellow curry paste
Juice of 1 lemon
¼ cup of water
1 teaspoon minced garlic
½ teaspoon salt

Directions:

In the slow cooker, mix the crab with the butter and the other ingredients. Close the lid and cook the crab legs for 3 hours on Low.
Nutrition Info:calories 165, fat 7.8, fiber 0, carbs 4.2, protein 5.6

523. Stevia Salmon

Servings: 3   Cooking Time: 4.5 Hours
Ingredients:
- 8 oz salmon fillet
- 1 tablespoon stevia
- 1 teaspoon saffron powder
- 1 teaspoon garam masala
- 2 tablespoons butter, melted
- ½ teaspoon ground black pepper
- ¼ teaspoon salt

Directions:
In the slow cooker mix the salmon with the stevia, saffron and the other ingredients, and close the lid. Cook the salmon steaks for 4.5 hours on Low.
Nutrition Info:calories 232, fat 14.7, fiber 3.1, carbs 5.4, protein 15.3

524. Mozzarella Shrimp Parcels

Servings: Makes 12 Parcels   Cooking Time: Approximately 3 Hours
Ingredients:
- 2 cups frozen shrimp (thawed)
- 12 slices streaky bacon, cut in half
- 2 cups grated mozzarella cheese
- Large bunch of Kale, washed and hard stalks removed
- 12 small skewers, (or 6 long ones, cut in half)

Directions:
Cut the kale into 12 large pieces – I usually just cut 6 large kale leaves in half, (they need to be large enough to be used as wraps). On a large board, lay out the kale halves. Lay 2 bacon half slices on the kale. Place a small handful of shrimp on top of the bacon. Place a small handful of grated mozzarella on top of the shrimp. Sprinkle with salt and pepper. Wrap the parcels up tightly by folding the sides up, then folding the top and bottom up, and use a skewer to secure them. Drizzle some olive oil into the Crock Pot. Place the parcels into the pot. Place the lid onto the pot and set the temperature to HIGH. Cook for 3 hours. Heat some olive oil into a frying pan. Take the parcels out of the Slow Cookeronce cooked and transfer them to the hot oil to cook on both sides to create a crisp and golden outer. Serve with your choice of sauces and dips!

525. Chocolate Covered Bacon Cupcakes

Servings: Makes 10 Cupcakes   Cooking Time: Approximately 3 Hours
Ingredients:
- 10 paper cupcake cases
- 5 slices streaky bacon, cut into small pieces, fried in a pan until crispy
- 1 cup ground hazelnuts
- 1 tsp baking powder
- 2 eggs, lightly beaten
- ½ cup full-fat Greek yogurt
- 1 tsp vanilla extract
- 5 ounces dark chocolate, melted

Directions:
In a small bowl, mix together the fried bacon pieces and melted chocolate, set aside. In a medium-sized bowl, mix together the ground hazelnuts, baking powder, eggs, yoghurt, vanilla, and a pinch of salt. Spoon the hazelnut mixture into the cupcake cases. Spoon the chocolate and bacon mixture on top of the hazelnut mixture. Place the cupcake cases into the Slow Cooker(careful not to spill!). Place the lid onto the Slow Cookerand set the temperature to HIGH. Cook for 3 hours. Remove the cupcakes from the pot and leave to cool on the bench before storing serving. Serve with whipped cream!

526. Salmon And Cauliflower Chowder

Servings: 2   Cooking Time: 2.5 Hours
Ingredients:
- 1-pound salmon fillet, boneless and cubed
- ¼ cup cauliflower florets
- 1 teaspoon turmeric powder
- 1 teaspoon basil, dried
- 1 cayenne pepper, chopped
- 1 teaspoon salt
- ½ teaspoon ground black pepper
- 2 tablespoon lemon juice
- 3 tablespoons coconut cream
- 1 ½ cup of water
- 2 tablespoons fresh parsley, chopped

Directions:
In the slow cooker, mix the salmon with cauliflower and the other ingredients and toss. Close the lid and cook the ingredients for 5 hours on High. Divide into bowls and serve.
Nutrition Info:calories 185, fat 6.9, fiber 2.1, carbs 7.5, protein 11.6

527. Marinara Shrimp

Servings: 2   Cooking Time: 1 Hour
Ingredients:
- 10 oz shrimp, peeled and deveined
- 3 tablespoons keto marinara sauce
- 2 tablespoons coconut flour
- 1 tablespoon coconut cream

Directions:
In the slow cooker, mix the shrimp with the other ingredients and close the lid. Cook the fish for 1 hour on High.
Nutrition Info:calories 212, fat 4.7, fiber 5.3, carbs 7.7, protein 26.9

528. Slow Cooked Sesame Prawns

Servings: 4   Cooking Time: Approximately 2 Hours
Ingredients:
- 3 cups large prawns, (if using frozen, thaw first)
- 4 garlic cloves, crushed
- 1 tbsp sesame oil
- 2 tbsp toasted sesame seeds
- ½ red chili, finely chopped
- ½ cup fish stock

Directions:
Drizzle the sesame oil into the Crock Pot.   Add the prawns, garlic, sesame seeds, chili, and fish stock to the pot, stir well to coat the prawns.   Place the lid onto the pot and set the temperature to HIGH. Cook for 2 hours.   Serve while hot, with fresh herbs and cauliflower rice!

529.   Parmesan Salmon

Servings: 3   Cooking Time: 2.5 Hours
Ingredients:

7 oz salmon fillets, boneless	3 oz Parmesan, grated
1 teaspoon cayenne pepper	2 tablespoons lime juice
1 teaspoon chili pepper	1 teaspoon minced garlic
½ cup coconut cream	¼ cup fresh chives, chopped

Directions:
In the slow cooker, mix the salmon with the coconut cream and the other ingredients and close the lid. Cook on High for 2 hours and 30 minutes and serve.
Nutrition Info:calories 279, fat 16.5, fiber 1.2, carbs 7.5, protein 18.8

530.   Fish Curry

Servings: 2   Cooking Time: 2 Hours
Ingredients:

1 curry leaves	1 teaspoon of ground coriander
½ tablespoon of olive oil	½ teaspoon of ground turmeric
½ teaspoon of red chili powder	1 cup of unsweetened coconut milk
½ small yellow onion, diced	1 cups of tomato, diced
1 garlic clove, minced	
1 tablespoon of curry powder	½ Serrano pepper, seeded and diced
1 teaspoon of cumin, ground	½ tablespoon of fresh lemon juice

Directions:
Start by throwing all the Ingredients: into your Crockpot.   Cover its lid and cook for 2 hours on High setting.   Once done, remove its lid and give it a stir.   Serve warm.
Nutrition Info: Calories 216 Total Fat 21.7 g Saturated Fat 6.1 g Cholesterol 16 mg Sodium 111 mg Total Carbs 7.1 g Sugar 2.4 g Fiber 0.6 g Protein 28.9 g

531.   Mozzarella Fish

Servings: 4   Cooking Time: 2 Hours
Ingredients:

1-pound salmon fillet	1 teaspoon butter
½ cup heavy cream	½ teaspoon ground black pepper
½ cup Mozzarella, shredded	
1 teaspoon oregano, dried	½ teaspoon smoked paprika
½ teaspoon turmeric powder	½ teaspoon ground nutmeg

Directions:
Put salmon fillet in the slow cooker.   Add the rest of the ingredients except the cheese.   Top the mix with the Mozzarella, and close the lid.   Cook fish gratin for 2 hours on High.
Nutrition Info:calories 241, fat 14.9, fiber 1.7, carbs 3.3, protein 24.2

532.   Salmon And Asparagus

Servings: 4   Cooking Time: 3.5 Hours
Ingredients:

1-pound salmon fillet, boneless	1 cup coconut cream
¼ pound asparagus, trimmed and halved	½ teaspoon salt
1 teaspoon dried basil	1 teaspoon dried parsley
	Cooking spray

Directions:
In the slow cooker, mix the salmon with the asparagus, cream and the other ingredients and close the lid.   Cook the fish loaf for 3.5 hours on Low.
Nutrition Info:calories 204, fat 9.2, fiber 2.8, carbs 6.7, protein 23

533.   Elegant Dinner Mussels

Servings: 4   Cooking Time: 2 Hours
Ingredients:

2 tablespoons of butter	½ teaspoon of rosemary, dried, crushed
1 medium yellow onion, diced	2 tablespoons of fresh lemon juice
1 garlic clove, minced	
1 cup of homemade chicken broth	½ cup of sour cream
	Salt and black pepper, to taste

Directions:
Start by throwing all the Ingredients: into your Crockpot except cream.   Cover its lid and cook for 2 hours on High setting.   Once done, remove its lid and give it a stir.   Stir in cream and mix it all gently   Serve warm.
Nutrition Info: Calories 245 Total Fat 16g Saturated Fat 10 g Cholesterol 16 mg Sodium 111 mg Total Carbs 2 g Sugar 1 g Fiber 1 g Protein 32 g

534.   Macadamia Fudge Truffles

Servings: Makes About 25 Small Truffles
Cooking Time: Approximately 4 Hours
Ingredients:

1 cup roasted macadamia nuts, finely chopped	½ cup ground almonds
2 ounces butter, melted	5 ounces dark chocolate, melted
	1 tsp vanilla extract
	1 egg, lightly beaten

Directions:
Place the macadamia nuts, almonds, melted butter, melted chocolate, vanilla, and egg into a large bowl, stir until combined.   Grease the bottom of the Slow Cookerby rubbing with butter.   Place the mixture into the Slow Cookerand press down. Place the lid onto the pot and set the temperature to

LOW.   Cook for 4 hours.   Remove the lid, turn the cooker off, and allow the mixture to cool until just warm.   Take a teaspoon and scoop the mixture out of the pot, and roll into balls until all mixture has been used.   Place the balls on a plate or in a container and refrigerate to harden slightly. If you like, you can roll the balls in unsweetened cocoa powder to finish!   Store the truffle balls in the fridge.

535.   Salmon And Radish Soup

Servings: 4   Cooking Time: 2.5 Hours
Ingredients:
- 1 cup radishes, halved
- 10 oz salmon, chopped
- 1 teaspoon lime juice
- 1 teaspoon lime zest, grated
- ½ cup of coconut milk
- 2 cups of water
- 1 teaspoon salt
- 1 teaspoon garlic, diced
- ½ teaspoon chives, chopped

Directions:
In the slow cooker, mix the salmon with radishes and the other ingredients.   Close the lid and cook the liquid for 5 hours on High.   Divide into bowls and serve.
Nutrition Info:calories 209, fat 11.6, fiber 1.7, carbs 5.4, protein 8.5

536.   Butter Salmon And Avocado

Servings: 1   Cooking Time: 1.5 Hours
Ingredients:
- 6 oz salmon fillet
- 2 avocados, peeled, pitted and cubed
- 1 teaspoon garam masala
- 1 teaspoon coriander, ground
- 1/3 cup butter
- 1 teaspoon lemon juice
- 1 teaspoon apple cider vinegar
- ¼ teaspoon salt

Directions:
In the slow cooker, mix the salmon with the butter and the other ingredients and close the lid.   Cook salmon for 1.5 hours on High.
Nutrition Info:calories 370, fat 11.9, fiber 0, carbs 0.2, protein 12.7

537.   Lemon Cheesecake

Servings: 8 – 10   Cooking Time: Approximately 6 Hours
Ingredients:
- 2 ounces butter, melted
- 1 cup pecans, finely ground in the food processor
- 1 tsp cinnamon
- 2 cups cream cheese
- 1 cup sour cream
- 2 eggs, lightly beaten
- 1 lemon
- Few drops of stevia
- 1 cup heavy cream

Directions:
Mix together the melted butter, ground pecans, and cinnamon until it forms a wet, sand-like texture. Press the butter/pecan mixture into a greased, heat-proof dish (make sure it fits in the Crock Pot) and set aside.   Place the cream cheese, eggs, sour cream, stevia, zest and juice of one lemon into a large bowl, beat with electric egg beaters until combined and smooth.   Pour the cream cheese mixture into the dish, on top of the base, smooth it out so that the top of the cheesecake is even.   Place the dish into the Slow Cookerand pour enough hot water into the pot so that it reaches half way up the side of the dish. Place the lid onto the pot and set the temperature to LOW.   Cook for 6 hours.   Set the cheesecake on the bench to cool and set.   Whip the cream until soft and pillowy, and spread over the cheesecake before serving.

538.   Slow Cooked Whole Fish With Ginger And Soy

Servings: Makes One Whole Fish, About 4 Servings
Cooking Time: Approximately 2 Hours
Ingredients:
- 1 fresh, whole fish
- 4 garlic cloves, crushed
- 2 tbsp grated fresh ginger
- 4 tbsp soy sauce

Directions:
Score the fish with a sharp knife by cutting diagonal lines through the skin.   Rub the fish with olive oil. Sprinkle the fish with sea salt and pepper. Sprinkle the grated ginger onto the fish and rub it into the scores.   Drizzle some olive oil into the Crock Pot.   Place the fish into the pot.   Pour the soy sauce over top of the fish.   Place the lid onto the pot and set the temperature to HIGH.   Cook for 2 hours.   Serve immediately! Garnish with fresh green herbs to give a pop of color.

539.   Creamy Sea Bass

Servings: 4   Cooking Time: 2 Hours
Ingredients:
- 1-pound sea bass fillets, boneless
- 1 teaspoon garlic powder
- ½ teaspoon salt
- ½ teaspoon Italian seasoning
- ¼ cup heavy cream
- 1 tablespoon butter

Directions:
In the slow cooker, mix the sea bass with the other ingredients.   Close the slow cooker lid and cook for 2 hours on High.
Nutrition Info:calories 231, fat 14.9, fiber 4.3 carbs 7.4, protein 24.2

540.   Mediterranean Cod Salad

Servings: 4   Cooking Time: 2 Hours
Ingredients:
- 6 tablespoons of capers
- 1 cup of fresh parsley, roughly diced
- 2 cups of jarred pimiento peppers, diced
- 1 cup of olives (Kalamata), pitted and roughly diced
- 2 lbs. salt cod
- ¾ cup of olive oil
- Salt and black pepper ground, to taste
- ½ teaspoon of red chili flakes
- Juice from 2 lemons
- 4 garlic cloves, peeled and minced
- 2 celery stalks, roughly diced

Directions:

Start by throwing all the Ingredients: into your Crockpot except escarole leaves.   Cover its lid and cook for 2 hours on High setting.   Once done, remove its lid and give it a stir.   Divide the seafood mixture into the escarole leaves.   Serve warm.
Nutrition Info: Calories 364 Total Fat 13.2 g Saturated Fat 3.4 g Cholesterol 141 mg Sodium 274 mg Total Carbs 10.8 g Sugar 2.8g Fiber 5.7 g Protein 47.7 g

541.	**Ginger Mackerel**

Servings: 6   Cooking Time: 1.5 Hours
Ingredients:

2-pound mackerel	1 teaspoon salt
1 teaspoon fresh ginger, minced	1 teaspoon lemon juice
1 teaspoon ground cumin	½ teaspoon lemon rind, grated
1 teaspoon black pepper	½ cup of coconut milk
1 teaspoon turmeric powder	1 teaspoon coconut oil

Directions:
In the slow cooker, mix the mackerel with the ginger, cumin and the other ingredients.   Close the slow cooker lid and cook fish for 1.5 hours on High. Divide between plates and serve.
Nutrition Info:calories 321, fat 25.8, fiber 1.1, carbs 2.7, protein 20.2

542.	**Coconut Fish Curry**

Servings: 4 – 6   Cooking Time: Approximately 4 Hours
Ingredients:

4 large fillets of fresh white fish, cut into chunks	2 tbsp yellow curry paste
4 garlic cloves, crushed	2 cups fish stock
1 small onion, finely chopped	2 cans full-fat coconut milk
1 tsp ground turmeric	1 lime
	Fresh coriander, roughly chopped

Directions:
Drizzle some olive oil into the Crock Pot.   Add the garlic, onion, turmeric, curry paste, fish, stock, coconut milk, salt, and pepper to the pot, stir to combine.   Place the lid onto the pot and set the temperature to HIGH.   Cook for 4 hours.   Serve while hot, with a small squeeze of fresh lime juice and fresh coriander!

543.	**Shrimp Salad**

Servings: 4   Cooking Time: 30 Minutes
Ingredients:

¼ cup cherry tomatoes	3 tablespoons butter
1 cup kale, chopped	1 tablespoon olive oil
½ cup avocado, peeled, pitted and cubed	1 tablespoon fresh parsley, chopped
7 oz shrimps, peeled and deveined	¾ cup heavy cream
	1 teaspoon ground black pepper
	½ teaspoon salt

1 teaspoon basil, dried
Directions:
In the slow cooker, mix the shrimp with tomatoes and the other ingredients, close the lid and cook for 30 minutes on High.   Divide into bowls and serve.
Nutrition Info:calories 249, fat 11.3, fiber 0.5, carbs 2.7, protein 8.3

544.	**Nutmeg Halibut**

Servings: 2   Cooking Time: 1 Hour
Ingredients:

2 halibut fillets	¾ teaspoon coriander, ground
1teaspoon lemon juice	1 tablespoon apple cider vinegar
1 teaspoon nutmeg, ground	¼ cup heavy cream
1 tablespoon butter, melted	

Directions:
In the slow cooker, mix the halibut with lemon juice, nutmeg and the other ingredients.   Close the lid and cook the fish for 1 hour on High.
Nutrition Info:calories 224, fat 6.8, fiber 0.1, carbs 5.1, protein 6.1

545.	**Crab Dip**

Servings: 3   Cooking Time: 2 Hours
Ingredients:

1 cup crabmeat	1 teaspoon paprika
1 cup Cheddar cheese, shredded	1 teaspoon oregano, dried
½ cup of coconut milk	½ teaspoon salt
2 spring onions, chopped	½ teaspoon dried cilantro
1 teaspoon olive oil	

Directions:
In the slow cooker, mix the crabmeat with the cheese and the other ingredients and whisk.   Close the lid and cook the dip for 2 hours on High.   Mix up it well with the help of the spoon.
Nutrition Info:calories 210, fat 13.1, fiber 1.2, carbs 4.2, protein 22.2

546.	**Keto Coconut Hot Chocolate**

Servings: 8   Cooking Time: Approximately 4 Hours
Ingredients:

5 cups full-fat coconut milk	1 tsp vanilla extract
2 cups heavy cream	1/3 cup cocoa powder
3 ounces dark chocolate, roughly chopped	½ tsp cinnamon
	Few drops of stevia to taste

Directions:
Add the coconut milk, cream, vanilla extract, cocoa powder, chocolate, cinnamon, and stevia to the Slow Cookerand stir to combine.   Place the lid onto the Slow Cookerand set the temperature to HIGH. Cook for 4 hours, whisking every 45 minutes. Taste the hot chocolate and if you prefer more sweetness, add a few more drops of stevia.   Enjoy with a dollop of whipped cream on top!

547. Lemon Salmon

Servings: 4   Cooking Time: 2 Hours

Ingredients:

Salt, to taste
Fresh black pepper to taste
1 lemon, sliced
¼ cup of onion
¼ cup of fennel
1 to 1 1/2 cups of water

Directions:

Start by throwing all the Ingredients: into your Crockpot.   Cover its lid and cook for 2 hours on Low setting.   Once done, remove its lid and give it a stir.   Serve warm.

Nutrition Info: Calories 238 Total Fat 9.5 g Saturated Fat 2.7 g Cholesterol 103 mg Sodium 403 mg Total Carbs 1.8 g Sugar 0.2 g Fiber 0.2 g Protein 34.2 g

548. Mustard Shrimp

Servings: 2   Cooking Time: 2 Hours

Ingredients:

1-pound shrimp, peeled and deveined
2 tablespoons Dijon mustard
½ teaspoon salt
½ cup of coconut water
1 teaspoon turmeric powder
1 teaspoon olive oil

Directions:

In the slow cooker, mix the shrimp with the mustard and the other ingredients.   Close the lid.   Cook the fish on Low for 2 hours.

Nutrition Info:calories 172, fat 4.4, fiber 0.6, carbs 1.3, protein 32.4

549. Vanilla And Strawberry Cheesecake

Servings: 8   Cooking Time: Approximately 6 Hours

Ingredients:

Base:
2 ounces butter, melted
1 cup ground hazelnuts
½ cup desiccated coconut
2 tsp vanilla extract
1 tsp cinnamon

Filling:
2 cups cream cheese
2 eggs, lightly beaten
1 cup sour cream
2 tsp vanilla extract
8 large strawberries, chopped

Directions:

Prepare the base: in a medium-sized bowl, combine the melted butter, hazelnuts, coconut, vanilla, and cinnamon.   Press the base into a greased heat-proof dish (make sure it fits into the Crock Pot). In a large bowl, place the cream cheese, eggs, sour cream, and vanilla extract, beat with electric egg beaters until thick and combined.   Fold the strawberries through the cream cheese mixture. Pour the cream cheese mixture into the dish, on top of the base, spread out until smooth.   Place the dish into the Slow Cookerand pour enough hot water around the dish so that it comes half way up the side of the dish.   Place the lid onto the pot and set the temperature to LOW.   Cook for 6 hours until just set but slightly wobbly.   Allow to cool slightly before placing in the fridge until cold.   Serve with a dollop of whipped cream!

550. Spicy Tuna

Servings: 3   Cooking Time: 1 Hour

Ingredients:

1 tablespoon olive oil
1 teaspoon hot paprika
1 red chili pepper minced
½ teaspoon black pepper
12 oz tuna fillet
½ teaspoon salt
1 jalapeno pepper, chopped
1/3 cup coconut oil
1 garlic clove, chopped

Directions:

Put the oil in the slow cooker.   Add the fish and the other ingredients and toss gently.   Close the lid and cook the oil mixture on High for 1 hour. Divide between plates and serve.

Nutrition Info:calories 309, fat 12.8, fiber 0.4, carbs 0.9, protein 19.1

551.Citrus Rich Octopus Salad

Servings: 2   Cooking Time: 2 Hours

Ingredients:

Juice of 1 lemon
21 oz. octopus, rinsed
4 celery stalks, roughly diced
Salt and black pepper ground, to taste
4 tablespoons of fresh parsley, roughly diced

Directions:

Start by throwing all the Ingredients: into your Crockpot.   Cover its lid and cook for 2 hours on Low setting.   Once done, remove its lid and give it a stir.   Serve warm.

Nutrition Info: Calories 225 Total Fat 17.7 g Saturated Fat 3.2 g Cholesterol 5 mg Sodium 386 mg Total Carbs 11.3 g Sugar 7.1 g Fiber 4.5 g Protein 7.4 g

552. Creamy Clam Chowder Luncheon

Servings: 4   Cooking Time: 2 Hours

Ingredients:

1 teaspoon of ground thyme
14 oz. canned baby clams
1 cup of celery stalks, roughly diced
2 cups of heavy cream
Salt and black pepper ground, to taste
1 cup of onion, peeled and roughly diced
12 bacon strips, roughly diced

Directions:

Start by throwing all the Ingredients: into your Crockpot.   Cover its lid and cook for 2 hours on High setting.   Once done, remove its lid and give it a stir.   Serve warm.

Nutrition Info: Calories 449 Total Fat 28.7 g Saturated Fat 14.9 g Cholesterol 163 mg Sodium 744 mg Total Carbs 8.4 g Sugar 2.6 g Fiber 1.9 g Protein 39.3 g

553. Rich Salmon Soup

Servings: 3   Cooking Time: 4 Hours

Ingredients:

1 tablespoon of coconut oil

1 cups of carrot, peeled and diced

½ cup of celery stalk, diced

½ cup of yellow onion, diced

1 cup of cauliflower, diced

2 cups of homemade chicken broth

Salt and black pepper, to taste

¼ cup of fresh parsley, chopped

Directions:
Start by throwing all the Ingredients: into your Crockpot. Cover its lid and cook for 4 hours on Low setting. Once done, remove its lid and give it a stir. Serve warm.

Nutrition Info: Calories 376 Total Fat 21.9 g Saturated Fat 7.8 g Cholesterol 110 mg Sodium 345 mg Total Carbs 57 g Sugar 4.6 g Fiber 5.7 g Protein 33.2 g

554. Shrimp And Green Beans

Servings: 5   Cooking Time: 3 Hours

Ingredients:

1-pound shrimp, peeled and deveined

¼ pound green beans, trimmed and halved

1 teaspoon salt

1 teaspoon chili flakes

1 teaspoon paprika

½ teaspoon garam masala

1 teaspoon coriander, ground

1 teaspoon basil, dried

¾ cup crushed tomatoes

1 tablespoon olive oil

3 spring onions, chopped

1 green bell pepper, chopped

1 cup of water

Directions:
In the slow cooker, mix the shrimp with green beans, salt and the other ingredients. Close the lid and cook for 3 hours on High. Divide into bowls and serve.

Nutrition Info:calories 202, fat 7.6, fiber 3, carbs 8.6, protein 12.4

555. Chocolate, Berry, And Macadamia Layered Jars

Servings: Makes 6 Jars (or Ramekins)   Cooking Time: Approximately 6 Hours

Ingredients:

½ cup mixed berries, (fresh) – any berries you like

3/4 cup toasted macadamia nuts, chopped

5 ounces dark chocolate, melted

7 ounces cream cheese

½ cup heavy cream

1 tsp vanilla extract

Directions:
In a medium-sized bowl, whisk together the cream cheese, cream, and vanilla extract. Spoon a small amount of melted chocolate into each jar or ramekin (only use half of the chocolate). Place a few berries on top of the chocolate (use half of the berries). Sprinkle some toasted macadamias onto the berries (use half of the nuts). Spoon a dollop of the cream cheese mixture into the ramekin (use all of the cream cheese mixture). Place another layer of chocolate, berries, and macadamia nuts on top of the cream cheese mixture. Place the jars into the Slow Cookerand pour enough hot water into the pot so that it reaches half way up the sides of the jars. Place the lid onto the pot and set the temperature to LOW. Cook for 6 hours. Remove the jars and leave them to cool and set on the bench for about 2 hours before serving.

556. Dark Chocolate And Peppermint Pots

Servings: Makes 6 Pots   Cooking Time: Approximately 3 Hours

Ingredients:

3 ounces dark chocolate, melted in the microwave

4 egg yolks, lightly beaten with a fork

2 ½ cups heavy cream

Few drops of stevia

Few drops of peppermint essence to taste

Directions:
Mix together the beaten egg yolks, cream, stevia, melted chocolate and peppermint essence in a medium-sized bowl. Prepare the pots by greasing 6 ramekins with butter. Pour the chocolate mixture into the pots, evenly. Place the pots into the Slow Cookerand very carefully pour hot water into the pot, (around the pots so it doesn't get into the chocolate mixture!) until it reaches just below half way up the pots. Place the lid onto the Slow Cookerand set the temperature to HIGH. Cook for 2 hours. Take the pots out of the Slow Cookerand leave to cool and set. Serve with a fresh mint leaf and a dollop of whipped cream on top!

557. Chili Shrimp And Okra

Servings: 4   Cooking Time: 2.5 Hours

Ingredients:

1 teaspoon chili pepper

½ teaspoon chili flakes

½ teaspoon salt

1-pound shrimp, peeled and deveined

1 cup okra, sliced

2 tablespoons lemon juice

2 tablespoons butter, soft

¾ cup of water

Directions:
In the slow cooker, combine the shrimp with chili pepper, flakes and the other ingredients. Cook the mix on Low for 5 hours.

Nutrition Info:calories 203, fat 11.6, fiber 3.9, carbs 8.1, protein 13.8

558. Flounder With Shrimp

Servings: 6   Cooking Time: 2 Hours

Ingredients:

A pinch of cinnamon ground

¼ teaspoon of ground nutmeg

½ teaspoon of allspice

¼ teaspoon of cloves, ground

2 cups of chicken stock

1 celery stalk, diced

1 tomato, cored and diced

2 shallots, peeled and roughly diced

8 oz. shrimp, peeled, deveined, and diced

4 garlic cloves, peeled and minced

1 tablespoon of

2 tablespoon of coconut flour
1 tablespoon of butter
8 oz. bacon, sliced
1 green bell pepper, seeded and diced

coconut milk
½ cup of fresh parsley, diced
2 tablespoons of butter
4 flounder fillets

Directions:
Start by throwing all the Ingredients: into your Crockpot except shrimp.   Cover its lid and cook for 2 hours on High setting.   Once done, remove its lid and give it a stir.   Stir in shrimp and continue cooking for 1 hour on low heat.   Serve warm.
Nutrition Info: Calories 202 Total Fat 9.5g Saturated Fat 2 g Cholesterol 62 mg Sodium 526 mg Total Carbs 11.5 g Sugar 5.8 g Fiber 2.6 g Protein 22 g

559.   Italian Shrimp Tortillas

Servings: 2   Cooking Time: 2 Hours
Ingredients:

2 keto tortillas
½ teaspoon Cajun seasoning
1 teaspoon Italian seasoning
1 tablespoon chives, chopped
2 tablespoons fresh cilantro, chopped

2 oz Cheddar cheese, shredded
7 oz shrimps, peeled
½ cup heavy cream
½ teaspoon ground coriander
1 teaspoon salt
1 jalapeno pepper, sliced

Directions:
In the slow cooker, mix the shrimp with the seasonings and the other ingredients and close the lid.   Cook shrimps on High for 2 hours.   After this, fill keto tortillas with shrimps and serve.
Nutrition Info:calories 220, fat 6.2, fiber 2.4, carbs 8.7, protein 6.5

560.   Avocado And Shrimp

Servings: 2   Cooking Time: 2 Hours
Ingredients:

1 avocado, peeled, pitted and cubed
8 oz shrimps, raw, peeled
1 teaspoon basil, dried
1 teaspoon coriander, ground
1/3 cup water

1 teaspoon butter, softened
½ teaspoon minced garlic
½ teaspoon chili flakes
½ teaspoon onion powder

Directions:
In the slow cooker, mix the shrimp with avocado, basil and the other ingredients and toss.   Close the lid and cook the meal on High for 2 hours.
Nutrition Info:calories 279, fat 13.9, fiber 6.8, carbs 12.1, protein 12.5

561.   Turmeric Calamari

Servings: 5   Cooking Time: 6 Hours
Ingredients:

1-pound calamari rings

1 teaspoon turmeric
1 tablespoon heavy

1 teaspoon hot paprika
2 tablespoons coconut cream
½ teaspoon minced garlic

cream
½ teaspoon ground coriander
½ teaspoon salt
½ teaspoon black pepper

Directions:
In the slow cooker, mix the calamari with the turmeric and the other ingredients and close the lid. Cook the seafood for 6 hours on Low.   When the time is over, stir the mix and serve.
Nutrition Info:calories 200, fat 4.8, fiber 2.2, carbs 3.6, protein 14.4

562.   Citrus Glazed Salmon

Servings: 2   Cooking Time: 2 Hours
Ingredients:

½ teaspoon of fresh ginger, minced
1 teaspoon of fresh orange zest, grated finely
½ cup of white wine

½ tablespoon of olive oil
1 tablespoon of fresh lemon juice
Black pepper, to taste

Directions:
Start by throwing all the Ingredients: into your Crockpot.   Cover its lid and cook for 2 hours on Low setting.   Once done, remove its lid and give it a stir.   Serve warm.
Nutrition Info: Calories 269 Total Fat 11.9 g Saturated Fat 5.5 g Cholesterol 36 mg Sodium 437 mg Total Carbs 8.6 g Sugar 1.4 g Fiber 3.4 g Protein 15 g

563.   Salmon With Mushroom

Servings: 4   Cooking Time: 3 Hours
Ingredients:

2 salmon fillets
2 cups of spinach, chopped
A drizzle of olive oil
¼ cup of macadamia nuts, toasted and roughly diced

6 mushrooms, diced
3 green onions, diced
Salt and black pepper ground, to taste
A pinch of nutmeg
5 oz. tiger shrimp, peeled, deveined, and diced

Directions:
Start by throwing all the Ingredients: into your Crockpot except shrimp   Cover its lid and cook for 2 hours on High setting.   Once done, remove its lid and give it a stir.   Stir in shrimp and continue cooking for 1 hour on low heat.   Serve warm.
Nutrition Info: Calories 282 Total Fat 4.6 g Saturated Fat 1.4 g Cholesterol 75 mg Sodium 560 mg Total Carbs 11.1 g Sugar 2.1 g Fiber 1.6 g Protein 22.2 g

564.   Scallops With Romanesco

Servings: 4   Cooking Time: 1 Hour
Ingredients:

3 tablespoon of olive oil
1 cup of chicken stock
1 tablespoon of butter
1 shallot, peeled and

1 lb. scallops
2 cups of spinach, chopped
¼ cup of walnuts,

diced
3 garlic cloves, peeled
and minced

toasted and diced
1½ cups of
pomegranate seeds
Salt and black pepper
ground, to taste

Directions:
Start by throwing all the Ingredients: into your Crockpot.   Cover its lid and cook for 1 hour on Low setting.   Once done, remove its lid and give it a stir. Serve warm.
Nutrition Info: Calories 307 Total Fat 29 g Saturated Fat 14g Cholesterol 111 mg Total Carbs 7 g Sugar 1 g Fiber 3 g Sodium 122 mg Potassium 78 mg Protein 6 g

565.	Lemon Cod

Servings: 4   Cooking Time: 2 Hours
Ingredients:

20 oz cod fillet
Juice of 1 lemon
Zest of 1 lemon, grated
1 tablespoon chives, chopped
1 teaspoon turmeric powder

2 oz Parmesan, grated
½ teaspoon salt
½ teaspoon ground black pepper
1 teaspoon butter

1/3 cup organic almond milk

Directions:
In the slow cooker, mix the cod with lemon juice, zest and the other ingredients.   Close the lid and cook the sauce for 2 hours on High.   Divide between plates and serve.
Nutrition Info:calories 212, fat 5.6, fiber 4.4, carbs 6.6, protein 30.2

566.	Wine Sauce Glazed Cod

Servings: 7   Cooking Time: 4 Hours
Ingredients:

1 tablespoon of fresh parsley
1/4 teaspoon of paprika

1 garlic clove, diced
1/2 cup of white wine
1 cup of water

Directions:
Start by throwing all the Ingredients: into your Crockpot.   Cover its lid and cook for 4 hours on Low setting.   Once done, remove its lid and give it a stir.   Serve warm.
Nutrition Info: Calories 434 Total Fat 36.4 g Saturated Fat 17.1 g Cholesterol 257 mg Sodium 1038 mg Total Carbs 2.5 g Sugar 0.9 g Fiber 0.2 g Protein 24.2 g

567. Spicy Pecans

Servings: 16   Cooking Time: 3 Hours
Ingredients:
- 2 tbsp. Cajun seasoning blend
- 2 tbsp. olive oil

Directions:
Add all ingredients to the slow cooker and stir well to combine.   Cover slow cooker with lid and cook on low for 1 hour.   Stir well. Cover again and cook for 2 hours more.   Serve and enjoy.
Nutrition Info: Calories 607 Fat 62.5 g Carbohydrates 12.2 g Sugar 3 g Protein 9.1 g Cholesterol 0 mg

568. Garlic Pork Slices

Servings: 10   Cooking Time: 8 Hours
Ingredients:
- 1-pound pork belly
- 2 teaspoons minced garlic
- 1 teaspoon garlic powder
- 1 teaspoon ground black pepper
- ½ teaspoon salt
- 1 tablespoon avocado oil
- 1/3 cup water
- 1 tablespoon apple cider vinegar

Directions:
In the slow cooker, mix the pork with garlic and the other ingredients and close the lid.   Cook the snack for 8 hours on Low.   Then remove the pork belly from the slow cooker and dry it gently with the help of the paper towel.   Slice the cooked pork belly into the slices.
Nutrition Info:calories 314, fat 12.4, fiber 5.2, carbs 12.7, protein 21

569. Tomato Chicken Wings

Servings: 4   Cooking Time: 6.5 Hours
Ingredients:
- 4 chicken wings
- 1 tablespoon lime juice
- 1 tablespoon Keto tomato sauce
- ½ teaspoon balsamic vinegar
- ½ teaspoon salt
- ½ teaspoon chili flakes
- ¾ teaspoon smoked paprika
- 1/3 cup water
- 1 teaspoon coconut butter

Directions:
In the slow cooker, mix the chicken wings with lime juice and the other ingredients   Close the lid and cook chicken wings for 6.5 hours on Low.   Serve the chicken wings as an appetizer.
Nutrition Info:calories 306, fat 15.2, fiber 4.9, carbs 12.9, protein 23.8

570. Cheddar Dip

Servings: 6   Cooking Time: 4 Hours
Ingredients:
- 3 spring onions, chopped
- 1 cup Cheddar cheese, shredded
- 1 teaspoon butter
- 1 teaspoon minced jalapeno pepper
- ½ cup of coconut cream
- 1 tablespoon Italian seasoning

Directions:
In the slow cooker, mix the cheese with the butter and the other ingredients and whisk.   Close the lid and cook the dip on Low for 4 hours.
Nutrition Info:calories 234, fat 9.6, fiber 3.4, carbs 8.3, protein 9.2

571. Garlic Chicken Wings

Servings: 4   Cooking Time: 6 Hours
Ingredients:
- 7 oz chicken wings
- 2 garlic cloves, peeled
- 1 teaspoon garlic powder
- 1 tablespoon paprika
- 2 tablespoons olive oil
- 3 tablespoons water

Directions:
Dice the garlic cloves and combine them with the paprika, garlic powder, olive oil, and water.   Then place the chicken wings in the slow cooker and sprinkle with the garlic mixture.   Stir the chicken wings and cook for 6 hours on Low.   Chill the cooked chicken wings slightly and serve!
Nutrition Info:calories 164, fat 10.9, fiber 0.8, carbs 2, protein 14.8

572. Zucchini Bread

Servings: 12   Cooking Time: 3 Hours
Ingredients:
- 1 c. almond flour
- 1/3 c. coconut flour
- ½ t. of each:
- Optional: xanthan gum
- Salt
- Baking soda
- 1 ½ t. baking powder
- 1/3 c. softened coconut oil/butter
- 3 eggs
- 2 t. vanilla
- 1 c. sweetener or ½ c. Pyure all-purpose
- 2 c. shredded zucchini
- ½ c. chopped pecans/walnuts
- Also Needed: 8x4 silicone bread pan

Directions:
Combine the coconut and almond flour, salt, baking soda and powder, cinnamon, and xanthan gum. Set aside for now.   Mix the oil, eggs, vanilla, and sugar in another dish. Combine the fixings.   Blend in the nuts and shredded zucchini. Scoop the batter into the prepared bread pan.   Arrange the cooker on the top rack (or on crunched up aluminum foil balls). You want it at least ½-inch from the bottom of the slow cooker.   Cover with the lid and cook for three hours on the high setting.   Cool, wrap in foil, and place in the fridge. It is best when refrigerated.
Nutrition Info: Calories: 174 Net Carbs: 13.8 g Fat: 15.7 g Protein: 5 g

573. Pizza

Servings: 4   Cooking Time: 3 Hours
Ingredients:
- Pizza seasoning – 1 tbsp.
- Tomatoes – ½ can
- Black olives – ½ cup
- Low carb pizza sauce

Mozzarella – 1 cup
Ground beef – ½ pound
Peppers – ½ cup

– ½ jar
Onions – ½ cup
Pepperoni – 15 slices
Mushrooms – ½ cup

Directions:
Brown both the meats.   Add them to the cooker. Add spices, mushrooms and vegetables.   Pour in the sauce and tomatoes.   Evenly distribute cheese. Add pepperoni.   Cook on low for 3 hours.
Nutrition Info: Calories: 441 Fat: 30g Carb: 6g Protein: 33g

---

574. Chili Dip

Servings: 8   Cooking Time: 1.5 Hour
Ingredients:

2 red chili peppers, minced
1 teaspoon hot paprika
1 teaspoon curry powder
1 teaspoon butter

1 tablespoon cream cheese
½ cup Cheddar cheese, shredded
¼ cup crushed tomatoes

Directions:
In the slow cooker, mix the chili peppers with the paprika and the other ingredients and whisk. Close the slow cooker lid and cook the dip for 1.5 hours on High.
Nutrition Info: calories 124, fat 3.4, fiber 3.6, carbs 3.6, protein 2.2

---

575. Applesauce

Servings: 6   Cooking Time: 2 Hours
Ingredients:

1/4 cup water
2 whole cinnamon sticks

2 tbsp fresh lemon juice

Directions:
Add all ingredients to the slow cooker and stir well. Cover slow cooker with lid and cook on high for 2 hours.   Discard cinnamon sticks and using potato masher mash until you get desired consistency.
Nutrition Info: Calories 59 Fat 0.2 g Carbohydrates 15.5 g Sugar 11.7 g Protein 0.3 g Cholesterol 0 mg

---

576. Pork Bites

Servings: 4   Cooking Time: 4 Hours
Ingredients:

1 cup pork stew meat, cubed
1 teaspoon keto tomato sauce
¼ cup heavy cream

1 teaspoon chili flakes
1 teaspoon olive oil
½ teaspoon salt

Directions:
In the slow cooker, mix the pork cubes with tomato paste and the other ingredients, close the lid and cook for 4 hours on High.   Divide into bowls and serve
Nutrition Info: calories 283, fat 20.2, fiber 3.3, carbs 1.4, protein 14.5

---

577. Cayenne Shrimps

Servings: 4   Cooking Time: 2 Hours
Ingredients:

¾ teaspoon cayenne pepper
1 teaspoon turmeric powder
1 teaspoon curry powder

1 oz Parmesan, grated
1 tablespoon butter
½ cup organic almond milk
9 oz shrimps, peeled

Directions:
In the slow cooker, mix the shrimp with the Parmesan and the other ingredients, stir and close the lid   Cook the shrimp for 2 hours on High. Divide into bowls and serve.
Nutrition Info: calories 184, fat 10.7, fiber 1.2, carbs 3.3, protein 19

---

578. Zucchini Bites

Servings: 6   Cooking Time: 1 Hour
Ingredients:

2 zucchinis, trimmed and roughly cubed
1 teaspoon turmeric powder
½ teaspoon salt

1 tablespoon yellow curry powder
1 tablespoon minced garlic
2 tablespoons butter

Directions:
In the slow cooker mix the zucchinis with the turmeric and the other ingredients and close the lid. Cook the zucchini rounds for 1 hour on High.
Nutrition Info: calories 46, fat 4, fiber 0.8, carbs 2.7, protein 0.9

---

579. Tofu Bites

Servings: 4   Cooking Time: 2 Hours
Ingredients:

3 oz firm tofu, cubed
1/3 cup coconut cream
1 tablespoon balsamic vinegar

½ teaspoon salt
1 teaspoon chili powder

Directions:
In the slow cooker, mix the tofu with the cream and the other ingredients, close the lid and cook for 5 hours on High.   Serve as a snack.
Nutrition Info: calories 214, fat 7.5, fiber 4.4, carbs 3.3, protein 11.1

---

580. Bacon Wrapped Duck Roll

Servings: 12   Cooking Time: 3 Hours
Ingredients:

1-pound duck breast
5 oz bacon, sliced
1 teaspoon salt
½ teaspoon ground black pepper

1 teaspoon butter
1 teaspoon cayenne pepper
4 tablespoons water

Directions:
Beat the duck breast gently to flatten.   Sprinkle the duck breast with the salt, ground black pepper, and cayenne pepper.   Spread the butter on the duck breast and roll it.   Wrap the duck breast in the bacon and put it in the slow cooker.   Add the water and cook the duck roll for 3 hours on High. When the duck roll is cooked, slice it and enjoy!

Nutrition Info:calories 116, fat 6.8, fiber 0.1, carbs 0.3, protein 12.7

581.   Molten Lava Cake

Servings: 24   Cooking Time: 4 Hours
Ingredients:

10 tablespoons cocoa powder, unsweetened, divided	6 whole eggs
2 teaspoons baking powder	1 cup almond flour
	1 teaspoon salt
6 egg yolks	1 cup butter, melted, cooled
2 teaspoons vanilla extract	2 teaspoons vanilla liquid stevia
8 ounces sugar free chocolate chips	4 cups hot water
	Butter for greasing

Directions:
Grease the inside of the pot with butter.   Add all the dry ingredients into a bowl and mix well.   Add all the wet ingredients into another bowl. Mix well. Pour the wet ingredient into the bowl of dry ingredients and mix until well combined.   Pour the batter into the slow cooker. Sprinkle chocolate chips on top.   Add remaining cocoa powder, swerve and hot water into a bowl and whisk well. Pour over the batter.   Close the lid. Cook on 'Low' for 4 hours.   Cool for a while. Slice and serve.
Nutrition Info: Calories194 Fat 17.4g Carbohydrate 5.2g Protein 4.8g

582.   Keto Bread Sticks

Servings: 4   Cooking Time: 1 Hour
Ingredients:

1 egg	2 oz Parmesan, grated
1 tablespoon Psyllium husk powder	
1 teaspoon cream cheese	2 tablespoons almond flour
	1 teaspoon olive oil
	¼ teaspoon thyme

Directions:
Beat the egg in the bowl and whisk.   Add Psyllium husk powder, cream cheese, almond flour, thyme, and grated cheese.   Stir the mixture until smooth and roll into medium sticks.   Freeze the sticks for 10 minutes and then place them in the slow cooker. Add olive oil and cook for 1 hour on High.   When the sticks are cooked, serve them hot!
Nutrition Info:calories 162, fat 12.6, fiber 3.3, carbs 5.7, protein 9

583.   Turkey Meatballs

Servings: 6   Cooking Time: 3 Hours
Ingredients:

1 teaspoon dried basil	10 oz ground turkey
1 teaspoon minced garlic	¾ cup almond milk, unsweetened
1 teaspoon ground black pepper	1 teaspoon oregano
	1 tablespoon almond flour

Directions:
Mix the ground turkey, dried basil, minced garlic, ground black pepper, oregano, and almond flour. Stir the mixture until well blended.   Pour the almond milk into the slow cooker.   Make medium meatballs from the turkey mix and put them in the slow cooker.   Cook the meatballs for 3 hours on High.   Let the cooked meatballs cool slightly. Serve!
Nutrition Info:calories 190, fat 14.7, fiber 1.4, carbs 3.2, protein 14.7

584.   Mini Muffins

Servings: 4   Cooking Time: 3 Hours
Ingredients:

4 tablespoons almond flour	¼ teaspoon baking powder
1 egg, beaten	
3 tablespoons coconut flour	¼ teaspoon paprika
	1 teaspoon butter, melted

Directions:
Whisk together the beaten egg and almond flour. Add coconut flour, baking powder, melted butter and paprika and stir until smooth.   Pour the muffin mixture into mini muffin molds.   Put the muffins in the slow cooker and cook for 3 hours on High.   Cool the cooked muffins slightly and serve!
Nutrition Info:calories 207, fat 16.6, fiber 5.3, carbs 10.1, protein 8.2

585.   Keto Crackers

Servings: 4   Cooking Time: 2 Hours
Ingredients:

1 teaspoon butter	½ teaspoon salt
¾ cup almond flour	1 teaspoon cumin
1 teaspoon ground black pepper	1 teaspoon olive oil

Directions:
Mix the butter, almond flour, salt, ground black pepper, and cumin.   Knead the dough until smooth   Make small balls and press them gently into cracker shapes.   Spray the olive oil inside the slow cooker.   Add the crackers and cook for 2 hours on High.   Cool the crackers and serve!
Nutrition Info:calories 52, fat 4.9, fiber 0.8, carbs 1.7, protein 1.3

586.   Pecans Bowls

Servings: 6   Cooking Time: 1 Hour
Ingredients:

6 pecans	1 tablespoon keto tomato sauce
1 teaspoon butter, melted	½ teaspoon olive oil

Directions:
In the slow cooker, mix the pecans with the keto tomato sauce and the other ingredients, toss and close the lid.   Cook pecans for 1 hour on High. Stir the pecans after 30 minutes of cooking and divide them into bowls at the end.
Nutrition Info:calories 126, fat 11.2, fiber 1.5, carbs 2, protein 1.5

587.   Paprika Almonds

Servings: 2   Cooking Time: 6 Hours
Ingredients:

1 cup almonds
1 tablespoon sweet paprika
1/3 cup water

½ teaspoon Vanilla extract
¾ teaspoon ground ginger

Directions:
In the slow cooker, mix the almonds with the other ingredients, toss and close the lid.   Cook the almonds for 6 hours on Low. Mix up the almonds every 1 hour.
Nutrition Info:calories 126, fat 4.3, fiber 2.1, carbs 9.1, protein 5.2

588.   Nacho Cheese Dip

Servings: 8   Cooking Time: 2 Hours
Ingredients:
¼ cup almond milk
½ cup chunky salsa

1 cup cheddar cheese, shredded

Directions:
Add all ingredients to the slow cooker and stir well. Cover slow cooker with lid and cook on low for 2 hours. Stir to mix.   Serve with fresh vegetables.
Nutrition Info: Calories 178 Fat 16.4 g Carbohydrates 2.4 g Sugar 0.9 g Protein 6.1 g Cholesterol 46 mg

589.   Marvelous Turkey Magic Sandwich

Servings: 12   Cooking Time: 5 Hours
Ingredients:
6 lb. turkey breast
¼ cup chili sauce
1 medium onion (chopped)
4 tsp beef Bouillon granules

3 tbsp white vinegar
2 tbsp Italian seasoning
12 ketogenic sandwich buns (sliced)

Directions:
Keep the turkey meat in the Slow Cookerand add the pepper and onion pieces.   Use a small bowl to mix the beef bouillon with chili sauce, seasoning mix and vinegar and pour the mixture over the meat in the pot.   Cook by covering the pot for 5 hours on low setting.   Allow cooling down and then shred the meat with two forks and return them to the pot for heating them up.   Prepare the sandwiches by placing spoonful of meat mixture in between each slices of bread.
Nutrition Info: Calories 200 Fat 16 g Carbohydrate 10 g Protein 5 g

590.   Ketogenic Chicken Sandwich From Crock Pot

Servings: 12   Cooking Time: 5 Hours
Ingredients:
6 lb. chicken breast
¼ cup chili sauce
1 medium onion (chopped)
4 tsp beef Bouillon granules

3 tbsp white vinegar
2 tbsp Italian seasoning
12 ketogenic sandwich buns (sliced)

Directions:
Keep the chicken meat in the Slow Cookerand add the pepper and onion pieces.   Use a small bowl to mix the beef bouillon with chili sauce, seasoning mix and vinegar and pour the mixture over the meat in the pot.   Cook by covering the pot for 5 hours on low setting.   Allow cooling down and then shred the chicken with two forks and return them to the pot for heating them up.   Prepare the sandwiches by placing spoonful of meat mixture in between each slices of bread.
Nutrition Info: Calories 230 Fat 20 g Carbohydrate 15 g Protein 6 g

591.   Cherry Marmalade

Servings: 6   Cooking Time: 3 Hours
Ingredients:
3 tbsps. Gelatin
4 c. pitted cherries

2 c. coconut sugar

Directions:
In your slow cooker, mix lemon juice with gelatin, cherries and coconut sugar, stir, cover and cook on High for 3 hours.   Divide into cups and serve cold. Enjoy!
Nutrition Info: Calories: 211 Total Fat: 3 g Net Carbs: 3 g Protein: 3 g

592.   Slow CookerSpecial Cheesy Steak Sandwich

Servings: 6   Cooking Time: 6 Hours
Ingredients:
2 onions (halved and sliced)
6 ketogenic sandwich buns (split)
2 sweet red or green peppers
14 oz beef broth

1 envelope onion soup mix
12 slices of provolone cheese (halved)
Pickled hot cherry peppers

Directions:
Keep the onions, peppers in the crockpot and add the beef along with soup mix and beef broth. Cover the pot and cook on low setting for 6 hours.   Keep the buns on baking sheet and place the meat mixture on the bottom of the buns and top with cheese. Broil the sandwiches for 6 minutes ensuring the cheese melts.   Serve with cherry peppers.
Nutrition Info: Calories 190 Fat 13 g Carbohydrate 12 g Protein 7 g

593.   Chicken Tenders

Servings: 7   Cooking Time: 2.5 Hours
Ingredients:
8 oz chicken fillet
¾ cup coconut flour
1 egg white

1 teaspoon ground black pepper
1 teaspoon olive oil

Directions:
Cut the chicken fillet into the medium tenders. Whisk the egg whites and dip the chicken tenders into the whites.   Remove the tenders from the egg white and sprinkle with the ground black pepper and coconut flour.   Place the chicken tenders in the slow cooker and drizzle with the olive oil. Cook the chicken tenders for 2.5 hours.   Let the cooked chicken tenders cool slightly.   Serve!
Nutrition Info:calories 122, fat 4.4, fiber 5.2, carbs 8.8, protein 11.6

594.	**Parmesan Cream Green Beans**

Servings: 2   Cooking Time: 2 Hours
Ingredients:
- A pinch of salt and black pepper
- 1/3 cup of parmesan (grated)
- 2 oz. cream cheese
- 1/3 cup of coconut cream
- 1 tablespoon of dill, diced

Directions:
Start by throwing all the ingredients into the Crockpot.   Cover its lid and cook for 2 hours on Low setting.   Once done, remove its lid of the crockpot carefully.   Mix well and garnish as desired.   Serve warm.
Nutrition Info: Calories 292 Total Fat 26.2 g Saturated Fat 16.3 g Cholesterol 100 mg Sodium 86 mg Total Carbs 8.2 g Sugar 6.6 g Fiber 0.2 g Protein 5.2 g

595.	**Keto Tortillas With Cheese**

Servings: 4   Cooking Time: 1 Hour
Ingredients:
- 4 egg whites
- 4 tablespoons almond flour
- 3 tablespoons water
- ¾ teaspoon baking soda
- 1 teaspoon olive oil
- ¼ teaspoon garlic powder
- ¼ teaspoon chili flakes
- 2 oz Parmesan, grated

Directions:
Whisk the egg whites gently then add almond flour and water.   Add baking soda, garlic powder, and chili flakes.   Knead the mix into a smooth dough. Roll out the dough into medium sized tortilla. Then pour the olive oil in the slow cooker and add the tortillas.   Sprinkle the tortilla with the grated cheese and close the lid.   Cook the tortilla for 1 hour on High.   Serve the cooked snack hot!
Nutrition Info:calories 233, fat 18.3, fiber 3, carbs 6.9, protein 14.2

596.	**Meatloaf Burger For Keto Diet**

Servings: 6   Cooking Time: 7 Hours
Ingredients:
- 2 lb. lean ground beef
- 2 cups of tomato juice
- 4 cloves of garlic, minced
- 1 celery rib, finely chopped
- 1 large onion, sliced
- 1 bay leaf
- 1 tsp + ½ tsp salt
- 1 tbsp ketchup
- 1 tsp Italian seasoning
- 6 ketogenic hamburger buns, split

Directions:
Keep the celery and onion in the crock pot. Mix the beef with 1 tsp salt and pepper to make 6 patties and then keep them over the vegetables in the pot. Use a bowl to mix the tomato juice with seasoning, ketchup, remaining salt and bay leaf and pour the mixture over the patties in the crock pot.   Cover the pot and cook on low setting for 7 hours, making sure that the meat is no longer pink in color. Serve the patties with the buns and your favorite sauce.
Nutrition Info: Calories 240 Fat 23 g Carbohydrate 16 g Protein 9 g

597.	**Oregano Dip**

Servings: 4   Cooking Time: 2 Hours
Ingredients:
- ½ cup Cheddar cheese, shredded
- 1 tablespoon dried oregano
- 2 tablespoon butter
- ½ teaspoon cayenne pepper
- 1 teaspoon smoked paprika
- ¼ cup coconut cream

Directions:
Put the cheese, oregano and the other ingredients in the slow cooker.   Close the lid and cook the dip of High for 2 hours.
Nutrition Info:calories 204, fat 12.4, fiber 1, carbs 2.9, protein 11.4

598.	**Radish Spinach Medley**

Servings: 2   Cooking Time: 2 Hours
Ingredients:
- 2 cups of radishes, sliced
- A pinch of salt and black pepper
- ¼ cup of vegetable broth
- 1 teaspoon of chili powder
- 1 tablespoon of parsley, chopped

Directions:
Start by throwing all the ingredients into the Crockpot.   Cover its lid and cook for 2 hours on Low setting.   Once done, remove its lid of the crockpot carefully.   Mix well and garnish as desired.   Serve warm.
Nutrition Info: Calories 244 Total Fat 24.8 g Saturated Fat 15.6 g Cholesterol 32 mg Sodium 204 mg Total Carbs 2.1 g Sugar 0.4 g Fiber 0.1 g Protein 24 g

599.	**Ginger Tea Drink**

Servings: 4   Cooking Time: 2 Hours
Ingredients:
- 15 individual green tea bags
- 4 cups of white grape juice
- 1 to 2 tablespoons of honey
- 1 tablespoon of minced fresh ginger root
- Crystallized ginger, optional

Directions:
Start by throwing all the ingredients into the Crockpot.   Cover its lid and cook for 2 hours on Low setting.   Once done, remove its lid of the crockpot carefully.   Strain the slow-cooked tea into the glasses.   Serve warm.
Nutrition Info: Calories 179 Total Fat 15.7 g Saturated Fat 8 g Cholesterol 0 mg Sodium 43 mg Total Carbs 4.8 g Sugar 3.6 g Fiber 0.8 g Protein 5.6 g

600.	Masala Hazelnuts

Servings: 4   Cooking Time: 2 Hours
Ingredients:
1 tablespoon avocado oil
1 cup hazelnuts
1 teaspoon garam masala
1 teaspoon coriander, ground
¼ cup water
1 teaspoon chili powder
1 teaspoon cayenne pepper
½ teaspoon salt
Directions:
In the slow cooker, mix the hazelnuts with the oil and the other ingredients and close the lid.   Cook the nuts for 2 hours on High.   Spread the hazelnuts on a lined baking sheet, cool down and serve as a snack.
Nutrition Info:calories 109, fat 5.1, fiber 1.3, carbs 2.2, protein 1.7

601.	Bacon Pepper Quiche

Servings: 12   Cooking Time: 4 Hours
Ingredients:
1 cup almond flour
3 tablespoons olive oil
1 teaspoon dried basil
1 teaspoon salt
4 eggs, beaten
1 green pepper, chopped
3 oz bacon, chopped
2 oz Parmesan, grated

Directions:
Whisk the eggs and combine them together with the dried basil, almond flour, salt, chopped green pepper, and grated cheese.   Stir the mixture and add chopped bacon.   Pour the olive oil in the slow cooker and add egg mixture.   Cook for 4 hours on High.   When the quiche is cooked, cool and slice into servings.   Enjoy!
Nutrition Info:calories 120, fat 10.1, fiber 0.4, carbs 1.3, protein 6.6

602.	Spiced Lemon Drink

Servings: 4   Cooking Time: 3 Hours
Ingredients:
2 cups of stevia
11/2 cups of lime juice
1/2 cup of plus 2 tablespoons of lemon juice
1/4 cup of cranberry juice
1 cinnamon stick (3 inches)
1/2 teaspoon of whole cloves
Directions:
Start by tying all the whole spices in a cheesecloth. Now place the tied spices along with all other Ingredients: into the Crockpot.   Cover its lid and cook for 3 hours on Low setting.   Once done, remove its lid of the crockpot carefully.   Strain the slow-cooked tea into the serving glasses.   Serve warm.
Nutrition Info: Calories 158 Total Fat 35.2 g Saturated Fat 15.2 g Cholesterol 69 mg Sodium 178 mg Total Carbs 7.4 g Sugar 1.1 g Fiber 3.5 g Protein 5.5 g

603.	Dairy-free Fudge

Servings: 15   Cooking Time: 2 Hours
Ingredients:
1 tablespoon coconut oil
1 teaspoon stevia drops
½ teaspoon vanilla extract
¼ cup coconut milk
2 tablespoons walnuts, chopped into small pieces (optional)
Directions:
Add all the ingredients to the slow cooker. Mix well. Close the lid. Cook on 'Low' for 2 hours. When done, open the lid and let it rest for 30 minutes. Do not stir at all.   Let it cool to room temperature. Now stir constantly for a few minutes.   Transfer the mixture into a greased tin. Cover and refrigerate until the fudge is set.   Cut into squares and serve.
Nutrition Info: Calories 71 Fat 5.1g Carbohydrate 7g Protein 1g

604.	Caprese Meatballs

Servings: 6   Cooking Time: 2 Hours
Ingredients:
7 oz ground turkey
1 egg
3 tablespoons almond flour
¼ teaspoon garlic powder
1 oz dried tomatoes, chopped
1 tablespoons dried basil
1 teaspoon butter
Directions:
Beat the egg into the ground turkey.   Add the almond flour and garlic powder.   Add the dried basil and stir the turkey mixture.   Roll into meatballs.   Place the meatballs in the slow cooker and add butter.   Close the lid and cook the meatballs for 2 hours on High.   Then slide the meatballs onto the skewers.   Add the dried tomatoes to the skewers and serve!
Nutrition Info:calories 162, fat 12, fiber 1.6, carbs 3.3, protein 13.1

605.	Bbq Beef Sandwich

Servings: 16   Cooking Time: 10 Hours
Ingredients:
1 can condensed beef broth
½ cup lemon juice
½ cup packed brown sugar
2 cloves of garlic, minced
3.5 lb. beef eye round roast
3 tbsp steak sauce
1 tsp Worcestershire sauce
1 tsp pepper
16 sandwich buns
Dill pickle spices
1 tsp salt
16 ketogenic sandwich bread roll, sliced

Directions:
Use a small bowl to blend ketchup with beef broth, brown sugar, lemon juice, steak sauce, minced cloves, pepper and Worcestershire sauce and pour half portion of it to the crock pot.   Sprinkle the beef roast with salt and keep it in the Slow Cookerand then pour the remaining liquid mixture from top.   Cover the pot and cook on low setting for 10 hours, making sure that the meat becomes tender.   Use two forks to shred the beef and then keep ½ cup beef in each sandwich.   Top the sandwiches with pickles and serve.
Nutrition Info: Calories 215 Fat 19 g Carbohydrate 12 g Protein 9 g

606. Delicious Custard

Servings: 6   Cooking Time: 2 Hours
Ingredients:
- 2 egg yolks
- 10 drops liquid stevia
- ½ cup almond milk
- 1 cup heavy cream

Directions:
Add all ingredients to the blender and blend until well combined.   Spray ramekins with cooking spray and pour batter into each ramekin.   Place ramekins into the slow cooker.   Cover slow cooker with lid and cook on high for 2 hours.   Serve and enjoy.
Nutrition Info: Calories 154 Fat 15.1 g Carbohydrates 2 g Sugar 0.8 g Protein 3.6 g Cholesterol 152 mg

607. Carrots Dessert

Servings: 4   Cooking Time: 1 Hour
Ingredients:
- 2 c. baby carrots
- 1 tbsp. melted ghee
- ½ c. water

Directions:
In your slow cooker, mix carrots with stevia, ghee and water, stir, cover and cook on High for 1 hour. Divide into dessert cups and serve them cold. Enjoy!
Nutrition Info: Calories: 120 Total Fat: 1 g Net Carbs: 2 g Protein: 2 g

608. Crockpot Milk Tea

Servings: 12   Cooking Time: 8 Hours
Ingredients:
- 3 cinnamon sticks (3 inches)
- 25 whole cloves
- 15 cardamom pods, lightly crushed
- 3 whole peppercorns
- 3 1/2 quarts water
- 8 black tea bags
- 1 cup of evaporated milk
- 2 tablespoons of stevia

Directions:
Start by tying all the whole spices in a cheesecloth. Now place the tied spices along with all other ingredients into the Crockpot.   Cover its lid and cook for 8 hours on Low setting.   Once done, remove its lid of the crockpot carefully.   Strain the slow-cooked tea into the serving glasses.   Serve warm.
Nutrition Info: Calories 214 Total Fat 19 g Saturated Fat 5.8 g Cholesterol 15 mg Sodium 123 mg Total Carbs 6.5 g Sugar 1.9 g Fiber 2.1 g Protein 6.5 g

609. Mini Chicken Meatballs

Servings: 4   Cooking Time: 2.5 Hours
Ingredients:
- 1 teaspoon hot sauce
- 7 oz ground chicken
- ½ onion, grated
- 1 teaspoon turmeric
- 1 teaspoon liquid stevia
- 1 teaspoon butter
- 1 egg white

Directions:
Mix the ground chicken and grated onion.   Add hot sauce, turmeric, liquid stevia, and egg white. Stir the mixture with a spoon.   Form the meatballs and place them in the slow cooker.   Add the butter and close the lid.   Cook the chicken meatballs for 2.5 hours on High.   Transfer the chicken meatballs onto a platter and serve!
Nutrition Info:calories 115, fat 4.7, fiber 0.4, carbs 1.7, protein 15.5

610. Almond Granola

Servings: 6   Cooking Time: 1.5 Hour
Ingredients:
- 1/3 cup coconut shred
- 1/4 cup almonds, chopped
- 1 tablespoon almond flour
- 2 eggs, whisked
- 1 teaspoon Erythritol
- 1 teaspoon ground cinnamon

Directions:
In the slow cooker, mix the almonds with the coconut and the other ingredients, stir and spread into the pot.   Cook granola on High for 1 hour. Then mix up the granola mixture well and cook it for 30 minutes more.   Chill the cooked granola well and store it in the glass jar.
Nutrition Info:calories 203, fat 12.3, fiber 3.1, carbs 5.9, protein 4.7

611. Eggplant Fries

Servings: 4   Cooking Time: 1.5 Hours
Ingredients:
- 1 eggplant
- 1 teaspoon paprika
- ½ teaspoon turmeric
- ½ teaspoon salt
- 1 tablespoon butter, melted
- ¼ cup coconut flour

Directions:
Cut the eggplant into medium sticks.   Sprinkle the eggplant sticks with the paprika, turmeric, and salt. Dip the eggplant sticks in the melted butter and coat in the coconut flour.   Place the eggplant sticks in the slow cooker and cook for 1.5 hours on High. Let the cooked eggplant fries cool slightly.   Enjoy!
Nutrition Info:calories 87, fat 4.2, fiber 6.8, carbs 11.2, protein 2.3

612. Chicken Bites

Servings: 4   Cooking Time: 4 Hours
Ingredients:
- 1-pound chicken fillet, roughly cubed
- 1 teaspoon turmeric powder
- 1 teaspoon yellow curry paste
- 1 oz Parmesan, grated
- ¼ cup butter

Directions:
In the slow cooker, mix the chicken with the curry paste and the other ingredients and toss.   Close the lid and the chicken tenders for 4 hours on High.
Nutrition Info:calories 336, fat 13.7, fiber 2.6, carbs 3.5, protein 16.5

613. Spicy & Salty Keto Nuts

Servings: 2   Cooking Time: 1 Hour
Ingredients:
- 1 oz walnuts, crushed
- 1 oz hazelnuts, crushed
- 1 oz pumpkin seeds
- 1 teaspoon salt
- 1 teaspoon olive oil
- 1 teaspoon garlic powder
- 1 Tablespoon Butter

1 teaspoon cayenne
pepper
Directions:
Place the walnuts, hazelnuts, and pumpkin seeds in the slow cooker.   Sprinkle them with the cayenne pepper, salt, olive oil, butter and garlic powder. Stir the mixture gently and close the lid.   Cook the nuts for 1 hour on High.   Then let the cooked mixture chill for 10 minutes.   Serve!
Nutrition Info:calories 292, fat 30, fiber 3.3, carbs 7.8, protein 9.4

614.   Flavorful Mexican Cheese Dip

Servings: 6   Cooking Time: 1 Hour
Ingredients:

¾ cup tomatoes with green chilies

8 oz. Velveeta cheese, cut into cube

Directions:
Add cheese into the slow cooker. Cover and cook on low for 30 minutes. Stir occasionally.   Add taco seasoning and tomatoes with green chilies and stir well.   Cover again and cook on low for 30 minutes more.   Stir well and serve.
Nutrition Info: Calories 159 Fat 12.6 g Carbohydrates 1.9 g Sugar 0.3 g Protein 9.6 g

615.   Bacon And Roasted Garlic Spinach Dip

Servings: 12   Cooking Time: 2 Hours
Ingredients:

1 cup sour cream
5 ounces parmesan cheese, grated
2 tablespoons roasted garlic
Salt to taste
16 ounces cream cheese, softened

Pepper to taste
10 ounces fresh spinach
3 tablespoons fresh parsley, chopped
2 tablespoons lemon juice

Directions:
Place a skillet over medium heat. Add bacon and cook until crisp.   Remove bacon with a slotted spoon and place on paper towels for a while to absorb excess grease.   Pour the bacon grease into the slow cooker.   Add all the ingredients including bacon into the slow cooker and stir.   Close the lid. Cook on 'Low' for 2 hours.   Serve warm, as it is or with keto crackers or vegetable sticks.
Nutrition Info: Calories322 Fat 27.8g Carbohydrate 4g Protein 15.1g

616.   Turkey Bites And Sauce

Servings: 3   Cooking Time: 3.5 Hours
Ingredients:

1-pound turkey breast, skinless, boneless and cubed
1 tablespoon butter
½ teaspoon ground coriander

1 teaspoon oregano, dried
1 teaspoon curry powder
1/3 cup keto tomato sauce

Directions:
In the slow cooker, mix the turkey with the butter, coriander and the other ingredients, stir and close the lid.   Cook the mix for 3.5 hours on High. Divide into bowls and serve.

Nutrition Info:calories 277, fat 11.2, fiber 5.3, carbs 8.4, protein 14.2

617.Chicken And Cauliflower Pizza

Servings: 6   Cooking Time: 5 Hours
Ingredients:

3 oz cauliflower, chopped
4 tablespoons almond flour
1 egg, beaten

¼ teaspoon salt
¼ teaspoon ground black pepper
2 oz ground chicken
1 teaspoon butter

Directions:
Mix the almond flour and beaten egg.   Add salt and ground black pepper.   Knead into a smooth dough.   Roll out the dough in the shape of pizza crust.   Rub the slow cooker bowl with the butter and place the pizza crust inside the bowl.   Place the ground chicken on top of the pizza crust. Sprinkle the ground chicken with the chopped cauliflower and close the lid.   Cook the pizza for 5 hours on Low.   Let the cooked pizza cool slightly then slice it into servings and enjoy!
Nutrition Info:calories 144, fat 11.4, fiber 2.4, carbs 4.9, protein 4.8

618.   Worcestershire Chicken

Servings: 5   Cooking Time: 4 Hours
Ingredients:

1 tablespoon Worcestershire sauce
1 tablespoon keto tomato sauce
1 teaspoon chili powder
1 teaspoon coriander, ground

1-pound chicken breast, skinless, boneless and cubed
1/3 teaspoon garlic powder
2 tablespoons butter, softened

Directions:
In the slow cooker, mix the chicken with the sauce and the other ingredients.   Close the lid and cook a snack for 4 hours on High.   Transfer the mix to bowls and serve.
Nutrition Info:calories 302, fat 20.7, fiber 4.3, carbs 12.7, protein 12.1

619.   Broccoli Balls

Servings: 4   Cooking Time: 2 Hours
Ingredients:

6 oz broccoli
1 egg
1 tablespoon almond flour

1 tablespoon butter
1 teaspoon dried parsley
2 oz Parmesan, grated

Directions:
Place the broccoli in a blender and blend until smooth.   Beat the egg into the broccoli.   Add almond flour, butter, and dried parsley.   Blend the mixture for 1 minute more at maximum speed. Transfer the broccoli mixture to a big bowl.   Add grated cheese and stir.   Make small balls from the mix and place them in the slow cooker.   Cook the broccoli balls for 2 hours on High.   Serve and enjoy!

Nutrition Info:calories 141, fat 10.7, fiber 1.9, carbs 4.9, protein 8.7

---

620. Sweet And Spicy Chicken Wings

Servings: 4   Cooking Time: 6 Hours
Ingredients:

4 chicken wings	1 tablespoon butter
1 tablespoon coconut flakes, unsweetened	½ teaspoon thyme
½ teaspoon chili flakes	½ teaspoon minced garlic
	1 teaspoon dried dill

Directions:
Mix the chili flakes, thyme, minced garlic, and dried dill together.   Sprinkle the chicken wings with the spices and coconut flakes.   Place the butter and chicken wings in the slow cooker and close the lid. Cook the chicken wings for 6 hours on Low.   Let the chicken wings cool a little.   Serve warm!
Nutrition Info:calories 33, fat 3.4, fiber 0.2, carbs 0.5, protein 0.4

---

621. Salsa Beef Dip

Servings: 20   Cooking Time: 1 Hour
Ingredients:

2 lbs. Velveeta cheese, cubed	2 lbs. ground beef

Directions:
Brown beef in a pan over medium heat. Drain well and transfer to the slow cooker.   Add cheese and salsa and stir well.   Cover slow cooker with lid and cook on high for 1 hour.   Stir well and serve.
Nutrition Info: Calories 279 Fat 17.9 g Carbohydrates 3.4 g Sugar 1.6 g Protein 25.8 g Cholesterol 88 mg

---

622. Sandwich With Roasted Pork

Servings: 15   Cooking Time: 8 Hours
Ingredients:

4 lb. pork roast	1 can of condensed cream of mushroom soup (undiluted)
6 oz. sliced mushrooms	
2 celery rib (finely chopped)	15 hard rolls (split)

Directions:
Cut the roast into two large pieces and keep in the crock pot.   Use a small bowl to mix the soup mixture along with the soup and celery and pour it over the meat in the pot and cook by covering it on low setting for 8 hours.   Just after 7 and half hours of cooking add the mushroom slices to the pot and continue cooking for the remaining time.   Take out the meat from the pot and allow a bit of cooling so that the meat can be easily shredded. Return them to the pot for heating up again.   Place the meat with the juices and vegetable in between the bread slices and serve.
Nutrition Info: Calories 203 Fat 18 g Carbohydrate 12 g Protein 7 g

---

623. Yummy Pumpkin Custard

Servings: 6   Cooking Time: 5 Hours
Ingredients:

2 tbsp coconut oil	¼ cup coconut milk
10 drops liquid stevia	6 eggs

Directions:
Pour 1 inch of water into the slow cooker.   Add all ingredients into the blender and blend until smooth. Spray ramekins with cooking spray.   Pour blended mixture into the prepared ramekins and place into the slow cooker.   Place ramekins into the slow cooker.   Cover slow cooker with lid and cook on high for 5 hours.   Serve warm and enjoy.
Nutrition Info: Calories 167 Fat 11.6 g Carbohydrates 10.8 g Sugar 4.7 g Protein 7.1 g Cholesterol 164 mg

---

624. Chili Walnuts

Servings: 3   Cooking Time: 2 Hours
Ingredients:

1 cup walnuts	1 egg white
1 teaspoon hot paprika	½ teaspoon chili powder
1 teaspoon salt	

Directions:
Whisk the egg white, paprika, salt and chili until you get foam.   Coat walnuts in the egg white mixture. Line the slow cooker bottom with baking paper and arrange coated walnuts.   Cook them for 2 hours on High.
Nutrition Info:calories 270, fat 10.1, fiber 4.7, carbs 6.3, protein 5.8

---

625. Fish Bites

Servings: 4   Cooking Time: 2.5 Hours
Ingredients:

1-pound salmon fillet, boneless and cubed	3 tablespoons coconut oil
½ teaspoon sweet paprika	½ cup keto tomato sauce

Directions:
In the slow cooker, mix the salmon with the paprika and the other ingredients.   Close the lid and cook the fish bites for 5 hours on High.
Nutrition Info:calories 224, fat 13.8, fiber 2.8, carbs 2.1, protein 8.1

---

626. Shrimp Skewers

Servings: 5   Cooking Time: 3 Hours
Ingredients:

1-pound shrimp, peeled and deveined	1 teaspoon Italian seasoning
2 tablespoons chives, chopped	1 teaspoon salt
1 tablespoon butter	¼ cup heavy cream

Directions:
In a bowl, mix the shrimp with chives, butter, seasoning and salt, toss and thread them on skewers Put the skewers in the slow cooker, add the cream on top and cook the appetizer for 3 hours on High.
Nutrition Info:calories 320, fat 18.9, fiber 3.1, carbs 10.8, protein 27.3

---

627. Cauliflower Popcorn

Servings: 4   Cooking Time: 6 Hours
Ingredients:

1 cup cauliflower florets

½ cup Parmesan, grated

1 teaspoon salt

1 teaspoon black pepper

1 teaspoon chili powder

1/3 cup heavy cream

Directions:
Put cauliflower florets in the slow cooker. Add the rest of the ingredients, toss and close the lid. Cook cauliflower popcorn for 6 hours on Low.

Nutrition Info:calories 210, fat 8.5, fiber 3.9, carbs 2.2, protein 4.3

628. Truffle Hot Chocolate

Servings: 4   Cooking Time: 2 Hours

Ingredients:

6 oz. 70% cacao dark baking chocolate, diced

3 tablespoons of stevia

1 teaspoon of instant espresso powder

Dash salt

1 teaspoon of vanilla extract

For Irish Whipped Cream:

1/2 cup of heavy whipping cream

1 tablespoon of Irish cream liqueur

Directions:
Start by throwing all the Ingredients: into the Crockpot except Irish whipped cream. Cover its lid and cook for 2 hours on Low setting. Once done, remove its lid of the crockpot carefully. Now mix whipping cream with Irish cream liqueur. Top the slow-cooked coffee with this cream mixture. Serve warm.

Nutrition Info: Calories 282 Total Fat 25.1 g Saturated Fat 8.8 g Cholesterol 100 mg Sodium 117 mg Total Carbs 9.4 g Sugar 0.7 g Fiber 3.2 g Protein 8 g

629. Lemon Blueberry Custard Cake

Servings: 6   Cooking Time: 3 Hours

Ingredients:

Lemon zest – 1 tsp.
Liquid stevia – 1 tsp.
Salt – ¼ tsp.
Blueberries – ¼ cup

Coconut flour – ¼ cup

Lemon juice – 3 tbsp.

Stevia – ¼ cup

Cream – 1 cup

Directions:
Separate eggs and whisk whites. Except for blueberries, mix all other ingredients with egg yolks. Slowly fold in egg whites. Put batter in the cooker. Pour in blueberries. Low cook for 3 hours. Cool and serve.

Nutrition Info: Calories: 140 Fat: 9g Carb: 5g Protein: 4g

630. Jalapeno Fritters

Servings: 4   Cooking Time: 3 Hours

Ingredients:

4 jalapeno peppers
1 egg, beaten
1 teaspoon cayenne pepper

½ teaspoon salt

1 teaspoon paprika

½ teaspoon garlic

2 tablespoons almond flour

powder

1 teaspoon butter

Directions:
Mix the beaten egg, cayenne pepper, salt, and almond flour. Add paprika and garlic powder and whisk the mixture until smooth. Melt the butter and place it in the slow cooker. Coat the jalapeno peppers in the egg batter well and transfer into the slow cooker. Cook the peppers for 3 hours on High. Let the cooked jalapenos cool slightly. Enjoy!

Nutrition Info:calories 114, fat 9.4, fiber 2.4, carbs 4.9, protein 4.8

631. Masala Green Beans Bowl

Servings: 4   Cooking Time: 3.5 Hours

Ingredients:

½ cup of water

½ teaspoon ground coriander

½ teaspoon garam masala

½ teaspoon salt

1 tablespoon butter

1 cup green beans, trimmed and halved

Directions:
In the slow cooker, mix the snap peas with the other ingredients. After this, close the slow cooker lid. Cook the mix for 5 hours on Low and serve.

Nutrition Info:calories 36, fat 3, fiber 0.6, carbs 3.5, protein 4.3

632. Bacon Dip

Servings: 4   Cooking Time: 4 Hours

Ingredients:

1 cup bacon, cooked and crumbled

1/4 cup spring onions, chopped

½ teaspoon salt

1 teaspoon ground black pepper

1 teaspoon smoked paprika

1/3 cup coconut cream

Directions:
In the slow cooker, mix the bacon with spring onions and the other ingredients. Close the slow cooker lid and cook meatballs for 4 hours on High.

Nutrition Info:calories 319, fat 22, fiber 4.3, carbs 12.3, protein 20.4

633. Herb Mixed Radish

Servings: 4   Cooking Time: 3 Hours

Ingredients:

½ cup of vegetable broth

2 tablespoons of basil, diced

1 tablespoon of oregano, diced

1 tablespoon of chives, diced

1 tablespoon of green onion, diced

A pinch of salt and black pepper

Directions:
Start by throwing all the ingredients into the Crockpot. Cover its lid and cook for 3 hours on Low setting. Once done, remove its lid of the crockpot carefully. Mix well and garnish as desired. Serve warm.

Nutrition Info: Calories 266 Total Fat 26.9 g Saturated Fat 15.8 g Cholesterol 18 mg Sodium 218 mg Total Carbs 2.5 g Sugar 0.4 g Fiber 0.2 g Protein 4.5 g

634.   Cheesecake

Servings: 6   Cooking Time: 2 Hours

Ingredients:

Butter – 2 tbsp.
Stevia to taste
Pecans – 1 cup
Egg – 1
Filling:
Cream cheese – 16 ounces

Stevia – 1 tsp.

Heavy cream – 4 tbsp.

Eggs – 2

Vanilla extract – 1 tsp.

Coconut flour – 1 tbsp.

Directions:
Grind nuts and mix with the remainder of the crust ingredients.   Shape into crust in the cooker. Mix filling ingredients.   Put in the crust.   Add one cup of water.   High cook for 2 hours.   Cool and serve.
Nutrition Info: Calories: 513 Fat: 49g Carb: 4.5g Protein: 14g

635.   Artichoke Hummus

Servings: 6   Cooking Time: 6 Hours

Ingredients:

10 oz artichoke, trimmed
1 tablespoon olive oil
3 tablespoons almond milk, unsweetened

2 tablespoons butter

¼ teaspoon salt
1 garlic clove
1 teaspoon ground black pepper

Directions:
Peel the garlic clove and place it in the slow cooker. Chop the artichoke and add into the slow cooker. Add the almond milk, salt, olive oil and ground black pepper. Stir well.   Cook the artichoke hummus for 6 hours on Low. Add water if you would like a softer hummus.   Transfer the mixture to a blender and blend until smooth.   Serve and enjoy!
Nutrition Info:calories 95, fat 8, fiber 2.8, carbs 5.8, protein 1.8

636.   Eggplant Bacon Fries

Servings: 7   Cooking Time: 2.5 Hours

Ingredients:

6 oz bacon, sliced
2 eggplants
¼ teaspoon ground nutmeg

1 teaspoon olive oil
1 teaspoon onion powder

Directions:
Cut the eggplant into the sticks and sprinkle them with the ground nutmeg and onion powder. Toss well.   Wrap the seasoned eggplant sticks in the sliced bacon.   Put the bacon fries in the slow cooker and add the olive oil.   Cook the bacon fries for 2.5 hours on High.   Serve the cooked meal immediately!
Nutrition Info:calories 178, fat 11.1, fiber 5.6, carbs 9.9, protein 10.6

637.   Mushroom Stuffed Meatballs

Servings: 4   Cooking Time: 3 Hours

Ingredients:

4 oz white mushrooms, chopped
1 oz Parmesan, grated
1 teaspoon olive oil
1 teaspoon onion powder

10 oz ground beef
1 tablespoon almond flour

½ teaspoon salt
1 teaspoon dried oregano

Directions:
Mix the ground beef, grated cheese, onion powder, almond flour, salt, and dried oregano and stir well. Make meatballs from the meat mixture and stuff them with the white mushrooms.   Place the meatballs in the slow cooker and add olive oil. Cook the meatballs for 3 hours on High.   Cool the cooked meatballs to room temperature and serve!
Nutrition Info:calories 214, fat 10.7, fiber 1.2, carbs 3.4, protein 26.3

638.   Creamy Dip

Servings: 6   Cooking Time: 1.5 Hours

Ingredients:

5 oz bacon, chopped
1 teaspoon turmeric powder
1/3 cup heavy cream
1 cup Mozzarella, shredded

1 teaspoon white pepper
½ teaspoon coriander, ground
1 teaspoon dried basil

Directions:
In the slow cooker, mix bacon with turmeric and the other ingredients, toss and close the lid.   Cook the cheese dip for 1.5 hours on High.
Nutrition Info:calories 220, fat 16.2, fiber 3, carbs 1.4, protein 8.8

639.   Herbed Cherry Tomatoes

Servings: 2   Cooking Time: 1 Hour

Ingredients:

A pinch of salt and black pepper
2 lbs. Cherry tomatoes halved
2 tablespoon of olive oil

1 tablespoon of dill, diced
½ cups of chicken stock
¼ cup of basil, diced

Directions:
Start by throwing all the ingredients into the Crockpot.   Cover its lid and cook for 1 hour on Low setting.   Once done, remove its lid of the crockpot carefully.   Mix well and garnish as desired. Serve warm.
Nutrition Info: Calories 145 Total Fat 13.1 g Saturated Fat 9.1 g Cholesterol 96 mg Sodium 35 mg Total Carbs 4 g Sugar 1.2 g Fiber 1.5 g Protein 3.5 g

640.   Lamb Steak Sandwich For Keto Diet

Servings: 8   Cooking Time: 7 Hours

Ingredients:

1 tbsp brown sugar
8 ketogenic French rolls (split)
1 clove of garlic, minced
2 tbsp water

Rings of pineapple
2 lb. boneless lamb chuck steak
1 tsp ground ginger
¼ cup melted butter

Chopped green
onions

Directions:
Lamb steak is to be cut into bite sized pieces and then placed into the crock pot. Mix the soy sauce with brown sugar, garlic and ginger and pour it over the steak pieces in the pot. Cook by covering the pot for 7 hours and then remove the meat from the pot. Skim out the fat from the cooking juice and add water to it to increase the volume. Pour the diluted juice in a saucepan and cook till it becomes bubbly and thick and then add the meat to it and hat up thoroughly. Bush the bread rolls with melted butter and then broil for 5 minutes to make them lightly roasted. Layer the sandwich with slices of onion and pineapple along with the cooked beef and serve.
Nutrition Info: Calories 210 Fat 19 g Carbohydrate 17 g Protein 9 g

641. Parmesan Green Beans

Servings: 2   Cooking Time: 3 Hours
Ingredients:

2 oz Parmesan, grated	5 oz green beans
¼ cup almond milk, unsweetened	1 teaspoon paprika

Directions:
Place the green beans in the slow cooker. Add almond milk and paprika. Stir and cook the green beans for 2 hours on High. Sprinkle the green beans with Parmesan cheese and cook for 1 hour more on High. Chill the cooked green beans slightly and serve!
Nutrition Info:calories 185, fat 13.5, fiber 3.5, carbs 8.3, protein 11.2

642. Peanut Butter Swirl Cake

Servings: 6   Cooking Time: 4 Hours
Ingredients:

Coconut flour – 2 tbsp.	Protein powder – 2 tbsp. whey and unflavored
Baking powder – 1 tsp.	Salt – ¼ tsp.
Peanut butter – 1/3 cup	Butter – ¼ cup
Eggs – 2	
Water – ¼ cup	Vanilla extract – ½ tsp.
Erythritol – 1/3 cup, powdered	Dark chocolate – 1 ounce, no sugar added

Directions:
Whisk coconut flour, almond flour, protein powder, salt, erythritol, and baking powder. Soften the peanut butter and melt the butter. Mix both of them into the dry mix. Add the eggs, water, and vanilla extract. Take .6 of the batter and put into the cooker. Add ½ ounce of chocolate and swirl. Add remaining batter and chocolate, and swirl. Low cook for 4 hours.
Nutrition Info: Calories: 335 Fat: 28g Carb: 6g Protein: 12g

643. Pulled Pork

Servings: 8   Cooking Time: 7 Hours
Ingredients:

1-pound pork shoulder	¼ teaspoon cayenne pepper
1 cup water	1 teaspoon tomato paste
¼ teaspoon peppercorn	1 tablespoon butter
¼ teaspoon ground ginger	
1 teaspoon paprika	

Directions:
Rub the pork shoulder with the cayenne pepper, peppercorns, ground ginger, paprika, cayenne pepper, and tomato paste. Let the pork shoulder marinate for 20 minutes in the fridge. Transfer the pork shoulder into the slow cooker. Add the butter and water. Close the lid and cook the pork shoulder for 7 hours on Low. Remove the pork shoulder from the slow cooker and shred it with two forks. Place the pork in a bowl and add ½ of the remaining liquid from the slow cooker. Stir the pulled pork and serve with keto bread, if desired.
Nutrition Info:calories 181, fat 13.6, fiber 0.2, carbs 0.5, protein 13.3

644. Pork Nuggets

Servings: 4   Cooking Time: 4 Hours
Ingredients:

8 oz pork loin	¼ teaspoon salt
1 egg white	1 teaspoon butter
1 teaspoon turmeric	¾ cup almond flour
1 teaspoon paprika	

Directions:
Cut the pork loin into one inch pieces. Whisk the egg and combine it with the paprika, turmeric, and salt. Dip the pork cubes into the egg mixture then coat the pork in the almond flour. Place the nuggets in the slow cooker and add butter. Close the lid and cook the nuggets for 4 hours on High. Cool the nuggets slightly. Serve!
Nutrition Info:calories 183, fat 11.6, fiber 0.9, carbs 1.9, protein 17.7

645. Pork Belly Bites

Servings: 4   Cooking Time: 3 Hours
Ingredients:

7 oz pork belly	¼ teaspoon ground coriander
¼ teaspoon thyme	
¼ teaspoon paprika	1 tablespoon butter

Directions:
Cut the pork belly into bite sized pieces and rub them with the thyme, paprika, and ground coriander. Place the butter in the slow cooker. Add the pork belly bites to the slow cooker and cook for 3 hours on High. Enjoy while hot!
Nutrition Info:calories 255, fat 16.3, fiber 0.1, carbs 0.1, protein 23

646. Mocha Pudding Cake

Servings: 6   Cooking Time: 3 Hours
Ingredients:

¾ c. butter – large chunks
½ c. heavy cream
2 oz. finely chopped chocolate - unsweetened
2 tbsp. instant coffee crystals
4 tbsp. unsweetened cocoa powder
1/3 c. almond flour

1/8 t. salt
1 t. vanilla extract
5 large eggs
2/3 c. stevia erythritol granulated sweetener
Low-carb whipped cream/ice cream – Optional Recommended: 4-6-quart slow cooker

Directions:
Grease the cooker with butter/spray.   Melt the unsweetened chocolate and butter in a small saucepan (medium heat). Whisk occasionally, remove from the heat, and cool.   Whisk the heavy cream, vanilla extract, and coffee crystals in a small container.   Mix together the almond flour, cocoa, and salt in another dish.   Whip the eggs using a mixer (high speed). Slowly add the sweetener when thickened. Beat on the high setting about five minutes.   Slowly, on the low setting, use the mixer to combine the unsweetened chocolate mixture and butter – adding it to the cake mixture.   Fold in the flour, salt, and cocoa mixture. Blend (medium speed), and add the coffee, cream, and vanilla ingredients.   Add the batter to the prepared slow cooker, and place a paper towel over the slow cooker top to absorb the moisture.   Secure the top and cook on low for 2 ½ to 3 ½ hours (4-quart cooker) or for 2-3 hours (6-quart cooker).   Test for doneness in the center at 160°F. The center will be a soft soufflé consistency with an outer cake-like appearance.
Nutrition Info: Calories: 413.5 Net Carbs: 3.76 g Fat: 29.81g Protein: 9.29 g

| 647. | **Savory Pine Nuts Cabbage** |

Servings: 2   Cooking Time: 2 Hours
Ingredients:

2 tablespoons of avocado oil
1 tablespoon of balsamic vinegar
¼ cup of pine nuts, toasted

½ cup of vegetable broth
Salt and black pepper- to taste

Directions:
Start by throwing all the ingredients into the Crockpot.   Cover its lid and cook for 2 hours on Low setting.   Once done, remove its lid of the crockpot carefully.   Mix well and garnish as desired.   Serve warm.
Nutrition Info: Calories 145 Total Fat 13.1 g Saturated Fat 9.1 g Cholesterol 96 mg Sodium 35 mg Total Carbs 4 g Sugar 1.2 g Fiber 1.5 g Protein 3.5 g

| 648. | **Pizza Dip** |

Servings: 4   Cooking Time: 5 Hours
Ingredients:

1 cup keto tomato sauce
½ cup Mozzarella, shredded

2 oz Parmesan, grated
1 teaspoon chili powder

1 teaspoon oregano, dried

½ teaspoon garlic powder
1 teaspoon butter

Directions:
In the slow cooker, mix the tomato sauce with the cheese and the other ingredients and close the lid. Cook the dip on Low for 5 hours.   Mix and serve.
Nutrition Info:calories 167, fat 4.9, fiber 2.3, carbs 3.1, protein 5.9

| 649. | **Spinach Rolls** |

Servings: 4   Cooking Time: 3 Hours
Ingredients:

1 cup spinach leaves
6 oz ground chicken
¼ teaspoon salt

¼ teaspoon paprika
¼ teaspoon turmeric
1 teaspoon butter

Directions:
Mix the ground chicken, salt, paprika, and turmeric. Place the ground chicken mixture in the slow cooker. Add the butter and cook on High for 3 hours.   Stir the cooked ground chicken mixture.   Place the ground chicken mixture in the spinach leaves and roll them up, enclosing the meat inside the leaf. Secure the rolls with the toothpicks and serve!
Nutrition Info:calories 92, fat 4.2, fiber 0.3, carbs 0.4, protein 12.6

| 650. | **Cheese Sticks** |

Servings: 8   Cooking Time: 2.5 Hours
Ingredients:

4 eggs, beaten
1 cup Cheddar cheese, shredded
1 tablespoon fresh dill, chopped
1 tablespoon chives, chopped

1 teaspoon turmeric powder
1 teaspoon butter, softened
1/3 cup almond flour
1 teaspoon salt

Directions:
In the mixing bowl, mix up together beaten eggs, cheese and the other ingredients. You should get a soft homogenous mixture.   Line the bottom of the slow cooker with the baking paper.   Transfer the cheese mixture in the slow cooker and flatten well. Close the lid and bake it for 2.5 hours on High. Then chill the cooked mixture very well and cut into the serving sticks.
Nutrition Info:calories 304, fat 8.3, fiber 4.5, carbs 1.6, protein 7

| 651. | **Chestnut Cream** |

Servings: 6   Cooking Time: 3 Hours
Ingredients:

11 oz. water

1 ½ lbs. chestnuts

Directions:
In your slow cooker, mix sugar with water and chestnuts, stir, cover and cook on Low for 3 hours. Blend using your immersion blender, divide into small cups and serve.   Enjoy!
Nutrition Info: Calories: 102 Total Fat: 1 g Net Carbs: 5 g Protein: 3 g

652.	Shrimp Meatballs

Servings: 4   Cooking Time: 3 Hours

Ingredients:
- 1 cup shrimp, cooked, peeled and minced
- 1 egg white
- 1 teaspoon salt
- ½ teaspoon ground black pepper
- ½ teaspoon turmeric
- 1 teaspoon oregano, dried
- ¼ cup of water
- 1 teaspoon avocado oil
- ¼ cup spring onions, chopped

Directions:
In the mixing bowl, combine the shrimp with egg white and the other ingredients except the oil and water, stir and make small meatballs.   Transfer the meatballs in the slow cooker.   Add coconut oil and water.   Close the lid and cook meatballs for 3 hours on Low.

Nutrition Info: calories 195, fat 7.3, fiber 2.5, carbs 1.4, protein 12.6

653.	Crab Dip With Mushrooms

Servings: 4   Cooking Time: 6 Hours

Ingredients:
- 3 oz crab meat
- 2 oz white mushrooms, chopped
- ¼ teaspoon minced garlic
- 5 oz Cheddar cheese, shredded
- ¾ cup almond milk
- ¼ teaspoon paprika

Directions:
Chop the crab meat and place it in the slow cooker. Add the chopped mushrooms, minced garlic, shredded cheese, and almond milk.   Add the paprika and stir the mixture.   Cook the dip for 6 hours on Low.   Then use the hand blender to puree the dip until smooth.   Transfer the dip into a bowl and enjoy!

Nutrition Info: calories 269, fat 22.9, fiber 1.2, carbs 3.9, protein 13

654.	Asian Pork With Keto Tortillas

Servings: 6   Cooking Time: 6 Hours

Ingredients:
- 6 keto tortillas
- 9 oz pork tenderloin
- 1 tablespoon apple cider vinegar
- 1 teaspoon olive oil
- ½ teaspoon thyme
- 1 teaspoon curry paste
- 1 teaspoon sesame seeds
- ¼ cup water

Directions:
Chop the pork tenderloins and sprinkle them with the apple cider vinegar, olive oil, thyme, curry paste, and sesame seeds.   Stir the meat well and let sit for 30 minutes to marinate.   Transfer the meat to the slow cooker and add water.   Close the lid and cook the meat for 6 hours on Low.   Place the cooked meat on the tortillas and roll. Serve warm!

Nutrition Info: calories 227, fat 11, fiber 4.1, carbs 8.4, protein 23.3

655.	Glazed Walnuts

Servings: 8   Cooking Time: 2 Hours

Ingredients:
- Keto sweetener – ¼ cup
- Butter – ¼ cup
- Vanilla extract – ½ tsp.

Directions:
Put all ingredients in the slow cooker.   Cook on low for 2 hours.   Cool and serve.

Nutrition Info: Calories: 264 Fat: 24g Carb: 8g Protein: 4g

656.	Bacon Chicken Chowder

Servings: 4   Cooking Time: 8 Hours

Ingredients:
- Leek – 1
- Mushrooms – 3 ounces
- Butter – 2 tbsp.
- Chicken – ½ pound
- Heavy cream – ½ cup
- Salt – ½ tsp.
- Garlic powder – ½ tsp.
- Shallot – 1
- Celery – 1 rib
- Sweet onion – ½
- Chicken stock – 1 cup
- Cream cheese – 4 ounces
- Bacon – ½ pound
- Black pepper – ½ tsp.
- Thyme – ½ tsp. dried

Directions:
Chop the onion, celery, shallot, bacon, chicken, mushrooms, leek, and dice the garlic.   Cook the chicken until done.   Add all the ingredients to the cooker.   Stir everything well.   Cook on low for 8 hours.

Nutrition Info: Calories: 355 Fat: 28g Carb: 6.4g Protein: 21g

657.	Crunchy Bacon

Servings: 6   Cooking Time: 1.5 Hours

Ingredients:
- 1 teaspoon liquid stevia
- 7 oz bacon, sliced
- ½ teaspoon butter

Directions:
Place the butter in the slow cooker.   Add the sliced bacon and sprinkle it with the liquid stevia.   Close the lid and cook the bacon for 1 hour on High. Turn the bacon over onto the other side and cook it for 30 minutes more on High.   Serve the bacon chilled.

Nutrition Info: calories 182, fat 14.1, fiber 0, carbs 0.5, protein 12.3

658.	Gingerbread

Servings: 10   Cooking Time: 3 Hours - 15 Minutes

Ingredients:
- 2 tbsp. coconut flour
- ¾ c. swerve sweetener
- 1 ½ tbsp. ground ginger
- 1 tbsp. dark cocoa powder
- ½ tbsp. ground
- ½ t. ground cloves
- ½ c. melted butter
- ⅔ c. water/almond milk
- 4 large eggs
- 1 t. vanilla extract
- 1 tbsp. freshly

cinnamon
¼ t. salt
2 t. baking powder

squeezed lemon juice
Recommended: 6-quart slow cooker

Directions:
Prepare the cooker with some cooking spray/oil. Whisk the all of the flour, salt, cloves, baking powder, cinnamon, ginger, sweetener, and cocoa powder in a large mixing bowl   Blend in the eggs, melted butter, almond milk/water, vanilla extract, and lemon juice.   Empty the batter into the slow cooker and cook until set - approximately   ½ to 3 hours.   Garnish as desired and enjoy, but count those carbs.

Nutrition Info: Calories: 223 Net Carbs: 8.58 g Fat: 24.79 g Protein: 9.07 g

659.   Salmon Spread

Servings: 6   Cooking Time: 2 Hours

Ingredients:

1 teaspoon hot paprika
6 oz salmon fillets, boneless, skinless and minced
¼ cup coconut cream

2 tablespoons Ricotta cheese
½ cup Cheddar cheese, shredded
½ teaspoon Italian seasoning

Directions:
In the slow cooker, mix the salmon with paprika, cream and the remaining ingredients, whisk and close the lid.   Cook the mass on Low for 2 hours. Divide into bowls and serve.

Nutrition Info:calories 209, fat 7.2, fiber 2.7, carbs 11.4, protein 4.3

660.   Ground Chicken Pepper Meatballs

Servings: 4   Cooking Time: 3 Hours

Ingredients:

11 oz ground chicken
1 bell pepper
1 teaspoon salt
1 teaspoon butter
1 teaspoon dried dill

1 teaspoon dried oregano
1 egg yolk
½ teaspoon ground ginger

Directions:
Chop the bell pepper and place it in a blender. Blend the bell pepper until smooth.   Mix the bell pepper puree with the ground chicken.   Add salt, dried dill, dried oregano, and ground ginger.   Add egg yolk and stir carefully.   Make small meatballs and place them in the slow cooker.   Add butter and close the lid.   Cook the meatballs for 3 hours. Serve the appetizer hot!

Nutrition Info:calories 182, fat 8, fiber 0.6, carbs 2.9, protein 23.6

661.   Spiced Punch

Servings: 4   Cooking Time: 3 Hours

Ingredients:

3 cups of apricot nectar
3 tablespoons of lemon juice
1/2 teaspoon of ground cardamom

1/4 cup of water
2 cinnamon sticks (3 inches)
1 teaspoon of diced fresh ginger root
1 teaspoon of grated

1/2 teaspoon of ground nutmeg

orange peel
8 whole cloves

Directions:
Start by throwing all the Ingredients: into the Crockpot.   Cover its lid and cook for 3 hours on Low setting.   Once done, remove its lid of the crockpot carefully.   Strain the slow-cooked tea into the serving glasses.   Serve warm.

Nutrition Info: Calories 331 Total Fat 38.5 g Saturated Fat 19.2 g Cholesterol 141 mg Sodium 283 mg Total Carbs 9.2 g Sugar 3 g Fiber 1 g Protein 2.1 g

662.   Beef & Mushroom – Super Combo Sandwich

Servings: 12   Cooking Time: 8 Hours

Ingredients:

4 lb. boneless beef chuck roast
1 tsp salt
½ lb. fresh mushrooms
2 medium carrots, cut into chunks
2 tbsp. olive oil
6 cloves of garlic, halved

1 medium onion, cut into wedges
2 tbsp. dried oregano
32 oz. beef broth
1 tbsp. beef base
16 oz. giardiniera, drained
12 Ketogenic Italian rolls, split

Directions:
Cut the roast into two equal pieces and sprinkle with pepper and salt, cook it in a skillet so that it becomes brown from all sides and then put it in the crock pot. Use a food processor to make the mixture of mushrooms, carrot, garlic, onion and oregano and pour the mixture into the slow crock pot.   Cover the pot and cook on low setting for 8 hours, making sure that the meat is tender.   Remove the meat from the pot and shred with forks. Skim out the fat from the cooking juices and return the shredded meat to the pot to heat up thoroughly.   Put the required amount of beef mixture on the buns and serve.

Nutrition Info: Calories 170 Fat 19 g Carbohydrate 9 g Protein 9 g

663.   Viennese Coffee

Servings: 2   Cooking Time: 2.5 Hours

Ingredients:

3 tablespoons of sugar-free chocolate syrup
1/3 cup of heavy whipping cream

1 teaspoon of stevia
1/4 cup of crème de cacao
Whipped cream, optional

Directions:
Start by throwing all the ingredients into the Crockpot.   Cover its lid and cook for 5 hours on Low setting.   Once done, remove its lid of the crockpot carefully.   Garnish with whipped cream. Serve warm.

Nutrition Info: Calories 231 Total Fat 32.9 g Saturated Fat 6.1 g Cholesterol 10 mg Sodium 18 mg Total Carbs 9.1 g Sugar 2.8 g Fiber 0.8 g Protein 4.4 g

664. Carrots And Cauliflower Spread

Servings: 4   Cooking Time: 7 Hours
Ingredients:
- 1½ c. cauliflower florets
- 1/3 c. cashews
- ½ c. chopped turnips
- 2½ c. water
- 1 c. coconut milk
- 1 tsp. garlic powder
- ¼ c. nutritional yeast
- ¼ tsp. smoked paprika
- ¼ tsp. mustard powder
- Salt
- Black pepper

Directions:
In your slow cooker, mix carrots with cauliflower, cashews, turnips and water, stir, cover and cook on Low for 7 hours.   Drain, transfer to a blender, add milk, garlic powder, yeast, paprika, mustard powder, salt and pepper, blend well, divide into bowls and serve as a party spread. Enjoy!
Nutrition Info: Calories: 291 Total Fat: 7 g Net Carbs: 14 g Protein: 3 g

665. Ketogenic Sloppy Joes From Crock Pot

Servings: 8   Cooking Time: 4 Hours
Ingredients:
- ½ cup ketchup
- 10 oz. condensed tomato soup (undiluted)
- 2 tbsp. prepared mustard
- 8 ketogenic hamburger buns, split
- 1 lb. lean ground turkey
- ¼ cup green pepper, chopped
- ½ cup chopped celery
- ¼ tsp pepper
- 1 tbsp. brown sugar

Directions:
Use a large skillet to cook the turkey with cooking spray along with onion, celery and pepper, making sure that the meat is no longer pink in color. Discard the excess juices and mix the tomato soup along with mustard, ketchup, pepper and brown sugar.   Pour the entire mixture into Slow Cookerand cook by covering for 4 hours on low setting.   Put the meat in between the bun and serve.
Nutrition Info: Calories 230 Fat 20 g Carbohydrate 16 g Protein 9 g

666. Eggplant Bread

Servings: 4   Cooking Time: 7 Hours
Ingredients:
- 2 eggplants, chopped
- 2 eggs, beaten
- 3 tablespoons coconut cream
- 1 teaspoon garam masala
- 2 tablespoons almond flour
- ½ teaspoon baking soda
- 1 teaspoon lime juice
- ½ teaspoon ground black pepper
- 1 teaspoon butter, melted

Directions:
Line the slow cooker bottom with the baking paper. In the mixing bowl, mix up together eggs with the eggplants and the other ingredients, and stir really well.   Transfer the eggplant bread mixture in the slow cooker and flatten it well.   Close the lid and cook zucchini bread for 7 hours on Low.
Nutrition Info:calories 186, fat 12.1, fiber 4.6, carbs 11.2, protein 7.5

667. Seasoned Mini Meatballs

Servings: 8   Cooking Time: 3 Hours
Ingredients:
- ¼ cup spinach
- 1 egg
- 1 tablespoon almond flour
- 1 tablespoon olive oil
- ½ teaspoon salt
- 1 teaspoon paprika
- 8 oz ground beef
- 1 teaspoon dried oregano

Directions:
Beat the egg in a mixing bowl.   Blend the spinach in a blender until smooth.   Add the blended spinach into the whisked egg.   Add almond flour, salt, paprika, ground beef, and dried oregano and mix well.   Make mini meatballs using 2 teaspoons to form the balls and place them in the slow cooker. Add olive oil and cook for 3 hours on High.   Chill the meatballs slightly and serve!
Nutrition Info:calories 97, fat 5.9, fiber 0.6, carbs 1.1, protein 10.1

668. Mozzarella Broccoli Bites

Servings: 8   Cooking Time: 4 Hours
Ingredients:
- 1-pound broccoli florets
- 1 cup Mozzarella, shredded
- 1 teaspoon turmeric powder
- 1 tablespoon butter, melted
- 1 teaspoon salt
- 1 teaspoon chili powder
- 2 egg, beaten

Directions:
In a bowl, mix the broccoli with the other ingredients except the butter and toss.   Grease the slow cooker with the butter and arrange the broccoli bites inside.   Close the lid and cook the appetizer for 4 hours on High.   Arrange on a platter and serve.
Nutrition Info:calories 264, fat 4.9, fiber 3.5, carbs 12.3, protein 4.6

669. Cocktail Shrimp

Servings: 4   Cooking Time: 2 Hours
Ingredients:
- 10 oz shrimp, peeled and deveined
- ½ cup crushed tomatoes
- 1 teaspoon sweet paprika
- 1 teaspoon olive oil
- 1 teaspoon chili pepper
- 1 teaspoon onion powder

Directions:
In the slow cooker, mix the shrimp with the other ingredients.   Close the lid and cook sausages for 2 hours on High.
Nutrition Info:calories 235, fat 11.3, fiber 1.1, carbs 3.1, protein 11.6

670. Garlic Bread With Cheese

Servings: 8   Cooking Time: 2 Hours

Ingredients:

2 c. Italian cheese blend/shredded mozzarella – divided	½ t. of each: Pepper & salt 2 minced garlic cloves
2 large eggs	Olive oil non-stick spray
3 tbsp. coconut flour/your choice	Recommended: 6-qt. cooker
¼ c. freshly chopped basil	

Directions:
Grease the sides and bottom of the cooker with the cooking spray. Process the cauliflower until it's rice-like in a food processor. Combine the cheese, eggs, flour, pepper, and salt. Mix well and press firmly into the slow cooker. Shake the rest of the cheese and garlic on top. Prepare on high for two to four hours. The cheese will be melted, and edges browned when it is done. Slice and sprinkle with the basil. Enjoy while warm.
Nutrition Info: Calories: 224 Net Carbs: 5.63 g Fat: 14.95 g Protein: 15.29 g

671. Mushroom Skewers

Servings: 4   Cooking Time: 4 Hours
Ingredients:

6 oz white mushrooms, roughly chopped	1 eggplant, peeled
1 tablespoon butter, melted	1 teaspoon dried parsley
1 teaspoon minced garlic	½ teaspoon ground black pepper

Directions:
Chop the eggplant roughly. Mix the white mushrooms, eggplant, minced garlic, dried parsley, and ground black pepper. Stir the vegetables and slide them onto skewers. Place the skewers in the slow cooker and add butter. Cook the skewers for 4 hours on Low. Serve the meal!
Nutrition Info:calories 65, fat 3.2, fiber 4.6, carbs 8.6, protein 2.6

672. Cauliflower Fritters

Servings: 6   Cooking Time: 2.5 Hours
Ingredients:

8 oz cauliflower	1 tablespoon butter
1 egg	1 teaspoon dried oregano
2 tablespoons almond flour	

Directions:
Chop the cauliflower roughly and place them in a blender. Blend the cauliflower until smooth and transfer into a mixing bowl. Add the almond flour and dried oregano. Add the beaten egg and stir it well. Make into medium fritters. Place the butter in the slow cooker and add the fritters. Cook the cauliflower fritters for 2.5 hours on High. Serve the meal!
Nutrition Info:calories 91, fat 7.4, fiber 2.1, carbs 4.2, protein 3.7

673. Nutmeg Fennel

Servings: 2   Cooking Time: 3 Hours
Ingredients:

2 tablespoon of olive oil	2 and ½ cups of baby spinach
4 garlic cloves, diced	½ teaspoon of nutmeg, ground
2 tablespoons of balsamic vinegar	¼ cup of vegetable broth

Directions:
Start by throwing all the ingredients into the Crockpot. Cover its lid and cook for 3 hours on Low setting. Once done, remove its lid of the crockpot carefully. Mix well and garnish as desired. Serve warm.
Nutrition Info: Calories 244 Total Fat 24.8 g Saturated Fat 15.6 g Cholesterol 32 mg Sodium 204 mg Total Carbs 2.1 g Sugar 0.4 g Fiber 0.1 g Protein 24 g

674. Sausage Bites And Sauce

Servings: 6   Cooking Time: 3 Hours
Ingredients:

1-pound smoked sausages, sliced	½ teaspoon minced garlic
½ cup keto tomato sauce	1 teaspoon coriander, ground
1 teaspoon butter	1 teaspoon sweet paprika
1 teaspoon chili powder	

Directions:
In the slow cooker, mix the sausages with tomato sauce and the other ingredients, toss, close the lid and cook for 3 hours on High. Transfer in the serving bowls serve.
Nutrition Info:calories 307, fat 22.9, fiber 4.8, carbs 12.5, protein 9.9

675. Sugar-free Fudge

Servings: 30   Cooking Time: 2 Hours
Ingredients:

1/3 c. coconut milk	2 t. vanilla liquid stevia - optional
Dash of salt	Recommended: 3-4-quart slow cooker
1 t. pure vanilla extract	

Directions:
Mix all of the goodies in the cooker. Close the lid and cook for two hours on the low setting. Take the lid off and unplug the unit. Don't stir for 30 minutes to one hour. Lastly, mix for five minutes until creamy smooth. Line a one-quart dish with some parchment paper. Spread the fudge into the dish, and chill until firm.
Nutrition Info: Calories: 65 Net Carbs: 2 g Fat: 5 g Protein: 1 g

676. Chicken Dip

Servings: 4   Cooking Time: 4 Hours
Ingredients:

1 teaspoon chives, chopped	1 cup ground chicken
½ cup keto tomato sauce	1 teaspoon basil, dried
1 tablespoon olive oil	¼ teaspoon minced garlic

3 oz Parmesan,
grated

Directions:
In the slow cooker, mix the chicken with the tomato sauce and the other ingredients, whisk and close the lid.   Cook the dip for 4 hours on High, divide into bowls and serve.
Nutrition Info:calories 236, fat 7.2, fiber 5.1, carbs 6.5, protein 17

677.   Cauliflower Bites

Servings: 4   Cooking Time: 2 Hours
Ingredients:

7 oz cauliflower florets	1 egg, beaten
1 tablespoon almond flour	¼ teaspoon chili pepper
	2 tablespoons butter

Directions:
Mix the almond flour and chili pepper together. Dip the cauliflower florets into the whisked egg. Then, coat them in the almond flour mixture. Toss the butter into the slow cooker.   Add the dipped cauliflower florets and close the lid   Cook the cauliflower for 2 hours on High.   When the cauliflower bites are cooked, let them cool slightly. Serve!
Nutrition Info:calories 119, fat 10.4, fiber 2, carbs 4.2, protein 3.9

678.   Coconut Mushrooms Caps

Servings: 4   Cooking Time: 6 Hours
Ingredients:

1 cup cremini mushroom caps	2 tablespoons olive oil
¼ cup spring onions, chopped	1 teaspoon salt
1 teaspoon sweet paprika	1 teaspoon black pepper
1 teaspoon garlic powder	½ teaspoon ground turmeric
	¾ cup coconut cream

Directions:
In the slow cooker, mix the mushroom caps with the spring onions, paprika and the other ingredients and toss.   Close the lid and cook mushroom caps for 6 hours on Low.
Nutrition Info:calories 246, fat 22.1, fiber 4.4, carbs 12.2, protein 1.3

679.   Cauliflower Bread

Servings: 6   Cooking Time: 4 Hours
Ingredients:

7 oz cauliflower	1 tablespoon Psyllium husk powder
1 egg, beaten	
3 tablespoons almond flour	1 teaspoon olive oil
¼ teaspoon salt	¼ teaspoon chili flakes
3 tablespoons coconut flour	¼ teaspoon ground black pepper

Directions:
Chop the cauliflower into tiny pieces and add the egg. Stir the mixture well and add the almond flour.

Sprinkle the mixture with the salt, coconut flour, Psyllium husk powder, olive oil, chili flakes, and ground black pepper.   Knead into a soft dough. Transfer the dough to a slow cooker and cook for 4 hours on High.   When the bread is cooked, cool it slightly then slice.   Enjoy!
Nutrition Info:calories 126, fat 8.9, fiber 8, carbs 8.7, protein 5.1

680.   Smoked Hazelnuts

Servings: 6   Cooking Time: 2. 5 Hours
Ingredients:

1 tablespoon smoked paprika	1 tablespoon butter
1 teaspoon turmeric powder	½ cup hazelnuts, chopped

Directions:
In the slow cooker, mix the hazelnuts with the paprika and the other ingredients and toss.   Close the lid and cook the mixture for 5 hours on Low. Divide into bowls and serve.
Nutrition Info:calories 218, fat 8.5, fiber 1.4, carbs 6.9, protein 3.9

681.   Zucchini Tots With Cheese

Servings: 6   Cooking Time: 3 Hours
Ingredients:

1 zucchini, grated	½ teaspoon salt
3 oz Parmesan, grated	1 egg
1 teaspoon dried dill	1 tablespoon almond flour
1 teaspoon dried oregano	1 tablespoon butter

Directions:
Mix the zucchini, Parmesan, dried dill, dried oregano, salt, almond flour, and beaten egg.   Stir the mixture until smooth.   Form small tots and place them in the slow cooker. The mixture should not be liquid so add more almond flour if needed in order to form the tots.   Add butter to the slow cooker and close the lid.   Cook the zucchini tots for 3 hours on High.   Chill the zucchini tots to room temperature and serve!
Nutrition Info:calories 106, fat 8.1, fiber 1, carbs 2.9, protein 7

682.   Citrus Rich Cabbage

Servings: 2   Cooking Time: 3 Hours
Ingredients:

½ cup of chicken stock	1 tablespoon of chives, diced
A pinch of salt and black pepper	1 tablespoon of lemon zest (grated)
1 tablespoon of lemon juice	

Directions:
Start by throwing all the ingredients into the Crockpot.   Cover its lid and cook for 3 hours on Low setting.   Once done, remove its lid of the crockpot carefully.   Mix well and garnish as desired.   Serve warm.
Nutrition Info: Calories 145 Total Fat 13.1 g Saturated Fat 9.1 g Cholesterol 96 mg Sodium 35

mg Total Carbs 4 g Sugar 1.2 g Fiber 1.5 g Protein 3.5 g

683. Creamy Mustard Asparagus

Servings: 2   Cooking Time: 3 Hours
Ingredients:

2 teaspoons of mustard	1 tablespoon of chives, diced
¼ cup of coconut cream	Salt and black pepper- to taste
2 garlic cloves, minced	

Directions:
Start by throwing all the ingredients into the Crockpot.   Cover its lid and cook for 3 hours on Low setting.   Once done, remove its lid of the crockpot carefully.   Mix well and garnish as desired.   Serve warm.
Nutrition Info: Calories 149 Total Fat 14.5 g Saturated Fat 8.1 g Cholesterol 56 mg Sodium 56 mg Total Carbs 10.6 g Sugar 0.3 g Fiber 0.2 g Protein 2.6 g

684. Butter Pork Ribs

Servings: 4   Cooking Time: 7 Hours
Ingredients:

10 oz pork ribs	1/3 cup coconut cream
3 tablespoons butter, soft	½ teaspoon salt
1 teaspoon turmeric powder	1 teaspoon garlic powder

Directions:
In the slow cooker, mix the pork with soft butter and the other ingredients.   Close the lid and cook the pork ribs for 7 hours on Low.
Nutrition Info:calories 321, fat 14.8, fiber 4.5, carbs 6.5, protein 19.7

685. Buffalo Chicken Wings

Servings: 4   Cooking Time: 7 Hours
Ingredients:

10 oz chicken wings	2 tablespoons butter
¾ cup hot sauce	1 teaspoon cayenne pepper
1 teaspoon minced garlic	1 teaspoon paprika

Directions:
Mix the hot sauce, minced garlic, butter, cayenne pepper, and paprika.   Mix the chicken wings with the sauce.   Place the chicken wings and all the sauce in the slow cooker.   Cook the chicken wings for 7 hours on Low.   Serve the chicken wings immediately!
Nutrition Info:calories 194, fat 11.3, fiber 0.5, carbs 1.5, protein 21

686. Wrapped Prawns In Bacon

Servings: 2   Cooking Time: 2 Hours
Ingredients:

6 oz prawns, peeled	¼ teaspoon minced garlic
2 oz bacon, sliced	
1 teaspoon butter	

Directions:
Mix the minced garlic and butter.   Rub the prawns in the butter mixture.   Wrap them in the sliced bacon.   Transfer the prawns to the slow cooker and cook for 2 hours on High.   Serve the cooked prawns and enjoy!
Nutrition Info:calories 272, fat 15.2, fiber 0, carbs 1.8, protein 29.9

687. Sweet Kahlua Coffee

Servings: 4   Cooking Time: 4 Hours
Ingredients:

1/2 cup of Kahlua (coffee liqueur)	1/4 cup of crème de cacao
3 tablespoons of instant coffee granules	1/4 cup of stevia
	1 teaspoon of vanilla extract
2 cups of heavy whipping cream, to garnish	2 tablespoons of sugar-free chocolate chips, to garnish

Directions:
Start by throwing all the Ingredients: into the Crockpot.   Cover its lid and cook for 4 hours on Low setting.   Once done, remove its lid of the crockpot carefully.   Garnish with whipping cream and chocolate chips.   Serve warm.
Nutrition Info: Calories 213 Total Fat 28.4 g Saturated Fat 12.1 g Cholesterol 27 mg Sodium 39 mg Total Carbs 9.2 g Sugar 3.1 g Fiber 4.6 g Protein 8.1 g

688. Onion Rings

Servings: 6   Cooking Time: 2 Hours
Ingredients:

1 big onion, peeled	1 tablespoon coconut flakes
1/3 cup almond flour	1 teaspoon ground black pepper
1 egg, beaten	1 teaspoon butter
2 tablespoons almond milk, unsweetened	

Directions:
Slice the onion and separate it into the rings.   Mix the almond milk and ground black pepper.   Add the beaten egg and whisk.   Dip the onion rings in the whisked egg mixture then coat the onion rings in the almond flour.   Toss the butter into the slow cooker and add the onion rings.   Cook the onion rings for 2 hours on High.   Serve the onion rings hot!
Nutrition Info:calories 50, fat 3.7, fiber 1, carbs 3.4, protein 1.7

689. Cinnamon Pecans

Servings: 6   Cooking Time: 3 Hours
Ingredients:

10 drops liquid stevia	1 ½ tsp vanilla extract
1 tbsp cinnamon	¾ tsp salt

Directions:
Spray slow cooker from inside with cooking spray. Add all ingredients to the slow cooker and stir well. Cover slow cooker with lid and cook on low for 2 hours. Stir after 1 hour.   Transfer pecans mixture onto a baking sheet.   Allow to cool completely then serve.

Nutrition Info: Calories 146 Fat 14.7 g Carbohydrates 3.7 g Sugar 0.8 g Protein 2.1 g Cholesterol 0 mg

690.	Hot Spiced Wine

Servings: 2   Cooking Time: 3 Hours

Ingredients:

- 3 whole cloves
- 3 medium pears, peeled and sliced
- 2 cups of sugar-free apple juice
- 1/2 cup of stevia
- 1 teaspoon of lemon juice
- 2 bottles (750 ml) dry red wine

Directions:

Start by tying the whole spices in cheesecloth. Now place the tied spices along with all the ingredients into the Crockpot.   Cover its lid and cook for 3 hours on Low setting.   Once done, remove its lid of the crockpot carefully.   Strain the slow-cooked tea into the serving glass.   Serve warm.

Nutrition Info: Calories 220 Total Fat 20.1 g Saturated Fat 7.4 g Cholesterol 132 mg Sodium 157 mg Total Carbs 3 g Sugar 0.4 g Fiber 2.4 g Protein 6.1 g

691.	Cheesy Zucchini Crisps

Servings: 2   Cooking Time: 2.5 Hours

Ingredients:

- 2 oz zucchini, sliced
- 1 oz Parmesan, grated
- 1 teaspoon olive oil
- ½ teaspoon chili flakes

Directions:

Place the olive oil in the slow cooker.   Place the zucchini slices in the slow cooker in one layer. Sprinkle the zucchini slices with chili flakes and grated Parmesan.   Close the lid and cook the zucchini for 2.5 hours on High.   Serve the cooked snack immediately!

Nutrition Info:calories 70, fat 5.4, fiber 0.3, carbs 1.5, protein 4.9

Dessert Recipes

692. Keto Brownies

Servings: 8   Cooking Time: 3 Hours

Ingredients:

1 teaspoon baking soda	1 oz dark chocolate
2 teaspoons liquid stevia	1 cup almond flour
1 teaspoon vanilla extract	3 tablespoons butter, melted
1 teaspoon ground cinnamon	1 egg, beaten
	1 tablespoon full-fat cream

Directions:

Melt the chocolate and mix it with the liquid stevia vanilla extract and ground cinnamon.   Add the butter and almond flour.   Add the egg and cream. Stir the mixture until smooth.   Transfer the mixture to the slow cooker. Flatten it gently and cook for 3 hours on High.   Cut the cooked dessert into the servings.   Enjoy!

Nutrition Info:calories 43, fat 3, fiber 0.3, carbs 2.6, protein 1.3

693. Tapioca Pudding

Servings: 2   Cooking Time: 4 Hours

Ingredients:

½ cup of small pearl tapioca	2 egg yolks
½ cup of erythritol	½ teaspoon of vanilla extract
Pinch of salt	
½ cup of almond milk	¼ cup of fresh raspberries

Directions:

Start by throwing all the Ingredients: into the Crockpot except berries.   Cover its lid and cook for 3-4 hours on Low setting.   Once done, remove its lid of the crockpot carefully.   Allow it to cool and refrigerate for 1 hour.   Garnish with berries. Serve.

Nutrition Info: Calories 320 Total Fat 27.4 g Saturated Fat 9.9 g Cholesterol 0.5 mg Sodium 122 mg Total Carbs 11 g Fiber 7.3 g Sugar 1.2 g Protein 4.3 g

694. Sunflower Seeds Cookies

Servings: 10   Cooking Time: 3 Hours

Ingredients:

3 oz sunflower seeds	6 tablespoons butter
2 tablespoons liquid stevia	1 teaspoon vanilla extract
10 tablespoons almond flour	1 teaspoon cocoa powder
1 teaspoon baking powder	¼ teaspoon ground cardamom

Directions:

Combine the sunflower seeds, butter, liquid stevia, almond flour, baking powder, vanilla extract, cocoa powder, and ground cardamom.   Knead into a smooth dough and make small cookies.   Put the cookies in the slow cooker and cook for 3 hours on High.   Chill the cookies well and serve!

Nutrition Info:calories 273, fat 25.3, fiber 3.8, carbs 8.1, protein 7.9

695. Blueberry Pie

Servings: 8   Cooking Time: 4 Hours

Ingredients:

2 oz blueberry	1 cup almond flour
1 cup almond milk, unsweetened	¼ cup Erythritol
1 teaspoon baking powder	1 teaspoon butter
	1 teaspoon vanilla extract

Directions:

Mix the almond flour and almond milk.   Add baking powder and Erythritol and stir   Add the butter and vanilla extract and stir until smooth. Place the dough in the slow cooker.   Add the blueberries and flatten the pie gently.   Close the lid and cook the pie for 4 hours on High.   Cool the pie and cut into the servings.   Enjoy!

Nutrition Info:calories 99, fat 9.4, fiber 1.2, carbs 11.3, protein 1.5

696. Pudding Cake

Servings: 6   Cooking Time: 3 Hours

Ingredients:

2 tablespoons butter	4 tablespoons coconut flour
1 oz dark chocolate	
2 oz full-fat cream	3 eggs, beaten
1 teaspoon vanilla extract	3 tablespoons Erythritol
1 tablespoon cocoa powder	1 teaspoon olive oil

Directions:

Melt the duck chocolate and combine it with the butter, cream, and vanilla extract.   Stir the mixture until smooth.   Add the cocoa powder and coconut flour.   Add the beaten eggs and Erythritol. Whisk the mixture until smooth.   Transfer the cake mixture to the slow cooker.   Cook for 3 hours on High.   Serve the cooked cake after 10 minutes of chilling!

Nutrition Info:calories 146, fat 10.9, fiber 2.4, carbs 15.6, protein 4.3

697. Lime Vanilla Bites

Servings: 4   Cooking Time: 2 Hours

Ingredients:

¾ cup butter, softened	2 tablespoons lime juice
½ teaspoon vanilla extract	½ teaspoon baking soda
1 tablespoon stevia	
1 teaspoon lime zest, grated	5 tablespoons coconut flour
	1 egg, beaten

Directions:

Mix up together the butter with vanilla, stevia and the other ingredients until smooth.   Then put the mixture into 4 ramekins and flatten gently. Transfer the ramekins in the slow cooker.   Cook the lemon bites for 2 hours on High.

Nutrition Info:calories 242, fat 7.4, fiber 0.4, carbs 5.2, protein 2.5

698.   Mini Pumpkin Cakes

Servings: 8   Cooking Time: 6 Hours
Ingredients:
- 6 tablespoons almond flour
- ½ teaspoon baking soda
- 1 teaspoon ground cinnamon
- ¼ teaspoon ground cardamom
- 2 oz pumpkin puree
- 1 teaspoon vanilla extract
- ¾ cup almond milk, unsweetened
- 1 tablespoon butter
- 1 oz walnuts, chopped

Directions:
Combine the pumpkin puree, almond flour, and baking soda.   Add the ground cinnamon, ground cardamom, and vanilla extract.   Stir the mixture gently and add almond milk and butter.   Add the chopped walnuts and stir the batter until smooth. Place the mixture into small cake molds and transfer them to a slow cooker.   Cook the cakes for 6 hours on Low.   Cool the cakes slightly and serve!
Nutrition Info:calories 211, fat 19.4, fiber 3.4, carbs 7, protein 6

699.   Spoon Cake

Servings: 6   Cooking Time: 2 Hours
Ingredients:
- ½ cup almond milk, unsweetened
- 1 teaspoon baking powder
- 1 cup almond flour
- 1 tablespoon butter
- 1 oz dark chocolate
- 2 tablespoons Erythritol
- 1 teaspoon ground cinnamon

Directions:
Mix the baking powder, almond milk, almond flour, butter, Erythritol, and ground cinnamon.   Chop the chocolate.   Stir the flour mixture until smooth, add the chopped chocolate.   Stir and transfer in the slow cooker.   Cook the cake for 2 hours on High.   Let the cake cool for 10 minutes and serve!
Nutrition Info:calories 117, fat 10.4, fiber 1.3, carbs 9.6, protein 1.9

700.   Mocha Brownie

Servings: 12.   Cooking Time: 3 Hours On Low.
Ingredients:
- 1 Tablespoon butter for the crock-pot
- ½ cup butter
- ½ cup double cream
- 2 Tablespoons instant coffee
- 1 Bourbon vanilla pod, scraped
- ½ teaspoon cinnamon
- 4 Tablespoons Dutch cocoa powder
- ⅓ cup ground almonds
- Pinch of salt
- 5 large eggs
- ⅔ cup granulated Swerve (or suitable substitute)

Directions:
Butter the crock-pot.   In a small pan, melt the butter and chocolate. Cool.   In another bowl, beat the cream, coffee, and vanilla together.   Combine the cocoa, almonds, and salt in a bowl.   Whisk the eggs and granulated Swerve together for 5 minutes.

Slowly add the chocolate mixture to the eggs, beat with a mixer.   Stir in the cocoa-almond mix. Slowly add the cream and coffee mixture.   Pour the batter in the buttered crock-pot.   Cover the pot with a paper towel to absorb the water.   Cover, cook on low for 3 hours.
Nutrition Info:net C 2g; P 4g; F 14g

701.   Zucchini And Pumpkin Pie

Servings: 8   Cooking Time: 4 Hours
Ingredients:
- 1 tablespoon pumpkin spices
- 1 tablespoon pumpkin puree
- ½ cup of coconut milk
- ½ cup zucchini, grated
- 2 tablespoons stevia
- 1 teaspoon almond extract
- 2 tablespoons butter, softened
- 2 cups almond flour
- ½ teaspoon lemon zest, grated
- 1 teaspoon baking soda
- 1 teaspoon apple cider vinegar

Directions:
In a bowl mix the pumpkin puree with zucchini and the other ingredients and stir.   When the mixture is smooth, pour it un the crockpot. Flatten it with the help of the spatula if needed.   Close the lid. Cook the zucchini for 4 hours on High.   Chill the cooked pie well and slice it.
Nutrition Info:calories 225, fat 10.1, fiber 3.3, carbs 7.1, protein 1.9

702.   Coffee Cream

Servings: 4   Cooking Time: 2 Hours
Ingredients:
- 1 cup of water
- 1 cup heavy cream
- 1 tablespoon cinnamon powder
- 1 oz brewed coffee
- 1 tablespoon coconut oil
- 2 teaspoons stevia

Directions:
In the crockpot, mix the water with cream and the other ingredients.   Close the lid and cook hot chocolate for 2 hours on High.   Then pour the cooked hot mix in the serving glasses.
Nutrition Info:calories 136, fat 5.2, fiber 0.9, carbs 5.1, protein 1.1

703.   Flax Seeds Balls

Servings: 4   Cooking Time: 2.5 Hours
Ingredients:
- 4 teaspoons flax seeds
- 2 tablespoons almond flour
- 1 tablespoon butter
- 1 tablespoon liquid stevia
- 1 teaspoon coconut flakes, unsweetened

Directions:
Combine all the ingredients in a mixing bowl. Knead the dough and then divide into small balls. Place the balls in the slow cooker and cook for 2.5 hours on High.   Chill the cooked balls and serve!
Nutrition Info:calories 119, fat 10.8, fiber 2.2, carbs 3.7, protein 3.5

704.	**Chocolate Walnut Pie**

Servings: Cooking Time: 2.5 Hours
Ingredients:

1 cup of coconut milk	3 tablespoons
1 ½ cup almond flour	walnuts chopped
1 teaspoon almond extract	1/3 cup peanut butter
1 tablespoon chocolate chips, melted	1 tablespoon Erythritol
	½ cup coconut flakes

Directions:
Mix up together coconut milk with the flour and the other ingredients and stir.   When the mixture is homogenous, pour it in the crockpot.   Add butter and close the lid.   Cook the mix for 2.5 hours.
Nutrition Info:calories 202, fat 12.5, fiber 3.1, carbs 10.1, protein 6.2

705.	**Tender Lime Cake**

Servings: 12   Cooking Time: 4 Hours
Ingredients:

1 lime, sliced	
1 cup almond milk, unsweetened	1 ½ cup coconut flour
1 teaspoon vanilla extract	1 teaspoon baking powder
	3 tablespoons Erythritol

Directions:
Combine the almond milk, coconut flour, vanilla extract, baking powder, and Erythritol.   Add the vanilla extract and stir until smooth.   Place the mixture in the slow cooker.   Then place the sliced lime over the cake.   Cook for 4 hours on High. Check if the cake is cooked and chill.   Slice the cake into servings and enjoy!
Nutrition Info:calories 109, fat 6.3, fiber 6.6, carbs 8, protein 2.5

706.	**Snowball Cookies**

Servings: 6   Cooking Time: 2.5 Hours
Ingredients:

2 tablespoons coconut flakes, unsweetened	2 tablespoons butter
1 egg, beaten	1 tablespoon Erythritol
4 tablespoons flour	1 tablespoon water

Directions:
Mix the egg, flour, butter, Erythritol, and water. Knead into a smooth dough.   Make small balls from the dough and coat them in the coconut flakes. Place the cookies in the slow cooker and cook for 2.5 hours on High.   Chill the cookies and serve!
Nutrition Info:calories 69, fat 5.2, fiber 0.3, carbs 6.8, protein 1.6

707.	**Almond Cocoa Cake**

Servings: 6.   Cooking Time: 3 Hours On Low.
Ingredients:

¾ cup butter, melted	Pinch of salt
1 ½ cups powdered sweetener	3 large eggs
⅔ cup Dutch cocoa powder	1 teaspoon vanilla
	½ cup dark chocolate chips

⅓ cup ground almonds
Directions:
Line the crock-pot with aluminium foil and butter it. In a bowl, mix all the ingredients.   Pour the batter into the buttered crock-pot.   Cover the pot with a paper towel to absorb the water.   Cover, cook on low for 3 hours.
Nutrition Info:net C 3g; P 6g; F 33g

708.	**Chocolate Cheese Cake**

Servings: 8   Cooking Time: 4 Hours
Ingredients:

3/4 tablespoon of cocoa powder	1 tablespoon of powdered peanut butter
1 egg	
8oz. cream cheese softened	½ teaspoon of pure vanilla extract

Directions:
Separately blend the wet and dry Ingredients: in the mixer while reserving the berries.   Mix both the mixtures together in a bowl until smooth.   Now spread the cake batter in a greased ramekin and place it in the Crockpot.   Cover its lid and cook for 3-4 hours on Low setting.   Once done, remove its lid of the crockpot carefully.   Allow it to cool and refrigerate for 1 hour.   Serve.
Nutrition Info: Calories 136 Total Fat 10.7 g Saturated Fat 0.5 g Cholesterol 4 mg Sodium 45 mg Total Carbs 1.2 g Sugar 1.4 g Fiber 0.2 g Protein 3.4 g

709.	**Espresso Cookie**

Servings: 6   Cooking Time: 3 Hours
Ingredients:

4 eggs, beaten	½ teaspoon fresh
2 cups almond flour	ginger, minced
1 teaspoon vanilla extract	2 tablespoons stevia
1 teaspoon ground ginger	2 tablespoons butter
2 tablespoons espresso powder	1 teaspoon of cocoa powder
	1 teaspoon baking soda

Directions:
Whisk together eggs, flour and the other ingredients and knead until you obtain a dough.   Line the crockpot with baking paper.   Put the dough in the crockpot and flatten it well.   Cook the cookie for 3 hours on High.
Nutrition Info:calories 173, fat 5.5, fiber 1.1, carbs 6.3, protein 4.8

710.	**Walnut Balls**

Servings: 6   Cooking Time: 2.5 Hours
Ingredients:

2 oz walnuts, chopped	4 tablespoons almond flour
4 tablespoons butter	1 teaspoon liquid stevia
1 teaspoon baking powder	1 egg, beaten
1 tablespoon Erythritol	

Directions:

Mix the chopped walnuts and butter. Add baking powder and Erythritol. Add almond flour, liquid stevia, and egg. Knead the dough until smooth. Make small balls from the dough. Cover the bottom of the slow cooker with the parchment and place the walnut balls inside. Cook the dessert for 2.5 hours on High. When the walnut balls are cooked, serve them immediately!
Nutrition Info:calories 166, fat 16.2, fiber 1.2, carbs 4.9, protein 4.3

711. Cinnamon Almonds

Servings: 4   Cooking Time: 3 Hours
Ingredients:

1 cup of brown swerve	2 teaspoons of vanilla
3 tablespoons of cinnamon ground	3 cups of almonds
⅛ teaspoon of salt	⅛ cup of water
1 egg white	

Directions:
Start putting all the Ingredients: into the Crockpot. Cover its lid and cook for 3 hours on Low setting with occasional stirring Once done, remove the pot's lid and give it a stir. Serve fresh.
Nutrition Info: Calories 261 Total Fat 7.1 g Saturated Fat 13.4 g Cholesterol 0.3 mg Sodium 10 mg Total Carbs 6.1 g Sugar 2.1 g Fiber 3.9 g Protein 1.8 g

712. Lemon Cake

Servings: 8.   Cooking Time: 3 Hours On High.
Ingredients:

1 ½ cup ground almonds	2 Tablespoons lemon juice
½ cup coconut flakes	Zest from two lemons
6 Tablespoons sweetener like Swerve (Erythritol, or suitable substitute)	2 eggs
2 teaspoons baking powder	Topping:
Pinch of salt	3 tablespoons Swerve (or suitable substitute)
½ cup softened coconut oil	½ cup boiling water
½ cup cooking cream	2 Tablespoons lemon juice
	2 Tablespoons softened coconut oil

Directions:
In a bowl, combine the almonds, coconut, sweetener, baking powder. Whisk until combined. In a separate bowl, blend coconut oil, cream, juice, and eggs together. Add the egg mixture to the dry ingredients. Mix thoroughly. Line the crock-pot with aluminium foil, pour in the batter. In a bowl, mix the topping. Pour it over the cake batter. Cover the top of the crock-pot with paper towels to absorb the water. Cover, cook on high for 3 hours. Serve warm.
Nutrition Info:net C 5g; P 7g; F 30g

713. Nutmeg Raspberry Crisp

Servings: 6   Cooking Time: 3 Hours
Ingredients:

2 teaspoons of cinnamon ground	¼ teaspoon of nutmeg ground
¼ teaspoon of ginger ground	¾ cup of walnut meal
1 tablespoon of sugar-free maple syrup	¼ cup of almond flour
½ cup of water	¼ cup of brown swerve
	¼ cup of unsalted butter, melted
	Pinch of salt

Directions:
Start by tossing all the Ingredients: together in a suitable bowl. Mix both the mixtures together in a bowl until smooth. Now spread the mixture in a grease Crockpot. Cover its lid and cook for 3 hours on Low setting. Once done, remove its lid of the crockpot carefully. Serve.
Nutrition Info: Calories 338 Total Fat 28.8 g Saturated Fat 32 g Cholesterol 21 g Sodium 24 mg Total Carbs 7.4 g Fiber 3.4 g Sugar 1.3 g Protein 3.2 g

714. Berry Brownies

Servings: 6   Cooking Time: 2.5 Hours
Ingredients:

1 cup coconut flour	1/3 cup butter, softened
½ cup blackberries	2 tablespoons stevia
1 teaspoon baking soda	½ teaspoon cinnamon powder
4 tablespoons cocoa powder	

Directions:
Line the slow cooker with baking paper. Blend together the flour with berries and the other ingredients and pour into the slow cooker. Flatten gently, close the lid and cook brownie for 2.5 hours on High. Then chill the cooked brownie well and remove it from the slow cooker. Cut it into the square serving pieces.
Nutrition Info:calories 213, fat 5,4, fiber 9.1, carbs 7.5, protein 4.8

715. Chocolate Cheesecake

Servings: 8.   Cooking Time: 2.5 Hours On High.
Ingredients:

3 cups cream cheese	3 eggs
Pinch of salt	1 teaspoon vanilla extract
1 cup powder sweetener of your choice, Swerve (or suitable substitute)	½ cup sugarless dark chocolate chips

Directions:
In a bowl, beat together the cream cheese, sweetener, and salt. Add the eggs one at a time. Combine thoroughly. Spread the cheesecake in a cake pan, which fits in the crock-pot you are using. Melt the chocolate chips in a small pot and pour over the batter. Using a knife, swirl the chocolate through the batter. Pour 2 cups of water in the crock-pot and set the cake pan inside. Attention: Careful the water does not exceed the level of the cake pan. Cover

the pot with a paper towel to absorb the water. Cover, cook on high for 2.5 hours. Remove from the crock-pot and let it cool in the pan for 1 hour. Refrigerate.
Nutrition Info:net C 3g; P 8g; F 33g

716.Chia Bites

Servings: 6   Cooking Time: 1 Hour
Ingredients:
1 tablespoon chocolate chips
3 tablespoons almond butter, softened
½ teaspoon almond extract
1 cup almond flour
1 tablespoon chia seeds
1 tablespoon liquid stevia
Directions:
Churn together butter with flour with chocolate chips, almond butter and the other ingredients and stir.   Then line the crockpot with baking paper. Scoop the dough and place it in the crockpot. You should get small bites. Press the scooped bites gently. Cook the dough bites for 1 hour on High.
Nutrition Info:calories 132, fat 4.6, fiber 5.3, carbs 7.7, protein 4.2

717. Cinnamon Swirls

Servings: 8   Cooking Time: 3 Hours
Ingredients:
1 teaspoon baking powder
1 cup almond flour
1 tablespoon ground cinnamon
1/3 cup butter
1 teaspoon vanilla extract
3 tablespoons Erythritol
Directions:
Combine the butter and almond flour.   Add Erythritol and baking powder.   Add vanilla extract and knead the dough.   Roll out the dough and sprinkle it with the ground cinnamon.   Then roll the dough into a spiral and cut into thick swirls. Place the swirls in the slow cooker and cook for 3 hours.   Chill the swirls and serve!
Nutrition Info:calories 92, fat 9.4, fiber 0.8, carbs 9, protein 0.9

718.   Chocolate Muffins

Servings: 4   Cooking Time: 2.5 Hours
Ingredients:
½ cup butter, softened
1 teaspoon baking soda
½ teaspoon ground cinnamon
1 tablespoon chocolate chips, softened
1 cup almond flour
4 teaspoons stevia
1 egg, beaten
Directions:
Make the muffin batter: in a bowl, mix the chocolate with the butter and the other ingredients and whisk. Pour it in the muffin molds (fill ½ part of every mold) and transfer in the crockpot.   Cook the muffins for 2.5 hours on High.
Nutrition Info:calories 225, fat 17.7, fiber 1.3, carbs 8.3, protein 3.3

719.Avocado And Walnuts Balls

Servings: 6   Cooking Time: 2.5 Hours
Ingredients:
1 avocado, pitted, peeled
1 oz dark chocolate
3 tablespoons almond butter
1 tablespoon stevia
2 tablespoons walnuts, chopped
½ teaspoon vanilla extract
Directions:
In the crockpot, mix the chocolate with almond butter and the other ingredients except the avocado. Close the lid and cook on Low for 5 hours. Meanwhile, place the avocado in the blender and blend until fluffy.   When the time is over, open the crockpot lid and transfer the walnuts mix in the mixing bowl.   Add blended avocado and stir until homogenous. Chill the mixture in the fridge for 15-20 minutes.   Make the small balls from the mixture, arrange on a platter and keep in the fridge until serving.
Nutrition Info:calories 212, fat 11.4, fiber 3.7, carbs 7.8, protein 2.5

720.   Avocado Bars

Servings: 6   Cooking Time: 3 Hours
Ingredients:
1 avocado, pitted
¾ cup coconut flour
1 teaspoon vanilla extract
2 tablespoons liquid stevia
4 tablespoons butter
3 tablespoons almond flour
½ teaspoon baking powder
Directions:
Peel the avocado and mash it.   Combine the mashed avocado and coconut flour.   Add vanilla extract and butter.   After this, add liquid stevia, baking powder and almond flour.   Stir the mix until smooth and transfer in the slow cooker. Flatten it gently and cook for 3 hours on High. Cut the cooked dessert into bars and serve!
Nutrition Info:calories 174, fat 15.1, fiber 5.8, carbs 6, protein 1.9

721.Pumpkin Pie Bars

Servings: 12   Cooking Time: 3 Hours
Ingredients:
3/4 cup of shredded coconut
1/4 cup of cocoa powder
1/2 cup of raw unsalted sunflower seeds
1/4 teaspoon of salt
1/4 cup of Swerve
4 tablespoons of butter softened
Filling
1 29 oz. can pumpkin puree
¼ cup of swerve
1 cup of heavy cream
6 eggs
1/2 teaspoon of salt
1 tablespoon of vanilla extract
1 tablespoon of pumpkin pie spice
1 teaspoon of cinnamon extract
Directions:
Start by coarsely blending all the Ingredients: for the crust together in a blender.   Spread this crust in the greased based on your Crockpot.   Now separately blend the filling mixture in a blender until smooth.   Spread this filling the crust-lined in the crockpot.   Cover its lid and cook for 3 hours on Low setting.   Once done, remove its lid of the

crockpot carefully. Garnish as desired. Slice into bars and serve.
Nutrition Info: Calories 198 Total Fat 19.2 g Saturated Fat 11.5 g Cholesterol 123 mg Sodium 142 mg Total Carbs 4.5 g Sugar 3.3 g Fiber 0.3 g Protein 3.4 g

722. Raspberry Cake

Servings: 12   Cooking Time: 3 Hours
Ingredients:

1 1/4 almond flour	2/3 cup of water
1/2 cup of Swerve	1/2 teaspoon of vanilla extract
1/4 cup of coconut flour	Filling
1/4 cup of Organic Valley Vanilla Fuel Protein Powder	8 oz. Organic Valley cream cheese
1 1/2 teaspoons of baking powder	1/3 cup of erythritol
1/4 teaspoon of salt	1 large egg
3 large eggs	2 tablespoons of Organic Valley whipping cream
6 tablespoons of Organic Valley Pasture Butter melted	1 1/2 cup of fresh raspberries

Directions:
Separately blend the cake mixture and the filling in the mixer while reserving the berries. Now spread the cake batter in the greased based on your crockpot. Top it with the prepared filling evenly and spread the berries over it. Cover its lid and cook for 3 hours on Low setting. Once done, remove its lid of the crockpot carefully. Allow it to cool and refrigerate for 1 hour. Serve.
Nutrition Info: Calories 114 Total Fat 9.6 g Saturated Fat 4.5 g Cholesterol 10 mg Sodium 155 mg Total Carbs 3.1 g Sugar 1.4 g Fiber 1.5 g Protein 3.5 g

723. Cinnamon Cake

Servings: 6   Cooking Time: 2.5 Hours
Ingredients:

1 cup coconut flour	1 teaspoon baking soda
2 eggs, beaten	1 tablespoon lime juice
2 teaspoons ground cinnamon	½ teaspoon almond extract
3/4 cup almond butter, melted	
2 tablespoons Swerve	

Directions:
In the mixing bowl combine the coconut flour with the eggs and the other ingredients and whisk. Mix up the mixture well and transfer it in the slow cooker. Make the swirls with the help of the fork and close the lid. Cook the cake for 2.5 hours on High. Chill the cooked cake well and cut into the servings. After this, remove the cake from the slow cooker.
Nutrition Info:calories 234, fat 5.3, fiber 1.3, carbs 2.8, protein 3.4

724. Red Berry Gummies

Servings: 5   Cooking Time: 1 Hour
Ingredients:

1 tablespoon gelatin	2 tablespoons blueberries puree
1 cup of water	1 tablespoon stevia
1 teaspoon red food coloring	

Directions:
Mix up together the gelatin and 5 tablespoons of water. Stir the mixture and leave it for 10 minutes. Meanwhile, pour the remaining water in the crockpot. Add stevia, berries puree and food coloring. Stir the liquid and cook it for 1 hour on High. Then switch off the crockpot and add gelatin mixture. Stir it well until homogenous. Pour the liquid in the gummy bear's molds and chill until solid. Discard the gummy bears from the molds and store them in the cool place.
Nutrition Info:calories 5, fat 0, fiber 0, carbs 3, protein 1

725. Zucchini Muffins

Servings: 4   Cooking Time: 2.5 Hours
Ingredients:

4 teaspoons butter, softened	1 cup almond flour
1 teaspoon baking powder	¼ cup heavy cream
1 teaspoon almond extract	4 teaspoons stevia
	1/2 cup zucchinis, grated

Directions:
In the crockpot, mix the butter with the zucchinis and the other ingredients. Stir it until smooth. Pour the muffin mixture in the muffin molds and transfer molds in the crockpot. Close the lid and cook muffins for 2.5 hours on High.
Nutrition Info:calories 215, fat 10.1, fiber 4.8, carbs 7.8, protein 3.7

726. Almond Cheese Cake

Servings: 8   Cooking Time: 4 Hours
Ingredients:

¼ cup of almonds, sliced	1 tablespoon of powdered peanut butter
1 egg	½ teaspoon of pure vanilla extract
8oz. cream cheese softened	

Directions:
Separately blend the wet and dry Ingredients: in the mixer while reserving the berries. Mix both the mixtures together in a bowl until smooth. Now spread the cake batter in a greased ramekin and place it in the Crockpot. Cover its lid and cook for 3-4 hours on Low setting. Once done, remove its lid of the crockpot carefully. Allow it to cool and refrigerate for 1 hour. Serve.
Nutrition Info: Calories 276 Total Fat 7.2 g Saturated Fat 6.4 g Cholesterol 134 mg Sodium 8 mg Total Carbs 42g Sugar 31 g Fiber 0.7 g Protein 2.2 g

727. Chocolate Cream Custard

Servings: 4   Cooking Time: 2 Hours
Ingredients:

3/4 cup of brown swerve	6 eggs
1 teaspoon of vanilla	¼ teaspoon of

extract
1 teaspoon of cocoa powder

cinnamon, ground
Sugar-free chocolate, grated
Whipped cream

Directions:
Start by blending all the Ingredients: together in a mixer.   Pour this mixture into 4 ramekins and place them in the Crockpot.   Cover its lid and cook for 2 hours on Low setting.   Once done, remove its lid of the crockpot carefully.   Allow it to cool and refrigerate for 1 hour.   Garnish with chocolate and whipped cream.   Serve.
Nutrition Info: Calories 117 Total Fat 21.2 g Saturated Fat 10.4 g Cholesterol 19.7 mg Sodium 104 mg Total Carbs 7.3 g Sugar 3.4 g Fiber 2 g Protein 8.1 g

728.	Sesame Cookies

Servings: 4   Cooking Time: 2 Hours
Ingredients:

2 tablespoons coconut flour
1 tablespoon butter
1 tablespoon sesame seeds

½ teaspoon baking powder
1 egg
1 teaspoon vanilla extract

Directions:
Mix the coconut flour and butter.   Add the baking soda and vanilla extract.   Beat the eggs into the mixture.   Add the sesame seeds and knead the dough.   Roll out the dough and cut out cookies with a cookie cutter.   Place the cookies in the slow cooker and cook them for 2 hours on High.   Chill the cookies and serve!
Nutrition Info:calories 73, fat 5.5, fiber 1.8, carbs 3.5, protein 2.3

729.	Red Velvet Cupcakes

Servings: 6   Cooking Time: 3 Hours
Ingredients:

1 cup almond flour
3 eggs
1 teaspoon baking powder
1 teaspoon vanilla extract

3 tablespoons butter
¼ cup full-fat whipped cream
3 tablespoons Erythritol
Red food coloring

Directions:
Beat the eggs in a bowl and whisk well.   Add butter, baking powder, vanilla extract, and whipped cream.   Add Erythritol and food coloring.   Stir the mixture until well blended and add almond flour. Stir until smooth.   Place the mixture in the muffin molds and transfer them to the slow cooker.   Cook for 3 hours on High.   Cool the cupcakes and serve!
Nutrition Info:calories 114, fat 10.3, fiber 0.5, carbs 9.5, protein 3.8

730.	Delicious Breakfast Cake

Servings: 6   Cooking Time: 6 Hours
Ingredients:

6 tablespoons of almond flour
¼ teaspoon of salt
½ teaspoon of baking soda
¼ teaspoon of baking powder
6 tablespoons of erythritol

½ cup of 2% vanilla yogurt
2 ½ eggs
¼ teaspoon of pure vanilla extract

Directions:
Separately blend the wet and dry Ingredients: in the mixer.   Mix both the mixtures together in a bowl until smooth.   Now spread the cake batter in a greased ramekin and place it in the Crockpot. Cover its lid and cook for 6 hours on Low setting. Once done, remove its lid of the crockpot carefully. Allow it to cool and refrigerate for 1 hour.   Serve.
Nutrition Info: Calories 107 Total Fat 9.3 g Saturated Fat 4.8 g Cholesterol 77 mg Sodium 135 mg Total Carbs 2.6 g Fiber 0.8 g Sugar 9.9 g Protein 3.9 g

731.	Orange Cheese Cake

Servings: 4   Cooking Time: 4 Hours
Ingredients:

¼ cup of erythritol
½ teaspoon of almond flour
2 tablespoons of sour cream
½ tablespoon of lemon Juice

¼ teaspoon of vanilla
zest of ¼ orange
1 ½ egg, room temp
½ jar Greek yogurt
3 raspberries
1 cup of water

Directions:
Separately blend the wet and dry Ingredients: in the mixer.   Mix both the mixtures together in a bowl until smooth.   Now spread the cake batter in a greased ramekin and place it in the Crockpot. Cover its lid and cook for 4 hours on Low setting. Once done, remove its lid of the crockpot carefully. Allow it to cool and refrigerate for 1 hour.   Serve.
Nutrition Info: Calories 173 Total Fat 13 g Saturated Fat 10.1 g Cholesterol 12 mg Sodium 67 mg Total Carbs 7.5 g Sugar 1.2 g Fiber 0.6 g Protein 3.2 g

732.	Keto Soufflé

Servings: 5   Cooking Time: 2.5 Hours
Ingredients:

1 tablespoon butter
¼ cup Erythritol
1 oz dark chocolate
4 egg yolks

2 egg whites
5 teaspoon whipped cream

Directions:
Whisk the butter with Erythritol.   Add the egg yolks and stir until well blended.   Whisk the eggs to stiff peaks.   Melt the chocolate and combine it with the egg yolk mixture.   Add the egg whites and whipped cream.   Stir gently to get a smooth batter. Place the mixture in ramekins and put the ramekins in the slow cooker.   Cook the soufflé for 2.5 hours on Low.   Serve it immediately!
Nutrition Info:calories 115, fat 9.2, fiber 0.2, carbs 16.1, protein 4.2

733. Chocolate Fudge

Servings: 12   Cooking Time: 2 Hours

Ingredients:

1/3 cup of almond milk

a dash of salt

1 teaspoon of pure vanilla extract

2 teaspoons of swerve

Directions:

Start by throwing all the Ingredients: into the Crockpot.   Cover its lid and cook for 2 hours on Low setting.   Once done, remove its lid of the crockpot carefully.   Now pour this mixture into a casserole dish lined with parchment paper. Refrigerate this fudge for 30 minutes until it is set. Slice and serve.

Nutrition Info: Calories 236 Total Fat 13.5 g Saturated Fat 4.2 g Cholesterol 541 mg Sodium 21 mg Total Carbs 7.6 g Sugar 1.4 g Fiber 3.8 g Protein 4.3 g

734. Vanilla Cake

Servings: 6   Cooking Time: 5 Hours

Ingredients:

4 tablespoons chocolate chips, softened

1 cup organic coconut milk

1 cup almond flour

1 teaspoon baking powder

1 teaspoon apple cider vinegar

2 tablespoons Erythritol

2 teaspoons vanilla extract

3 eggs, beaten

Directions:

In the big bowl combine together the coconut milk with the flour and the other ingredients and whisk. Line the slow cooker with the baking paper.   Pour the batter in the slow cooker. Flatten it with the help of the spatula if needed.   Cook the cake for 5 hours on Low.   Then chill the cake well and remove it from the slow cooker.   Discard the baking paper and cut the cake into the servings.

Nutrition Info:calories 239, fat 14.6, fiber 4.5, carbs 10.4, protein 5.4

735. Almond Coffee Cream

Servings: 5   Cooking Time: 40 Minutes

Ingredients:

2 tablespoons almonds, chopped

2 oz dark chocolate, melted

1 cup brewed coffee

½ cup coconut cream

1 tablespoon coconut oil

Directions:

In your crockpot, mix the chocolate with coffee and the other ingredients, close the lid and cook on High for 40 minutes.   Divide into bowls and serve cold.

Nutrition Info:calories 141, fat 7.9, fiber 4.1, carbs 4.9, protein 3.9

736. Vanilla Cream

Servings: 6   Cooking Time: 2 Hours

Ingredients:

2 egg whites

4 tablespoons Erythritol

1 cup almond milk, unsweetened

1 teaspoon ground

1 teaspoon vanilla extract

cinnamon

½ teaspoon turmeric

Directions:

Whisk the egg whites until soft peaks and add Erythritol.   Add the vanilla extract and almond milk.   Keep whisking the mixture for 2 minutes more.   Then add the ground cinnamon and turmeric.   Stir the mixture gently and transfer to the slow cooker.   Cook the cream for 2 hours on Low.   Transfer the cooked dessert into ramekins and enjoy!

Nutrition Info:calories 101, fat 9.6, fiber 1.1, carbs 12.8, protein 2.2

737. Lemon Cheese Cake

Servings: 4   Cooking Time: 6 Hours

Ingredients:

¼ cup of erythritol

½ teaspoon of almond flour

2 tablespoons of sour cream

½ tablespoon of Lemon Juice

¼ teaspoon of vanilla

zest of half lemon

1 ½ egg, room temp

½ jar lemon curd

3 raspberries

1 cup of water

Directions:

Separately blend the wet and dry Ingredients: in the mixer while reserving the berries   Mix both the mixtures together in a bowl until smooth.   Now spread the cake batter in a greased ramekin and place it in the Crockpot.   Cover its lid and cook for 6 hours on Low setting.   Once done, remove its lid of the crockpot carefully.   Allow it to cool and refrigerate for 1 hour.   Garnish with the berries Serve.

Nutrition Info: Calories 334 Total Fat 28.9 g Saturated Fat 25 g Cholesterol 51 mg Sodium 30 mg Total Carbs 10.8 g Fiber 5.9 g Sugar 1.4 g Protein 4.3 g

738. Maple Custard

Servings: Cooking Time: 2 Hours

Ingredients:

1 cup of heavy cream horizon organic

1/2 cup of almond milk

1/4 cup of swerve

1 teaspoon of maple extract

1/4 teaspoon of salt

1/2 teaspoon of cinnamon

Directions:

Start by blending all the Ingredients: together in a mixer.   Pour this mixture into a 4 oz. ramekin and place it in the Crockpot.   Cover its lid and cook for 2 hours on Low setting.   Once done, remove its lid of the crockpot carefully.   Allow it to cool and refrigerate for 1 hour.   Garnish as desired. Serve.

Nutrition Info: Calories 215 Total Fat 20 g Saturated Fat 7 g Cholesterol 38 mg Sodium 12 mg Total Carbs 8 g Sugar 1 g Fiber 6 g Protein 5 g

739. Keto Cobbler

Servings: 4   Cooking Time: 2 Hours

Ingredients:

1 cup blackberries	5 tablespoons almond flour
1 tablespoon liquid stevia	1 egg, beaten
1 teaspoon Psyllium Husk	1 tablespoon butter

Directions:
Whisk the egg and combine them with the almond flour and Psyllium Husk.   Add the liquid stevia and butter and knead into a smooth dough.   Chop the dough into small pieces.   Cover the bottom of the slow cooker with parchment.   Place a small amount of the dough in the bottom of the slow cooker.   Sprinkle the dough with a small amount of the blackberries.   Add a second layer of the chopped dough followed by more blackberries. Continue layering until you use all the ingredients. Close the lid and cook the cobbler for 2 hours on High.   Let the cooked cobbler cool slightly. Serve it!

Nutrition Info:calories 264, fat 21.7, fiber 8, carbs 13.9, protein 9.4

740.   Raspberry Custard Trifle

Servings: 4   Cooking Time: 3 Hours

Ingredients:

6 eggs	1 pinch salt
3/4 cup of erythritol	4 tablespoons of brown swerve
1 teaspoon of vanilla extract	2 tablespoons of water
¼ teaspoon of cinnamon, ground	1 cup of raspberries

Directions:
Start by blending all the Ingredients: together in a mixer except raspberries, brown swerve, and water. Pour this mixture into 4 ramekins and place them in the Crockpot.   Cover its lid and cook for 3 hours on Low setting.   Once done, remove its lid of the crockpot carefully.   Allow it to cool and refrigerate for 1 hour.   Meanwhile, boil brown swerve with water in a saucepan and cook until it is caramelized. Garnish the custard with raspberries then pour the caramel mixture on top.   Serve.

Nutrition Info: Calories 197 Total Fat 19.2 g Saturated Fat 10.1 g Cholesterol 11 mg Sodium 78 mg Total Carbs 7.3 g Sugar 1.2 g Fiber 0.8 g Protein 4.2 g

741.Lavender Cookies

Servings: 6   Cooking Time: 2 Hours

Ingredients:

1 teaspoon lavender extract	¼ cup butter
1 teaspoon vanilla extract	1 egg, whisked
1 cup coconut flour	1 teaspoon baking powder
	½ teaspoon olive oil

Directions:
Mix the lavender extract and vanilla extract.   Add the coconut flour and butter.   Add the whisked egg and baking powder.   Knead into a smooth dough.   Roll out the dough and cut the cookies with a cookie cutter.   Pour the olive oil in the slow cooker.   Transfer the cookies to the slow cooker and cook them for 2 hours on High.   Cool the cookies and serve!

Nutrition Info:calories 165, fat 10.8, fiber 8, carbs 13.9, protein 3.7

742.   Pecan Pie

Servings: 8   Cooking Time: 3.5 Hours

Ingredients:

1 tablespoon chocolate chips	1 tablespoon lemon juice
4 tablespoons peanut butter	2 cups almond flour
4 pecans, chopped	3 tablespoons Erythritol
1 teaspoon baking powder	1 teaspoon vanilla extract

Directions:
Make the dough: in the mixing bowl, mix up together chocolate chips, peanut butter, chopped pecans, baking powder, lemon juice, almond flour, Erythritol, and vanilla extract.   Knead the smooth and non-sticky dough.   Then line the crockpot with baking paper.   Make the shape of bun from the dough and put it in the crockpot.   Flatten it well with the help of the fingertips.   Close the lid and cook pecan pie for 3.5 hours on High.   Chill the cooked pie well and then remove from the crockpot.   Slice it into the servings.

Nutrition Info:calories 145, fat 12.9, fiber 2, carbs 7.2, protein 4.4

743.   Mint Cake

Servings: 6   Cooking Time: 3 Hours

Ingredients:

1 teaspoon dried mint	1 teaspoon butter, melted
1 teaspoon mint extract	1 teaspoon baking soda
1 teaspoon almond extract	1 cup almond flour
1 cup almond flour	½ cup Monk fruit
½ cup of coconut milk	

Directions:
Line the crockpot with baking paper.   In the big mixing bowl mix up together all ingredients. When you get a smooth batter, pour it in the crockpot.   Flatten it gently and close the lid. Cook the mint cake on High for 3 hours.   When the cake is cooked, chill it well and only then remove from the crockpot.   Slice it into the servings.

Nutrition Info:calories 215, fat 11.1, fiber 5.4, carbs 4.6, protein 5.5

744.   Carrot Walnut Cake

Servings: 6   Cooking Time: 6 Hours

Ingredients:

1/3 cup of Brown swerve	½ cup of almond flour
½ teaspoon of baking powder	¼ cup of heavy whipping cream
3/4 teaspoons of apple pie spice	½ cup of carrots shredded
2 tablespoons of coconut oil	¼ cup of walnuts diced

Directions:

Separately blend the wet and dry Ingredients: in the mixer.   Mix both the mixtures together in a bowl until smooth.   Now spread the cake batter in a greased ramekin and place it in the Crockpot. Cover its lid and cook for 6 hours on Low setting. Once done, remove its lid of the crockpot carefully. Allow it to cool and refrigerate for 1 hour.   Serve.
Nutrition Info: Calories 101 Total Fat 15.5 g Saturated Fat 4.5 g Cholesterol 12 mg Sodium 18 mg Total Carbs 4.4 g Sugar 1.2 g Fiber 0.3 g Protein 4.8 g

745.   Ricotta And Pecan Cupcakes

Servings: 4   Cooking Time: 3 Hours
Ingredients:
- 1 teaspoon almond extract
- 1 teaspoon ground nutmeg
- 4 tablespoons butter, frozen
- 1 cup almond flour
- 1 teaspoon Ricotta cheese
- 2 tablespoons pecans, chopped
- 1 tablespoon stevia

Directions:
Mix up together the flour with almond extract and the other ingredients and stir until you obtain a dough   After this, transfer the dough in the freezer for 20 minutes.   Remove the dough from the freezer and grated it.   Divide the dough into muffin molds.   After this, arrange the cupcakes in the crockpot.   Close the lid and cook them on High for 3 hours.
Nutrition Info:calories 209, fat 15.1, fiber 5.1, carbs 6.1, protein 3.8

746.   Keto Sweet Bread

Servings: 8   Cooking Time: 4 Hours
Ingredients:
- 1 cup coconut flour
- ¼ cup Erythritol
- 1 teaspoon baking powder
- ¼ cup almond milk
- 3 tablespoons butter
- 1 oz pumpkin seeds

Directions:
Mix the coconut flour and Erythritol.   Add the baking powder and almond milk.   Add butter and stir it gently.   Add the pumpkin seeds and knead the dough.   Place the dough in the slow cooker and cook the bread for 4 hours on High.   Slice the cooked bread and enjoy!
Nutrition Info:calories 135, fat 9.2, fiber 6.3, carbs 18.9, protein 3.1

747.   Strawberry Jam

Servings: 4   Cooking Time: 15 Hours
Ingredients:
- ¼ teaspoon ground nutmeg
- 1 cup strawberries
- ½ cup Monk fruit

Directions:
Put berries in the bowl and mash until smooth with the help of the spoon.   Then add ground nutmeg and Monk fruit.   Mix up the mixture well and transfer in the crockpot.   Cook the jam for 5 hours on Low.   Then transfer the cooked jam in the glass jar and store it in the fridge.
Nutrition Info:calories 30, fat 0.2, fiber 2, carbs 2.6, protein 0.5

748.   Green Tea Cupcakes

Servings: 4   Cooking Time: 3.5 Hours
Ingredients:
- 1 teaspoon green tea powder
- 4 eggs, beaten
- 1 teaspoon baking soda
- 1 teaspoon lemon juice
- 1 cup coconut flour
- 1 tablespoon stevia
- ½ teaspoon almond extract
- 1 tablespoon peanut butter, softened

Directions:
In the mixing bowl whisk together the green tea powder with the eggs and the other ingredients and whisk.   Fill ½ part of every cupcake mold with matcha batter and transfer in the crockpot.   Close the lid and cook cupcakes for 5 hours on High.
Nutrition Info:calories 233, fat 11.9, fiber 3.3, carbs 8.2, protein 4.1

749.   Cocoa Pudding Cake

Servings: 10.   Cooking Time: 2.5-3 Hours On Low.
Ingredients:
- 1 Tablespoon butter for greasing the crock-pot
- 1 ½ cups ground almonds
- ¾ cup sweetener, Swerve (or a suitable substitute)
- ¾ cup cocoa powder
- ¼ cup whey protein
- 2 teaspoons baking powder
- ¼ teaspoon salt
- 4 large eggs
- ½ cup butter, melted
- ¾ cup full-fat cream
- 1 teaspoon vanilla extract

Directions:
Butter the crock-pot thoroughly.   In a bowl, whisk the dry ingredients together.   Stir in the melted butter, eggs, cream, and vanilla. Mix well.   Pour the batter into the crock-pot and spread evenly. Cover, cook on low for 2½ to 3 hours. If preferred — more like pudding, cook cake shorter; more dry cake, cook longer.   Cool in the crock-pot for 30 minutes. Cut and serve.
Nutrition Info:net C 6.5g; P 7g; F 17g

750.   Dessert Pancakes

Servings: 2   Cooking Time: 2 Hours
Ingredients:
- ¼ cup almond milk, unsweetened
- 1 teaspoon vanilla extract
- 1 teaspoon ground cinnamon
- 1 teaspoon baking powder
- 1 cup almond flour
- 1 egg, beaten
- 1 tablespoon butter
- 1 teaspoon olive oil

Directions:
Whisk the egg and combine it with the almond milk, vanilla extract, ground cinnamon, baking powder, and almond flour.   Add the butter and stir it until smooth.   Spray the slow cooker with the olive oil. Pour the pancake batter into the slow cooker and cook for 2 hours on High.   Cut the pancake into servings and enjoy!
Nutrition Info:calories 263, fat 24.5, fiber 2.8, carbs 7.2, protein 6.6

751. Peanut Butter Bars

Servings: 7   Cooking Time: 4 Hours
Ingredients:

4 tablespoons peanut butter
1 teaspoon ground ginger
½ teaspoon almond extract
1 teaspoon nutmeg, ground
2 tablespoons almonds, chopped
1 teaspoon cinnamon powder
1 tablespoon coconut shred
¾ cup heavy cream
2 tablespoons stevia
Cooking spray

Directions:
In the crockpot, mix the peanut butter with almond extract and the other ingredients except the cooking spray and close the lid   Cook the mixture on Low for 4 hours.   Then stir it carefully.   Grease a baking sheet with cooking spray and spread the peanut butter mix inside.   Spread well, freeze for 1.5 hours, cut into bars and serve.
Nutrition Info:calories 128, fat 8.1, fiber 3.8, carbs 7.3, protein 3.1

752.   Lavender Crème Brule

Servings: 4   Cooking Time: 2 Hours
Ingredients:

5 egg yolks
½ cup of swerve
2 cups of heavy cream
½ tablespoon of lavender buds
1 tablespoon of vanilla extract

Directions:
Start by blending all the Ingredients: except lavender in a blender until smooth.   Now divide the batter into 4 ramekins and place them in the Crockpot.   Cover its lid and cook for 2 hours on Low setting.   Once done, remove its lid of the crockpot carefully.   Allow it to cool and refrigerate for 1 hour.   Garnish with lavender.   Serve.
Nutrition Info: Calories 188 Total Fat 3 g Saturated Fat 2.2 g Cholesterol 101 mg Sodium 54 mg Total Carbs 3 g Sugar 1.3 g Fiber 0.6 g Protein 5 g

753.   Sweet Zucchini Muffins

Servings: 6   Cooking Time: 3 Hours
Ingredients:

1 teaspoon baking powder
2 oz zucchini, grated
1 teaspoon vanilla extract
1 cup almond flour
3 teaspoons Erythritol
3 tablespoons butter
1 tablespoon almond milk, unsweetened

Directions:
Mix all the ingredients together.   Stir them well to get a smooth batter.   Place the muffins in the muffin molds and transfer them to the slow cooker. Cook the muffins for 3 hours on High.   When the muffins are cooked cool slightly.   Enjoy!
Nutrition Info:calories 88, fat 8.7, fiber 0.7, carbs 4.4, protein 1.2

754.   Keto Peanut Butter Cookies

Servings: 6   Cooking Time: 2 Hours

Ingredients:

4 tablespoons peanut butter, unsweetened
1 teaspoon liquid stevia
4 tablespoons almond flour
1 tablespoon coconut flakes, unsweetened
1 teaspoon vanilla extract

Directions:
Mix the peanut butter, almond flour, vanilla extract, and liquid stevia.   Mix until smooth.   Knead the dough with the coconut flakes.   Make the small balls from the dough and flatten them gently. Place the cookies in the slow cooker and cook them for 2 hours on High.   Chill the cooked cookies and store them in the paper bags to prevent them from drying out.
Nutrition Info:calories 174, fat 15, fiber 2.7, carbs 6.3, protein 6.7

755.   Almond Cookies

Servings: 6   Cooking Time: 2 Hours
Ingredients:

1 oz almonds, chopped
1 teaspoon baking powder
3 tablespoons butter
2 tablespoons Erythritol
½ cup almond flour
1 teaspoon vanilla extract

Directions:
Combine the almond flour, vanilla extract, baking powder, and Erythritol.   Stir the mixture and add butter.   Knead into a smooth dough.   Make small balls from the dough and sprinkle the balls with the almonds.   Press the almond into the cookies gently.   Transfer the cookies to the slow cooker.   Cook the cookies for 2 hours on High. Cool the cookies.   Enjoy!
Nutrition Info:calories 94, fat 9.3, fiber 0.9, carbs 7, protein 1.6

756.   Keto Cheesecake

Servings: 6   Cooking Time: 6 Hours
Ingredients:

3 tablespoons almond flour
3 tablespoons butter
½ teaspoon ground cinnamon
1 teaspoon vanilla extract
1 tablespoons liquid stevia
1 tablespoon full-fat cream
6 oz full-fat cream cheese
3 tablespoons Erythritol
2 eggs, whisked

Directions:
Mix the butter, almond flour, and ground cinnamon. Add the liquid stevia, cream cheese, and vanilla extract and stir well.   Add the cream and Erythritol.   Add the whisked eggs and stir it well. Pour 1 cup of water in the slow cooker.   Transfer the batter into a cheesecake mold.   Place the cheesecake mold in the slow cooker and cook it for 6 hours on Low.   Cool the cooked cheesecake a little. Serve it!
Nutrition Info:calories 195, fat 19, fiber 0.5, carbs 1.9, protein 4.9

| **757.** | **Rutabaga Cake** |

Servings: 6   Cooking Time: 4.5 Hours
Ingredients:

1 cup coconut flour	1 tablespoon stevia
¾ cup butter, softened	1 cup rutabaga, chopped
1 teaspoon almond extract	1 tablespoon coconut oil
½ teaspoon vanilla extract	Cooking spray

Directions:
For the pie crust: mix up together coconut flour, butter, and knead the soft dough.   Then cut the dough into 2 parts.   Spray the crockpot bottom with cooking spray from inside.   Roll up first dough part with the help of the rolling pin and place it in the crockpot.   Then mix up together rutabaga with the other ingredients and arrange this over the crust.   Then roll up the second dough part and cover the rutabaga.   Close the crockpot lid and cook the cake for 4.5 hours on Low.   When the pie is cooked, chill it well and only them cut into the pieces.
Nutrition Info:calories 260, fat 27.7, fiber 1.3, carbs 5.8, protein 1.5

| **758.** | **Super Fudgy Brownies** |

Servings: 8   Cooking Time: 4 Hours
Ingredients:

2 tablespoons of water	1/2 teaspoon of espresso powder
1/2 teaspoon of salt	2 large eggs
1 cup of almond flour	1/3 cup of coconut oil, melted
1/2 cup of cocoa powder	1 teaspoon of vanilla extract
1/2 cup of swerve	1/3 cup of sugar-free chocolate chips
1 teaspoon of baking powder	

Directions:
Blend bok choy with all the wet Ingredients: in a blender.   Gradually add the dry Ingredients: and mix well.   Fold in chocolate chips then spread this mixture in the Crockpot.   Cover its lid and cook for 4 hours on Low setting.   Once done, remove its lid of the crockpot carefully.   Slice and serve.
Nutrition Info: Calories 167 Total Fat 5.1 g Saturated Fat 1.1 g Cholesterol 121 mg Sodium 48 mg Total Carbs 8.9 g Sugar 1.8 g Fiber 2.1 g Protein 6.3 g

| **759.** | **Lava Cake** |

Servings: 6   Cooking Time: 2.5 Hours
Ingredients:

1 oz dark chocolate	¼ cup almond milk, unsweetened
1 tablespoon cocoa powder	
6 tablespoons almond flour	3 tablespoons liquid stevia

Directions:
Combine the cocoa powder and almond flour. Add almond milk and liquid stevia.   Stir the mixture until smooth.   Place the batter in ramekins and place the dark chocolate in the center of the cake.   Cook the lava cake for 2.5 hours on High.   Serve the cake immediately while hot!
Nutrition Info:calories 210, fat 17.9, fiber 3.7, carbs 9.8, protein 6.8

| **760.** | **Rhubarb Crumble** |

Servings: 8   Cooking Time: 3 Hours
Ingredients:

8 oz rhubarb, chopped	½ cup almond flour
1/3 cup Erythritol	4 tablespoons butter
1 teaspoon vanilla extract	2 oz walnuts, chopped

Directions:
Mix the vanilla extract, almond flour, and butter. Add walnuts and knead the dough.   Chop the dough into small pieces.   Cover the bottom of the slow cooker with parchment.   Sprinkle it with the small amount of the chopped dough.   Add some of the rhubarb and sprinkle it with some Erythritol. Add a layer of the dough again and repeat all the steps until you finish all the ingredients.   Cook the crumble for 3 hours on High.   Cool the crumble and serve!
Nutrition Info:calories 112, fat 10.9, fiber 1.2, carbs 12.4, protein 2.4

| **761.** | **Avocado Mousse** |

Servings: 2   Cooking Time: 2 Hours
Ingredients:

2 avocados, peeled, pitted and mashed	3 egg yolks
¼ cup heavy cream	2 tablespoons monk fruit
½ teaspoon almond extract	¼ cup organic almond milk

Directions:
In the crockpot, mix the avocados with the cream and the other ingredients, whisk and close the lid. Cook the mixture for 2 hours in Low.   Divide into cups and serve cold.
Nutrition Info:calories 217, fat 14.7, fiber 3.4, carbs 5.8, protein 5

| **762.** | **Blackberry Pancake** |

Servings: 6   Cooking Time: 1 Hour
Ingredients:

1 cup almond flour	½ cup coconut flour
1 teaspoon vanilla extract	3 eggs, beaten
¼ teaspoon ground nutmeg, ground	1 tablespoon stevia
	1 teaspoon butter
½ cup blackberries, pureed	¼ cup coconut cream
	Cooking spray

Directions:
In the mixing bowl, combine the flour with vanilla, nutmeg and the other ingredients except the cooking spray and whisk.   Spray the crockpot bottom with the cooking spray.   Pour pancake batter in the crockpot and flatten it gently.   Cook the pancake for 50 minutes on High.   Then open the lid and add butter.   Let the pancake rest for 10 minutes.
Nutrition Info:calories 131, fat 4.7, fiber 4.7, carbs 4.8, protein 5.9

763. Almond Spread

Servings: 10   Cooking Time: 40 Minutes

Ingredients:

1/3 cup almonds, chopped	1 cup almond butter
2 tablespoons cocoa powder	½ teaspoon almond extract
	¼ cup stevia

Directions:
In the crockpot, mix the almonds with almond butter and the other ingredients and whisk   Close the lid and the mixture for 40 minutes in High. Then whisk the mixture with the help of the hand mixer/blender.   Divide into bowls and serve.
Nutrition Info:calories 100, fat 2.6, fiber 0.7, carbs 4.3, protein 0.9

764. Coconut Bars(1)

Servings: 8   Cooking Time: 2 Hours

Ingredients:

1 cup coconut flour	1 teaspoon baking powder
2 tablespoons coconut flakes, unsweetened	1 teaspoon vanilla extract
3 tablespoons butter	
1 egg, beaten	

Directions:
Mix the coconut flour and coconut flakes.   Add the butter and beaten egg.   Add baking powder and vanilla extract.   Stir the dough until smooth. Place the dough in the slow cooker, press down to flatten and cook it for 2 hours on High.   Cut the dessert into the bars and serve!
Nutrition Info:calories 113, fat 6.8, fiber 6.1, carbs 10.6, protein 2.8

765. Chewy Seed And Nut Bars

Servings: 6   Cooking Time: 1 Hour

Ingredients:

2 tablespoons swerve	1 tablespoon butter
1 tablespoon Erythritol	2 tablespoons flour
1 oz pumpkin seeds	1 teaspoon coconut flakes, unsweetened
1 oz almonds, chopped	

Directions:
Mix the swerve, Erythritol, pumpkin seeds, almond, butter, flour, and coconut flakes.   Stir the mix well. Place it in the slow cooker and flatten the surface. Cook the dessert for 1 hour on High.   Let the bars cool slightly.   Cut it into the bars and serve!
Nutrition Info:calories 82, fat 6.6, fiber 0.9, carbs 7, protein 2.5

766. Pineapple Cheese Cake

Servings: 8   Cooking Time: 6 Hours

Ingredients:

8oz. ricotta cheese	¼ cup of sour cream
1 tablespoon of sugar-free pineapple extract	2 cups of mixed nuts, crushed
¼ cup of erythritol	2 tablespoons of unsalted butter,
2 eggs	
1 tablespoon of vanilla extract	

melted

¼ cup of raspberries

Directions:
Start by blending the Nuts with butter in the mixer. Spread this Nuts mixture in the greased Crockpot firmly.   Now beat the remaining filling Ingredients: except berries in a blender until smooth. Add this cream filling to the Nutty crust and spread evenly.   Cover its lid and cook for 6 hours on Low setting.   Once done, remove its lid of the crockpot carefully.   Allow it to cool and refrigerate for 12 hours.   Garnish with berries.   Serve.
Nutrition Info: Calories 213 Total Fat 19 g Saturated Fat 15.2 g Cholesterol 13 mg Sodium 52 mg Total Carbs 5.5 g Sugar 1.3 g Fiber 0.5 g Protein 6.1 g

767. Peanut Pie

Servings: 10   Cooking Time: 6 Hours

Ingredients:

1 cup peanut butter	¼ cup hazelnuts
1 tablespoon chocolate chips	¾ cup organic coconut milk
1 teaspoon avocado oil	2 cups coconut flour
1 teaspoon vanilla extract	1/3 cup Monk fruit
	¼ cup almond, chopped

Directions:
In the big mixing bowl mix up together the peanut butter with hazelnuts and the other ingredients. Line the crockpot with baking paper and place pie dough on it.   Flatten the dough with the help of the wet fingertips and close the lid.   Cook the nut pie for 6 hours on Low.   Chill the cooked pie well and cut into the servings.
Nutrition Info:calories 248, fat 11.3, fiber 10.8, carbs 17.9, protein 8.6

768. Soft Bacon Cookies

Servings: 6   Cooking Time: 3 Hours

Ingredients:

½ cup almond flour	1 egg, beaten
3 tablespoons butter, melted	1 teaspoon olive oil
3 oz bacon, chopped cooked	1 teaspoon stevia extract

Directions:
Whisk the egg and mix it with the butter and olive oil.   Add the stevia extract and stir the mixture gently.   Add the almond flour and knead the dough.   When the dough is smooth, add the chopped bacon and knead it again.   Make medium cookies by rolling the dough into small balls with your hands.   Place the cookies in the slow cooker and cook for 3 hours on Low.   Check if the cookies are cooked and remove them from the slow cooker. Cool slightly.   Serve!
Nutrition Info:calories 198, fat 17.9, fiber 1, carbs 2.3, protein 8.2

769. Cinnamon And Blackberry Pie

Servings: 12   Cooking Time: 7.5 Hours

Ingredients:

1 tablespoon cinnamon powder

1 teaspoon baking soda

1 teaspoon apple cider vinegar

1 cup almond flour

½ cup coconut flour

3 tablespoons coconut shred

½ cup blackberries, mashed

1/3 cup Erythritol

5 eggs, beaten

1 teaspoon avocado oil

Directions:

Mix up together the flour with the cinnamon and the other ingredients except the oil.   Then brush the crockpot with the oil from inside.   Pour the batter in the crockpot and flatten it gently.   Close the lid and cook per for 7.5 hours on Low.

Nutrition Info:calories 130, fat 4.7, fiber 4.1, carbs 8.8, protein 2.9

770. Candied Almonds

Servings: 6   Cooking Time: 3 Hours

Ingredients:

1 cup almonds

1/3 cup granulated monk fruit sweetener

4 tablespoons water

¼ teaspoon ground cinnamon

Directions:

Mix the sweetener and water.   Add the ground cinnamon and stir.   Place the almonds in the slow cooker.   Add the sweetener mix and stir.   Cook the almonds for 3 hours on High.   Cool the dessert a little.   Enjoy!

Nutrition Info:calories 92, fat 7.9, fiber 2, carbs 3.5, protein 3.4

771. Keto Almond Scones

Servings: 4   Cooking Time: 4 Hours

Ingredients:

½ teaspoon baking soda

½ cup almond flour

¼ cup coconut milk

2 eggs, beaten

1 teaspoon vanilla extract

3 tablespoons coconut flour

1 oz almonds, chopped

Directions:

Combine the baking soda and almond flour.   Add the coconut milk and beaten eggs,   Add the vanilla extract and stir the mixture gently.   Add the coconut flour and almonds.   Stir the mixture and knead into a dough.   Make into small scones and put them in the slow cooker.   Cook the scones for 4 hours on High.   Chill the cooked scones and then remove them from the slow cooker to col slightly.   Enjoy!

Nutrition Info:calories 153, fat 11.6, fiber 3.9, carbs 7.2, protein 6.1

772. Mascarpone Fudge

Servings: 8   Cooking Time: 40 Minutes

Ingredients:

2 tablespoons coconut cream

2 tablespoons Mascarpone cheese, soft

1 teaspoon Erythritol

1 teaspoon almond extract

1/3 cup sugar-free chocolate chips

1 teaspoon coconut butter

Directions:

In the slow cooker, mix the mascarpone with the cream and eth other ingredients and close the lid. Cook it for 40 minutes on High.   Meanwhile, line the baking tray with baking paper.   Transfer in the baking tray.   Cover it with the second sheet of baking paper.   With the help of the rolling pin, roll up the fudge into the square.   Cool it in the fridge for 10 minutes.   Then discard the baking paper and cut fudge into the serving squares.   Store dessert in the cool place.

Nutrition Info:calories 56, fat 3.5, fiber 0.1, carbs 7, protein 0.9

773. Pumpkin Cake

Servings: 6   Cooking Time: 4 Hours

Ingredients:

6 tablespoons of unbleached almond flour

¼ teaspoon of salt

½ teaspoon of baking soda

¼ teaspoon of baking powder

¼ teaspoon of pumpkin pie spice

6 tablespoons of swerve

½ medium banana mashed

1 tablespoon of canola oil

¼ cup of Greek yogurt

¼ (15 oz.) can pumpkin puree

½ egg

¼ teaspoon of pure vanilla extract

¼ cup of sugar-free chocolate chips

Directions:

Separately blend the wet and dry Ingredients: in the mixer.   Mix both the mixtures together in a bowl until smooth.   Now spread the cake batter in a greased ramekin and place it in the Crockpot. Cover its lid and cook for 4 hours on Low setting. Once done, remove its lid of the crockpot carefully. Allow it to cool and refrigerate for 1 hour.   Serve.

Nutrition Info: Calories 153 Total Fat 13 g Saturated Fat 9.2 g Cholesterol 6.5 mg Sodium 81 mg Total Carbs 4.5 g Sugar 1.4 g Fiber 0.4 g Protein 5.8 g

774. Walnut Muffins

Servings: 8   Cooking Time: 3 Hours

Ingredients:

2 oz walnuts, chopped

5 tablespoons butter

1 cup coconut flour

1 teaspoon vanilla extract

1 egg

2 tablespoons liquid stevia

3 tablespoons almond milk, unsweetened

1 teaspoon baking powder

Directions:

Mix the butter, flour, vanilla extract, liquid stevia, almond milk, and baking powder.   Beat the egg

into the mixture and whisk it well until smooth. Add the chopped walnuts and stir well.   Place the dough in the muffin molds and transfer into the slow cooker.   Cook the muffins for 3 hours on High. Cool the cooked muffins and enjoy!
Nutrition Info:calories 190, fat 14.8, fiber 6.6, carbs 11.4, protein 4.6

775.   Chocolate Crème Brule

Servings: 4   Cooking Time: 2 Hours
Ingredients:

5 egg yolks	2 cups of heavy cream
1 tablespoon of vanilla extract	½ cup of swerve
½ tablespoon of cocoa powder	½ tablespoon of grated sugar-free chocolate

Directions:
Start by thoroughly blending all the Ingredients: in a blender until smooth.   Now divide the batter into 4 ramekins and place them in the Crockpot. Cover its lid and cook for 2 hours on Low setting. Once done, remove its lid of the crockpot carefully. Allow it to cool and refrigerate for 1 hour.   Serve.
Nutrition Info: Calories 183 Total Fat 15 g Saturated Fat 12.1 g Cholesterol 11 mg Sodium 31 mg Total Carbs 9.2 g Sugar 1.6 g Fiber 0.8 g Protein 4.5 g

776.   Almond Roll

Servings: 6   Cooking Time: 3.5 Hours
Ingredients:

1 teaspoon baking powder	1/3 cup coconut oil
1 cup almond flour	1 teaspoon almond extract
1 tablespoon ground cinnamon	1 egg, beaten
2 tablespoons stevia	¾ cup Mascarpone cream

Directions:
In a bowl mix the flour with coconut oil and the other ingredients except the cinnamon and stevia. Mix up together ground cinnamon with stevia Roll up the dough with the help of the rolling pin. Spread the surface of the dough with ground cinnamon mixture and roll it into the log.   Cut the log into 6 buns and secure the edges of every bun. Line the crockpot with baking paper.   Place the buns in the crockpot and close the lid.   Cook the cinnamon roll for 3.5 hours on High.   Check if the rolls are cooked with the help of the toothpick – if it is dry, the buns are cooked.   Chill the dessert well and then remove from the crockpot in the serving plate.
Nutrition Info:calories 208, fat 15.3, fiber 1.1, carbs 8.2, protein 4.2

777.Caramel Cheesecake

Servings: 6   Cooking Time: 6 Hours
Ingredients:

¼ cup of erythritol	¼ cup of sour cream
2 eggs	
1 tablespoon of vanilla extract	Toppings:
2 cups of mixed nuts, crushed	10 caramels, unwrapped
2 tablespoons of unsalted butter, melted	2 tablespoons of heavy cream
	¼ cup of melted sugar-free chocolate

Directions:
Start by blending the Nuts with butter in the mixer. Spread this Nuts mixture in the greased Crockpot firmly.   Now beat the remaining filling Ingredients: except berries in a blender until smooth. Add this cream filling to the Nutty crust and spread evenly.   Cover its lid and cook for 6 hours on Low setting.   Once done, remove its lid of the crockpot carefully.   Allow it to cool and refrigerate for 1 hour.   Garnish with berries and other toppings. Serve.
Nutrition Info: Calories 252 Total Fat 17.3 g Saturated Fat 11.5 g Cholesterol 141 mg Sodium 153 mg Total Carbs 7.2 g Sugar 1.3 g Fiber 1.4 g Protein 5.2 g

778.   Cinnamon Cup Cake

Servings: 6   Cooking Time: 3 Hours
Ingredients:

1 teaspoon ground cinnamon	½ teaspoon baking soda
2 eggs	2 tablespoon stevia extract
1 cup almond milk, unsweetened	1 oz walnuts, chopped
½ cup coconut flour	

Directions:
Beat the eggs in a big bowl and whisk well.   Add ground cinnamon and almond milk and stir gently. Then add baking soda and stevia extract.   Whisk the mixture until smooth and add chopped walnuts. Stir the batter and place it in small ramekins.   Put the ramekins in the slow cooker and cook for 3 hours on High.   Serve the dessert immediately!
Nutrition Info:calories 183, fat 14.8, fiber 5.4, carbs 9.8, protein 5.3

779.   Strawberries Cake

Servings: 4   Cooking Time: 4.5 Hours
Ingredients:

1/3 cup strawberries, chopped	1 teaspoon vanilla extract
1 cup coconut flour	¾ teaspoon cinnamon powder
¼ cup butter, softened	1 teaspoon coconut oil
¾ cup stevia	

Directions:
Spread the slow cooker bottom with coconut oil. Place the chopped strawberries in the slow cooker and flatten them to get the layer shape.   In a bowl mix the rest of the ingredients, stir and knead the dough a bit.   Then place the dough over the strawberries. Flatten it well and close the lid. Cook the cake for 4.5 hours on Low.   When the cake is cooked, transfer it in the serving plates and eat hot.
Nutrition Info:calories 160, fat 16.2, fiber 1.1, carbs 3.2, protein 1.7

780.	**Keto Flan**

Servings: 3   Cooking Time: 10 Hours
Ingredients:

1 cup heavy cream	¼ cup Swerve
3 eggs, beaten	
½ teaspoon vanilla extract	½ teaspoon butter
	½ cup water, for cooking

Directions:
Put butter in the skillet and melt it.   Add Swerve and simmer the liquid over the medium heat for 3 minutes.   Then pour the butter sweet mixture into the ramekins.   Mix up together beaten eggs, vanilla extract, and heavy cream.   When the liquid is smooth, pour it over the sweet butter mixture in the ramekins.   Pour water in the crockpot. Place the ramekins with flan in the water and close the lid.   Cook flan for 10 hours on Low.   Chill the flan little and turn the ramekins over in the plates to get flan.
Nutrition Info:calories 209, fat 19.8, fiber 0, carbs 1.7, protein 6.4

781.	**Avocado Muffins**

Servings: 4   Cooking Time: 2.5 Hours
Ingredients:

1 egg, beaten	1 tablespoon butter
1 teaspoon baking powder	2 teaspoons liquid stevia
1 avocado, mashed	1 teaspoon coconut flour
3 tablespoons almond flour	

Directions:
Whisk together the egg and mashed avocado. Add the baking powder and almond flour.   Add the butter and liquid stevia.   Sprinkle the mixture with the coconut flour and knead the dough. Place the dough in 4 muffin molds.   Transfer the muffins to the slow cooker and cook for 2.5 hours on High.   Cool the cooked muffins and serve!
Nutrition Info:calories 265, fat 24.3, fiber 5.7, carbs 9.5, protein 6.9

782.	**Coconut Bars(2)**

Servings: 7   Cooking Time: 3 Hours
Ingredients:

¼ cup coconut flakes, unsweetened	1 teaspoon baking powder
1 cup coconut flour	1 teaspoon vanilla extract
½ cup almond milk, unsweetened	1 teaspoon butter

Directions:
Mix the coconut flakes and coconut flour.   Add the baking soda and stir the mixture.   Add the butter and vanilla extract.   Add the almond milk and stir it until smooth.   Transfer the mixture to the slow cooker.   Flatten it with a spatula and cook for 3 hours on High.   Cut the cooked dessert into bars and serve!
Nutrition Info:calories 125, fat 7.3, fiber 7.5, carbs 13.2, protein 2.8

783.	**Walnut Cake**

Servings: 8   Cooking Time: 4.5 Hours
Ingredients:

1 cup almond flour	2 tablespoons walnuts, chopped
4 tablespoons butter, softened	
1 teaspoon almond extract	3 eggs, beaten
	1/3 cup coconut milk
½ cup stevia	2 egg yolks
3 tablespoons Ricotta cheese	1 teaspoon peanut butter

Directions:
In a bowl, mix the coconut milk with the flour and the other ingredients and whisk well.   Line the slow cooker with baking paper, pour the cake mix inside and close the lid.   Cook the mix for 4.5 hours on Low.   Cool down and serve.
Nutrition Info:calories 214, fat 4.3, fiber 0.6, carbs 2.3, protein 6.8

784.	**Spiced Strawberry Pudding**

Servings: 6   Cooking Time: 4 Hours
Ingredients:

2 cups of strawberries, cored	2 eggs
1 tablespoon of vanilla	2 cups of almond flour
1 tablespoon of apple pie spice	1 tablespoon of baking powder

Directions:
Separately blend the wet and dry Ingredients: in the mixer.   Mix both the mixtures together in a bowl until smooth.   Now spread the cake batter in a greased ramekin and place it in the Crockpot. Cover its lid and cook for 4 hours on Low setting. Once done, remove its lid of the crockpot carefully. Allow it to cool and refrigerate for 1 hour.   Serve.
Nutrition Info: Calories 254 Total Fat 09 g Saturated Fat 10.1 g Cholesterol 13 mg Sodium 179 mg Total Carbs 7.5 g Sugar 1.2 g Fiber 0.8 g Protein 7.5 g

785.	**Rhubarb Bars**

Servings: 4   Cooking Time: 3 Hours
Ingredients:

5 oz rhubarb, chopped	4 tablespoons butter
2 tablespoons liquid stevia	4 tablespoons coconut flour
1 teaspoon swerve	¼ teaspoon ground cinnamon
1 teaspoon vanilla extract	

Directions:
Combine the liquid stevia, swerve, vanilla extract, butter, coconut flour, and ground cinnamon. Knead into a smooth dough.   Place the dough in the slow cooker and flatten it into the shape of a pie crust.   Sprinkle with the chopped rhubarb and press gently.   Close the lid and cook the dessert for 3 hours.   Cool and cut into the bars.   Enjoy!
Nutrition Info:calories 42, fat 0.8, fiber 3.7, carbs 7.4, protein 1.3

786.	**Walnut Squares**

Servings: 6   Cooking Time: 3 Hours
Ingredients:

- 1 cup walnuts, chopped
- 2 tablespoons stevia
- 1 teaspoon vanilla extract
- 2 eggs, beaten
- 1 cup
- ½ cup coconut flour
- 1 teaspoon baking soda
- 1 tablespoon butter, softened
- Cooking spray

Directions:
Spray the crockpot with cooking spray from inside. In the mixing bowl, combine the walnuts with stevia and the other ingredients and stir until you obtain a dough.   Transfer the dough in the crockpot and flatten it well with the help of the spatula.   Close the lid and cook the dough for 3 hours on High. The time of cooking depends on the dough thicknesses. When the dough is cooked, carefully transfer it on the chopping board and let chill to the room temperature.   Cut it into the squares.
Nutrition Info:calories 230, fat 11.4, fiber 4.5, carbs 11.9, protein 7.9

787.	**Keto Chocolate Bars**

Servings: 8   Cooking Time: 3 Hours
Ingredients:

- 1 oz dark chocolate
- 1 tablespoons chia seeds
- 1 cup almond flour
- 1 tablespoons liquid stevia
- 1 egg, beaten
- 1 teaspoon vanilla extract
- ½ cup almond milk, unsweetened

Directions:
Melt the dark chocolate and mix it with the beaten egg.   Whisk the mixture until smooth.   Add the liquid stevia, vanilla extract, and almond milk. Whisk the mixture until smooth.   Add almond flour and stir the dough with a spatula.   When the dough is smooth, add the chia seeds and stir it well. Transfer the dough to the slow cooker and flatten it gently.   Close the lid and cook the dessert for 3 hours on High or until the bar is set in the middle. Let the cooked dessert cool.   Cut into bars and place on a serving platter.   Serve!
Nutrition Info:calories 100, fat 8, fiber 2.1, carbs 5.3, protein 2.6

788.	**Slow-cooked Cranberry Custard**

Servings: 4   Cooking Time: 2 Hours
Ingredients:

- 1 tablespoon of lemon zest
- 5 large egg yolks
- 2 cups of whipping cream or coconut cream
- 1 teaspoon of vanilla extract
- 1/4 cup of cranberries
- ½ cup of erythritol

Directions:
Start by blending all the Ingredients: together in a mixer.   Pour this mixture into 4 ramekins and place them in the Crockpot.   Cover its lid and cook for 2 hours on Low setting.   Once done, remove its lid of the crockpot carefully.   Allow it to cool and refrigerate for 1 hour.   Garnish as desired. Serve.
Nutrition Info: Calories 151 Total Fat 14.7 g Saturated Fat 1.5 g Cholesterol 13 mg Sodium 53 mg Total Carbs 1.5 g Sugar 0.3 g Fiber 0.1 g Protein 23.8 g

789.	**Crème Brûlée**

Servings: 6.   Cooking Time: 2 Hours On High.
Ingredients:

- 5 large egg yolks
- 6 Tablespoons sweetener, Erythritol
- 2 cups double cream
- 1 Bourbon vanilla pod, scraped
- Pinch of salt

Directions:
In a bowl, beat the eggs and sweetener together. Add the cream and vanilla. Whisk together, Divide the mixture between 6 small ramekin dishes or one big dish.   Set them in the crock-pot and pour hot water around them - so the water reaches half way up the ramekins.   Cover, cook on high for 2 hours.   Take the dishes out, let them cool. Refrigerate for 6-8 hours.
Nutrition Info:net C 2g; P 2g; F 34g

790.	**Low Carb Sweet Pecans**

Servings: 4   Cooking Time: 3 Hours
Ingredients:

- 1 cup of swerve
- 1 cup of brown swerve
- 3 tablespoons of cinnamon ground
- ⅛ teaspoon of salt
- 1 egg white
- 2 teaspoons of vanilla
- ⅛ cup of water

Directions:
Start putting all the Ingredients: into the Crockpot. Cover its lid and cook for 3 hours on Low setting with occasional stirring   Once done, remove the pot's lid and give it a stir.   Serve fresh.
Nutrition Info: Calories 266 Total Fat 25.7 g Saturated Fat 1.2 g Cholesterol 41 mg Sodium 18 mg Total Carbs 9.7 g Sugar 1.2 g Fiber 0.5 g Protein 2.6 g

791.	**Traditional Egg Custard**

Servings: 4   Cooking Time: 3 Hours
Ingredients:

- 6 eggs
- 3/4 cup of erythritol
- 1 teaspoon of vanilla extract
- 1 pinch salt
- ¼ teaspoon of cinnamon, ground
- Nutmeg, grated
- Fresh fruits, diced

Directions:
Start by blending all the Ingredients: together in a mixer.   Pour this mixture into 4 ramekins and place them in the Crockpot.   Cover its lid and cook for 2-3 hours on Low setting.   Once done, remove its lid of the crockpot carefully.   Allow it to cool and refrigerate for 1 hour.   Garnish as desired. Serve.
Nutrition Info: Calories 172 Total Fat 10.7 g Saturated Fat 7.4 g Cholesterol 62 mg Sodium 121 mg Total Carbs 10.9 g Fiber 0.6 g Sugar 1.5 g Protein 12 g

792. Zucchini Cake

Servings: 8   Cooking Time: 4 Hours

Ingredients:

1 cup almond flour
3 tablespoons coconut flour
1 teaspoon baking soda
½ teaspoon apple cider vinegar
1 teaspoon cocoa powder
2 zucchinis, grated
2 tablespoons pecans, chopped
1/3 cup organic coconut milk
2 eggs, beaten
1/3 cup stevia
1 teaspoon coconut oil
2 tablespoons cream cheese

Directions:
In the mixing bowl mix up together the flour with the baking soda and the other ingredients and whisk. Line the slow cooker with baking paper and transfer the cake mixture inside.   Flatten it gently.   Cook the cake for 4 hours on Low.   Cut the cake into the servings.

Nutrition Info:calories 215, fat 6.2, fiber 4.3, carbs 4.7, protein 5.4

793. Blueberry Crisp

Servings: 2   Cooking Time: 5 Hours

Ingredients:

1/2 cup blueberries
¼ cup coconut flakes
2 tablespoons almond butter, softened
1 teaspoon almond extract
¾ teaspoon ground nutmeg
1 tablespoon Erythritol
1 egg, beaten

Directions:
In the mixing bowl, combine the berries with the flakes and the other ingredients and whisk.   Put the homogenous berries mixture in the crockpot and flatten well.   Flatten the crisp gently.   Close the lid.   Cook the crisp 5 hours on Low.

Nutrition Info:calories 202, fat 7.5, fiber 2.8, carbs 5.3, protein 4.5

794. Pound Cake

Servings: 8   Cooking Time: 3 Hours

Ingredients:

1 cup almond flour
¼ cup coconut flour
1 teaspoon vanilla extract
3 tablespoons butter
2 egg, beaten
1 teaspoon baking powder
2 teaspoons full-fat cream cheese

Directions:
Whisk the eggs and combine them with the baking powder and cream cheese.   Stir and add vanilla extract and coconut flour.   Add the almond flour and stir the mixture until smooth.   Place the cake in the slow cooker and cook for 3 hours on High. Cool the cooked cake and cut into the servings. Enjoy!

Nutrition Info:calories 92, fat 7.6, fiber 1.9, carbs 3.8, protein 2.9

795. Vanilla Avocado Cookies

Servings: 3   Cooking Time: 1 Hour

Ingredients:

½ cup almond flour
1 avocado, peeled, pitted and mashed
½ teaspoon vanilla extract
1 tablespoon stevia
1 tablespoon butter
½ teaspoon avocado oil
Cooking spray

Directions:
In the mixing bowl, mix up together flour with avocado and the other ingredients except the cooking spray and stir until you obtain a dough Knead the soft but non-sticky dough.   Brush the crockpot bowl with cooking spray from inside. Make the small balls from the dough and press them gently with the help of the fork.   Put the cookies in the crockpot and cook for 1 hour on High.

Nutrition Info:calories 124, fat 6.3, fiber 2.5, carbs 6.1, protein 2.1

796. Chocolate Mousse

Servings: 4   Cooking Time: 4 Hours

Ingredients:

2 oz dark chocolate
1 cup almond milk, unsweetened
2 egg whites
1 tablespoon full-fat cream cheese

Directions:
Melt the chocolate and combine it with the almond milk.   Whisk the egg whites until soft peaks and combine it together with the cream cheese. Whisk it gently for 1 minute more.   Combine chocolate mixture and egg white mixture.   Stir and transfer into ramekins.   Place the ramekins in the slow cooker and cook on Low for 4 hours. Serve the cooked mousse!

Nutrition Info:calories 231, fat 6.719.4, fiber 1.8, carbs 11.9, protein 4.4

797. Sweet Sesame Buns

Servings: 8   Cooking Time: 3 Hours

Ingredients:

1 tablespoon sesame seeds
2 tablespoons butter
1 egg, beaten
1 egg white
1 cup almond flour
1 tablespoon coconut flakes, sesame
¼ cup Erythritol
1 teaspoon vanilla extract

Directions:
Whisk the egg and egg whites.   Add the butter and almond flour.   Add Erythritol, vanilla and coconut flakes and knead into a smooth dough.   Form small buns from the dough and place them in the slow cooker.   Sprinkle the buns with the sesame seeds and cook for 3 hours on High.   Cool the cooked buns until room temperature and transfer onto a platter.   Enjoy!

Nutrition Info:calories 66, fat 6, fiber 0.6, carbs 20.8, protein 2.1

798. Crockpot Lemon Custard

Servings: 4   Cooking Time: 2 Hours

Ingredients:

1/4 cup of freshly squeezed lemon juice
1 tablespoon of lemon zest
1 teaspoon of vanilla extract
½ cup of erythritol
2 cups of whipping cream or coconut cream
Lightly sweetened whipped cream

Directions:

Start by blending all the Ingredients: together in a mixer. Pour this mixture into 4 ramekins and place them in the Crockpot. Cover its lid and cook for 2 hours on Low setting. Once done, remove its lid of the crockpot carefully. Allow it to cool and refrigerate for 1 hour. Garnish as desired. Serve.

Nutrition Info: Calories 195 Total Fat 14.3 g Saturated Fat 10.5 g Cholesterol 175 mg Sodium 125 mg Total Carbs 4.5 g Sugar 0.5 g Fiber 0.3 g Protein 3.2 g

799. Lemon Scones

Servings: 6   Cooking Time: 2.5 Hours
Ingredients:

2 cups almond flour	½ cup of coconut oil
2 tablespoons lemon juice	1 teaspoon baking powder
1 teaspoon cinnamon powder	1 egg, beaten
	4 tablespoons Swerve

Directions:
In the mixing bowl, combine the flour with the coconut oil and the other ingredients and stir well. Line the slow cooker with baking paper. Make the ball from the dough and place it in the slow cooker. Cut the dough into 6 scones and close the lid. Cook the scones for 2.5 hours on High. Then chill the cooked dessert well and cut the dough into scones again.
Nutrition Info:calories 221, fat 14.4, fiber 1, carbs 6.6, protein 3.1

800. Chocolate Pudding

Servings: 3   Cooking Time: 15 Minutes
Ingredients:

½ cup heavy cream	½ teaspoon vanilla extract
1 oz dark chocolate	
1 tablespoon Truvia	

Directions:
Put dark chocolate and vanilla extract in the slow cooker. Close the lid and cook the chocolate for 15 minutes on High. Meanwhile, whip the heavy cream. Add Truvia and stir it well. Gradually start to add the melted dark chocolate. Stir it until smooth. Transfer the cooked pudding in the serving cups.
Nutrition Info:calories 124, fat 10.7., fiber 0.7, carbs 7.5, protein 0.8

801. Vanilla Bars

Servings: 6   Cooking Time: 5 Hours
Ingredients:

1 cup almond flour	1 tablespoon stevia
¼ cup coconut butter, softened	1 teaspoon vanilla extract
4 eggs, beaten	Cooking spray
½ cup coconut cream	

Directions:
In the bowl, combine together eggs with almond flour and the other ingredients and stir. Transfer this to the lined and sprayed crockpot, and cook on Low for 5 hours. Cool down, cut into bars and serve.
Nutrition Info:calories 207, fat 7.7, fiber 0.5, carbs 4.5, protein 6.2

802. Granola

Servings: 6   Cooking Time: 2 Hours
Ingredients:

1 teaspoon of vanilla extract	1/2 cup of hazelnuts
1/2 cup of raw almonds	1 cup of shredded coconut
1/2 cup of walnuts	1/2 cup of Swerve
1/2 cup of pecans	1 teaspoon of cinnamon, ground
1 cup of sunflower seeds	1 teaspoon of salt
1 cup of pumpkin seeds	1 cup of whipped cream

Directions:
Start by putting everything in the Crockpot and mix well. Cover its lid and cook for 2 hours on Low setting. Once done, remove its lid of the crockpot carefully. Spread the mixture on a baking sheet and leave for 30 minutes. Slice and serve.
Nutrition Info: Calories 175 Total Fat 16 g Saturated Fat 2.1 g Cholesterol 0 mg Sodium 8 mg Total Carbs 2.8 g Sugar 1.8 g Fiber 0.4 g Protein 9 g

803. Raspberry & Coconut Cake

Servings: 10.   Cooking Time: 3 Hours On Low.
Ingredients:

2 cups ground almonds	4 large eggs
1 cup shredded coconut	½ cup melted coconut oil
¾ cup sweetener, Swerve (or suitable substitute)	¾ cup coconut milk
2 teaspoon baking soda	1 cup raspberries, fresh or frozen
¼ teaspoon salt	½ cup sugarless dark chocolate chips

Directions:
Butter the crock-pot. In a bowl, mix the dry ingredients. Beat in the eggs, melted coconut oil, and coconut milk. Gently fold in the raspberries and chocolate chips. Combine the cocoa, almonds, and salt in a bowl. Pour the batter into the buttered crock-pot. Cover the crock-pot with a paper towel to absorb the water. Cover, cook on low for 3 hours. Let the cake cool in the pot.
Nutrition Info:net C 8g; P 7g; F 43g

804. Delightful Crème Brule

Servings: 4   Cooking Time: 2 Hours
Ingredients:

5 egg yolks	2 cups of heavy cream
1 tablespoon of vanilla extract	½ cup of swerve
½ tablespoon of cocoa powder	¼ cup of superfine swerve

Directions:
Start by thoroughly blending all the Ingredients: in a blender until smooth. Now divide the batter into 4 ramekins and place them in the Crockpot. Cover its lid and cook for 2 hours on Low setting. Once done, remove its lid of the crockpot carefully. Allow it to cool and refrigerate for 1 hour. Serve.
Nutrition Info: Calories 243 Total Fat 21 g Saturated Fat 18.2 g Cholesterol 121 mg Sodium 34 mg Total Carbs 7.3 g Sugar 0.9 g Fiber 0.1 g Protein 4.3 g

805. Strawberry Cobbler

Servings: 2   Cooking Time: 4 Hours
Ingredients:

¼ cup strawberries	1 cup almond flour
¾ teaspoon almond extract	3 tablespoons coconut butter
1 teaspoon vanilla extract	1 teaspoon liquid stevia
1 tablespoon Monk fruit	1 egg, beaten
	Cooking spray

Directions:
Mix up together strawberries almond extract and vanilla extract. Mash the mixture gently.   Then spray the crockpot bottom with cooking spray. Place the berry mixture inside the crockpot and flatten it gently.   After this, mix up together Monk fruit with the remaining ingredients.   Stir the mixture until homogenous.   Then transfer the prepared almond flour mixture over the berry mixture and flatten gently.   Cook the cobbler for 4 hours on High.
Nutrition Info:calories 241, fat 6.7, fiber 3.1, carbs 4.6, protein 5.3

806. Almond Blondies

Servings: 14   Cooking Time: 3.5 Hours
Ingredients:

½ cup almond butter, softened	1 egg, beaten
1 cup stevia	1 cup almond flour
1 teaspoon almond extract	1 oz white chocolate, melted

Directions:
In the mixing bowl combine the butter with the stevia and the other ingredients and whisk.   Line the crockpot with baking paper and pour blondies mixture inside.   Flatten it and cook for 5 hours. Then remove the blondies from the crockpot and cut into the servings.
Nutrition Info:calories 145, fat 2.5, fiber 3.1, carbs 5.2, protein 1.7

807. Gingerbread Cookies

Servings: 6   Cooking Time: 2.5 Hours
Ingredients:

1 teaspoon ground ginger	1 cup almond flour
1 teaspoon ground cinnamon	4 tablespoons butter
1 teaspoon vanilla extract	1 egg, whisked
	1 teaspoon baking powder

Directions:
Add the ground ginger, ground cinnamon, vanilla extract, almond flour, and baking powder into a large bowl.   Stir and add the butter and whisked the egg.   Knead into a soft dough.   Roll it out with a rolling pin and make the cookies.   Place the cookies in the slow cooker and cook them for 2.5 hours on High.   Chill the cookies and serve!
Nutrition Info:calories 195, fat 17.3, fiber 2.3, carbs 5.1, protein 5.1

808. Pumpkin Custard

Servings: 4   Cooking Time: 4 Hours
Ingredients:

1 cup of pumpkin purée	6 eggs
	1 pinch salt
3/4 cup of brown swerve	¼ teaspoon of cinnamon ground
1 teaspoon of pumpkin spice	1 cup of heavy cream
	Walnuts, to serve

Directions:
Start by blending all the Ingredients: together in a mixer.   Pour this mixture into 4 ramekins and place them in the Crockpot.   Cover its lid and cook for 4 hours on Low setting.   Once done, remove its lid of the crockpot carefully.   Allow it to cool and refrigerate for 1 hour.   Garnish with walnuts and cream.   Serve.   Serve.
Nutrition Info: Calories 174 Total Fat 12.3 g Saturated Fat 4.8 g Cholesterol 32 mg Sodium 597 mg Total Carbs 10.5 g Fiber 0.6 g Sugar 1.9 g Protein 12 g

809. Toffee Pudding

Servings: 4   Cooking Time: 4 Hours
Ingredients:

¼ cup of sugar-free maple syrup	1 pinch salt
¼ cup of boiling water	6 tablespoons of brown swerve
3/4 cup of almond flour	1/6 cup of unsalted butter
½ teaspoon of baking powder	½ egg
	½ teaspoon of vanilla extract

Directions:
Start by blending all the Ingredients: together in a mixer.   Pour this mixture into 4 ramekins and place them in the Crockpot.   Cover its lid and cook for 4 hours on Low setting.   Once done, remove its lid of the crockpot carefully.   Allow it to cool and refrigerate for 1 hour.   Serve.
Nutrition Info: Calories 113 Total Fat 9 g Saturated Fat 0.2 g Cholesterol 1.7 mg Sodium 134 mg Total Carbs 6.5 g Sugar 1.8 g Fiber 0.7 g Protein 7.5 g

810. Berry & Coconut Cake

Servings: 8.   Cooking Time: 2 Hours On High.
Ingredients:

1 Tablespoon butter for greasing the crock	1 large egg, beaten with a fork
1 cup almond flour	¼ cup coconut flour
¾ cup sweetener of your choice	¼ cup coconut milk
1 teaspoon baking soda	2 Tablespoons coconut oil
¼ teaspoon salt	4 cups fresh or frozen blueberries and raspberries

Directions:
Butter the crock-pot well.   In a bowl, whisk the egg, coconut milk, and oil together.   Mix the dry ingredients. Slowly stir in the wet ingredients. Do not over mix.   Pour the batter in the crock-pot, spread evenly.   Spread the berries on top. Cover, cook on high for 2 hours. Cool in the crock for 1-2 hours.
Nutrition Info:net C 7g; P 7g; F 17g

811. Biscuits

Servings: 6   Cooking Time: 2 Hours
Ingredients:

1 cup coconut flour
1/3 cup almond butter, softened
1 teaspoon almond extract
1 teaspoon baking powder
¼ cup coconut flakes
1 teaspoon lemon juice
2 tablespoons Erythritol
Cooking spray

Directions:
Knead the dough: mix up together flour with the coconut flakes and the other ingredients except the cooking spray. The dough should be very soft but non-sticky. After this, roll the dough into a log and cut into pieces. Roll up the dough pieces into the round biscuits with the help of the rolling pin. Line the crockpot bottom with baking paper and spray with cooking spray. Carefully place the almond biscuits in the crockpot and cook them for 2 hours on High. Chill the biscuits well before serving.
Nutrition Info:calories 203, fat 14.6, fiber 1, carbs 5.4, protein 2

812.   Vanilla Rolls

Servings: 8   Cooking Time: 3 Hours
Ingredients:
1 tablespoon vanilla extract
3 tablespoons Erythritol
½ cup almond milk, unsweetened
1 cup almond flour
1 tablespoon cocoa powder
1 tablespoon coconut flour
1 teaspoon butter

Directions:
Mix the butter, coconut flour, cocoa powder, almond flour, almond milk, and vanilla extract. Add the Erythritol and knead into a smooth dough. Roll out the dough it into a log. Cut the log into slices and place them in the slow cooker. Cook the vanilla rolls for 3 hours on High. Chill the rolls to room temperature and serve!
Nutrition Info:calories 69, fat 6, fiber 1.3, carbs 8.4, protein 1.4

813.   Cream Cheese Cookies

Servings: 4   Cooking Time: 4.5 Hours
Ingredients:
1 teaspoon baking soda
1 tablespoon apple cider vinegar
3 tablespoons sugar-free chocolate chips
¼ cup stevia
1/3 cup avocado oil
1 cup almond flour
1 egg, beaten
1 teaspoon cream cheese
1 teaspoon almond extract

Directions:
In a bowl, mix the egg with flour, cream cheese and the other ingredients and whisk. Transfer the cookies mixture in the slow cooker. Flatten the surface of the cookie dough with the help of the spatula. Cook the chip cookies for 5 hours on Low.
Nutrition Info:calories 245, fat 14.3, fiber 0.8, carbs 6.4, protein 3.2

814.   Keto Fudge

Servings: 12   Cooking Time: 3 Hours
Ingredients:
5 tablespoons butter
1 oz dark chocolate
3 tablespoons almond flour
1 teaspoon vanilla extract
½ cup Erythritol
4 tablespoons cocoa powder
1 tablespoon cream cheese

Directions:
Combine the butter and dark chocolate and preheat the mixture. When the mixture is melted, add the almond flour, Erythritol, vanilla extract, and cocoa powder. Add the cream cheese and stir. Place the fudge mixture in the slow cooker and cook it for 3 hours on High. Serve the cooked fudge hot!
Nutrition Info:calories 103, fat 9.5, fiber 1.4, carbs 14 protein 2.1

815.   Cherry Cheese Cake

Servings: 8   Cooking Time: 6 Hours
Ingredients:
8oz. ricotta cheese
¼ cup of erythritol
2 eggs
¼ cup of sour cream
1 tablespoon of vanilla extract
2 cups of mixed nuts, crushed
2 tablespoons of unsalted butter, melted
2 tablespoons of erythritol
¼ cup of fresh cherries pitted

Directions:
Start by blending the Nuts with butter in the mixer. Spread this Nuts mixture in the greased Crockpot firmly. Now beat the remaining filling Ingredients: except cherries in a blender until smooth. Add this cream filling to the Nutty crust and spread evenly. Cover its lid and cook for 6 hours on Low setting. Once done, remove its lid of the crockpot carefully. Allow it to cool and refrigerate for 1 hour. Garnish with cherries. Serve.
Nutrition Info: Calories 220 Total Fat 2.8 g Saturated Fat 0.1 g Cholesterol 5 mg Sodium 177 mg Total Carbs 47.7 g Fiber 3 g Sugar 24.2 g Protein 3.7 g

816.   Vanilla Pudding

Servings: 2   Cooking Time: 4 Hours
Ingredients:
1 cup organic coconut milk
1 teaspoon vanilla extract
4 tablespoons coconut flakes
2 tablespoons stevia

Directions:
In the crockpot, mix the coconut milk and vanilla and the other ingredients. Close the lid. Cook the pudding for 4 hours on Low.
Nutrition Info:calories 149, fat 5.8, fiber 7.8, carbs 6.2, protein 4

817. Balsamic Beef Pot Roast

Servings: 10   Cooking Time: 4 Hours
Ingredients:

1 tbsp. of each:
-Kosher salt
- Black ground pepper
- Garlic powder
¼ c. balsamic vinegar

½ c. chopped onion
2 c. water
¼ t. xanthan gum
For the Garnish:
Fresh parsley

Directions:
Season the chuck roast with garlic powder, pepper, and salt over the entire surface.   Use a large skillet to sear the roast until browned.   Deglaze the bottom of the pot using balsamic vinegar. Cook one minute. Add to the slow cooker.   Mix in the onion, and add the water. Once it starts to boil, secure the lid, and continue cooking on low for three to four hours.   Take the meat out of the slow cooker, and place it in a large bowl where you will break it up carefully into large chunks.   Remove all fat and anything else that may not be healthy such as too much fat.   Whisk the xanthan gum into the broth, and add it back to the slow cooker.   Serve and enjoy with a smile!
Nutrition Info: Calories: 393 Net Carbs: 3 g Protein: 30 g Fat: 28 g

818. Pork Mexican Wraps

Servings: 4   Cooking Time: 9 Hours
Ingredients:

2 tablespoons / 28 gr of ghee
2 tablespoons / 28 gr of vegetable broth
1 pinch of red hot pepper
1 pinch of chili powder

1 dash of tabasco
1 pinch of sweet paprika
1 pinch of cayenne powder
½ / 100 gr of ripe avocado for garnishing, sliced

Directions:
Mix all of the ingredients in your Slow Cooker pot Close the pot and cook on LOW for 9 hours   Serve hot with avocado slices on top
Nutrition Info: Calories: 640 Fat: 56 gr Total carbs: 8.15 Net carbs: 1.8 Protein 25.5 g

819. Crockpot Carnitas Taco

Servings: 12   Cooking Time: 8 Hours And 30 Minutes
Ingredients:

1 envelop taco seasoning
2 tablespoon green chilies, chopped

1 cup tomatoes, diced
2 cups Monterey Jack cheese, shredded

Directions:
Place the roast in the slow cooker and sprinkle with taco seasoning all over.   Pour the tomatoes and green chilies around the pork roast.   Cook on low for 8 hours or until the meat is very tender.   Use two forks to shred the meat. Return the shredded meat back to the slow cooker and sprinkle cheese on

top.   Cook for another 30 minutes on high or until the cheese has slightly melted.   Garnish with sour cream or cilantro if preferred.
Nutrition Info: Calories: 435 Carbohydrates: 0.7g Protein: 42.1g Fat: 28.9g Sugar: 0g; Sodium: 271mg Fiber: 0g

820. Herbed Green Beans

Servings: 2   Cooking Time: 2 Hours
Ingredients:

½ teaspoon of chili powder
1 lb. green beans, trimmed and halved
1 and ½ cups of chicken stock
1 tablespoon of rosemary, diced

1 tablespoon of basil, diced
1 tablespoon of dill, diced
A pinch of salt and black pepper
½ cup of almonds, diced

Directions:
Start by throwing all the Ingredients: into the Crockpot.   Cover its lid and cook for 2 hours on Low setting.   Once done, remove its lid of the crockpot carefully.   Mix well and garnish as desired.   Serve warm.
Nutrition Info: Calories 149 Total Fat 14.5 g Saturated Fat 8.1 g Cholesterol 56 mg Sodium 56 mg Total Carbs 10.6 g Sugar 0.3 g Fiber 0.2 g Protein 2.6 g

821. Spiced Nut "snackers"

Servings: Makes 2 Large Jars Of Spiced Nuts Cooking Time: Approximately 4 Hours
Ingredients:

4 cups mixed nuts, the best Keto-friendly nuts are almonds, pecans, and macadamia nuts
2 tbsp coconut oil, melted

2 tbsp butter, melted
2 tsp cinnamon
½ tsp ground nutmeg
1 tsp sea salt
Small pinch of curry powder

Directions:
Place the butter, coconut oil, cinnamon, nutmeg, sea salt, and curry powder into the Slow Cookerand stir to combine.   Add the nuts to the pot and stir until the nuts are coated.   Place the lid onto the Slow Cookerand set the temperature to LOW.   Cook for 3 hours.   If you prefer crispier nuts, toss the cooked nuts in a hot skillet with the remaining liquid from the Slow Cookerbefore serving in small bowls, otherwise, remove from the Slow Cookerand place in bowls.   Serve once slightly cooled.

822. Low Carb Taco Soup

Servings: 6   Cooking Time: 2 Hours
Ingredients:

2, 8-ounce packages of cream cheese
2, 10-ounce cans of Rotel tomatoes
1 2 tablespoons of

2 tablespoons of taco seasonings
4 cups of chicken broth
1/2 cup of shredded

cilantro fresh or dried   cheese for garnish
optional   optional

Directions:
Start by throwing all the Ingredients: into your Crockpot.   Mix well and cover the Crockpot with its lid.   Select the High settings for 2 hours. Serve warm.
Nutrition Info: Calories 538 Total Fat 23.2 g Saturated Fat 13 g Cholesterol 61 mg Total Carbs 6.8 g Sugar 0 g Fiber 0.9 g Sodium 115 mg Potassium 303 mg Protein 21.3 g

823.   Shrimp Soup

Servings: 4   Cooking Time: 3 Hours
Ingredients:

1-pound shrimp, peeled and deveined
1 ½ cup organic almond milk
½ teaspoon turmeric powder

¼ cup cauliflower, chopped
½ teaspoon salt
1 teaspoon minced garlic
1 cup water

Directions:
In the slow cooker, mix the shrimp with milk and the other ingredients, close the lid and cook on Low for 3 hours.   When the soup is cooked, divide into bowls and serve.
Nutrition Info:calories 117, fat 6, fiber 0.9, carbs 6.7, protein 6.2

824.   Spinach Soup

Servings: 4   Cooking Time: 6-8 Hours
Ingredients:

¼ cup cream cheese
1 onion, diced
1 garlic clove, minced

2 cups heavy cream
2 cups water
salt, pepper, to taste

Directions:
Pour water into the slow cooker. Add spinach, salt and pepper.   Add cream cheese, onion, garlic and heavy cream.   Close the lid and cook on Low for 6-8 hours.   Puree soup with blender and serve.
Nutrition Info: Calories 322 Fats 28.2g Net carbs 10.1g Protein 12.2g

825.   Spiced Chicken

Servings: 3   Cooking Time: 3.5 Hours
Ingredients:

3 chicken thighs, boneless, skinless
1 teaspoon cumin, ground
1 teaspoon coriander, ground
1 teaspoon nutmeg, ground
1/3 cup water

1 jalapeno pepper, sliced
1 teaspoon minced garlic
1 teaspoon ground cinnamon
½ teaspoon chili flakes
1 teaspoon olive oil

Directions:
In the slow cooker, mix the chicken with cumin, coriander and the rest of the ingredients.   Close the lid and cook chicken for 3.5 hours on High. Divide into bowls and serve.
Nutrition Info:calories 301, fat 12.4, fiber 1.5, carbs 8.8, protein 22.8

826.   Mashed Broccoli

Servings: 2   Cooking Time: 3 Hours
Ingredients:

1 broccoli, florets separated
A pinch of salt and black pepper
1 tablespoon of butter, melted

½ cup of chicken stock
1 tablespoon of chives, diced

Directions:
Start by throwing all the Ingredients: into the Crockpot.   Cover its lid and cook for 3 hours on Low setting.   Once done, remove its lid of the crockpot carefully.   Puree this mixture using an immersion blender.   Mix well and garnish as desired.   Serve warm.
Nutrition Info: Calories 124 Total Fat 13.4 g Saturated Fat 7 g Cholesterol 20 mg Sodium 136 mg Total Carbs 6.4 g Sugar 2.1 g Fiber 4.8 g

827.   Garlicky Shrimp

Servings: 4   Cooking Time: 2 Hours
Ingredients:

5 cloves of garlic, minced
Salt and pepper, to taste

½ cup olive oil
1 ½ lb. jumbo shrimp, shelled and deveined

Directions:
Place all ingredients in the Slow Cookerand stir well. Close the lid and cook on high for 2 hours. Garnish with chopped fresh parsley if desired.
Nutrition Info: Calories: 473 Carbohydrates: 1.3g Protein: 34.4g Fat: 36.7g Sugar: 0.1g Sodium: 242mg Fiber: 0.1g

828.   Chard Chicken Soup

Servings: 8   Cooking Time: 5 Hours
Ingredients:

4 cups of chicken breast, cooked and shredded
1 cup of mushrooms, sliced
1/4 cup of onion, diced
8 cups of chicken stock
2 tablespoons of vinegar
1/4 cup of basil, diced

2 cups of water
1 tablespoon of garlic, minced
4 bacon strips, diced
1/4 cup of sundried tomatoes, diced
1 cup of green beans, cut into medium pieces
1 tablespoon of coconut oil, melted
Salt and black pepper- to taste

Directions:
Start by throwing all the Ingredients: except cilantro into your Crockpot.   Mix well and cover the Crockpot with its lid.   Select the Low settings for 5 hours.   Garnish with cilantro.   Serve warm.
Nutrition Info: Calories 238 Total Fat 16.9 g Saturated Fat 16.9 g Cholesterol 32 mg Total Carbs 3.5 g Sugar 0.1 g Fiber 7.2 g Sodium 469 mg Potassium 0 mg Protein 10.8 g

829.	**Carrots With Mushroom Sauce**

Servings: 4   Cooking Time: 4 Hours
Ingredients:

2 garlic cloves, minced	¼ cup of heavy cream
1 tablespoon of fresh sage leaves, diced	1 scallion, diced
1 lb. fresh mushrooms, sliced	3 large carrots, spiralized with blade C
Salt and black pepper, to taste	1 cup of whipping cream

Directions:
Start by throwing all the Ingredients: into your Crockpot.   Cover its lid and cook for 4 hours on Low setting.   Once done, remove its lid and give it a stir.   Garnish as desired.   Serve warm.
Nutrition Info: Calories 376 Total Fat 12.1 g Saturated Fat 14.2 g Cholesterol 195 mg Sodium 73 mg Total Carbs 4.6 g Fiber 3.1 g Sugar 2.1 g Protein 5.7 g

830.	**Broccoli Mushroom Hash**

Servings: 2   Cooking Time: 3 Hours
Ingredients:

1 broccoli head, florets separated	1 yellow onion, diced
1 tablespoon of olive oil	1 avocado, peeled and pitted
1 garlic clove, minced	A pinch red pepper flake
1 teaspoon of basil, dried	salt and black pepper –to taste
1 tablespoon of balsamic vinegar	¼ cup of vegetable stock

Directions:
Start by throwing all the Ingredients: into your Crockpot except avocado.   Cover its lid and cook for 3 hours on Low setting.   Once done, remove its lid and give it a stir.   Garnish with avocado. Serve warm.
Nutrition Info: Calories 431 Total Fat 27.6 g Saturated Fat 2.4 g Cholesterol 44 mg Sodium 65 mg Total Carbs 4.1 g Fiber 0.7 g Sugar 1.3 g Protein 5.4 g

831.	**Creamy Smoked Salmon Soup**

Servings: 6   Cooking Time: Approximately 3 Hours
Ingredients:

½ lb smoked salmon, roughly chopped	1 small onion, finely chopped
4 garlic cloves, crushed	1 leek, finely chopped
2 cups heavy cream	1 fish stock cube

Directions:
Drizzle some oil into the Crock Pot.   Add the onion, garlic, salmon, leek, stock cube, and 1 cup of water into the pot.   Place the lid onto the pot and set the temperature to LOW.   Cook for 2 hours.   Stir the cream through the soup and continue to cook for a further 1 hour.   Serve with a sprinkling of freshly cracked pepper, I don't add extra salt because the smoked salmon is salty enough for me.

832.	**Lamb Chops**

Servings: 2   Cooking Time: 6 Hours
Ingredients:

1/2 tsp dried oregano	1/4 tsp dried thyme

Directions:
Prepare the seasonings: oregano and thyme with some garlic powder, salt and pepper to taste.   Rub the seasonings on the lamb chops.   Place onion slices in a crock-pot and place chops over the onion slices. Top with garlic, too.   Cover and cook for 6 hours on low.
Nutrition Info: Calories: 201 Fat: 8g Net Carbs: 3g Protein: 26g Cholesterol: 79mg Sodium: 219mg

833.	**Thai Turkey Legs**

Servings: 4   Cooking Time: 4 Hours
Ingredients:

1 lime, halved	15 oz. coconut milk, full-fat
2 1/2 teaspoon lemon- garlic seasoning	

Directions:
Pour the coconut milk into a 4-quart slow-cooker and stir in lemon-garlic seasoning.   Juice one half of the lime, and stir the juice into the slow-cooker. Slice the other half of lime, and add to the slow-cooker.   Add the turkey legs, cover and seal the slow-cooker with its lid.   Set the cooking timer for 3 to 4 hours, and allow to cook at a high heat setting. Carve the meat from the bone, and serve warm.
Nutrition Info: Energy: 275.8 Kcal Carbohydrates: 4 g Net Carbs: 2.8 g Fats: 12.4 g Protein: 35.5 g

834.	**Ground Turkey And Mushrooms**

Servings: 2   Cooking Time: 3 Hours
Ingredients:

1/2 cup chopped green onions	1/4 cup beef gravy mix
6 oz. white mushrooms, sliced	1/2 cup water

Directions:
Grease a 4-quart slow-cooker with a non-stick cooking spray and add the ground turkey.   Stir in the mushrooms, gravy mix, and water, and mix until well-combined.   Cover and seal slow-cooker with its lid, then set the cooking timer for 2 to 3 hours. Allow to cook at a high heat setting.   To serve, season with salt and ground black pepper, and garnish with green onions.   Serve in lettuce wraps.
Nutrition Info: Energy: 314.1 Kcal Carbohydrates: 0.5 g Net Carbs: 0.4 g Fats: 24.7 g Protein: 20.5 g

835.	**Chicken Soup**

Servings: 8   Cooking Time: 6 Hours
Ingredients:

14 oz. canned whole tomatoes, diced	2 tablespoon of tomato puree
5 cups of chicken broth	1 tablespoon of chili powder

¼ cup of cheddar cheese, shredded
2 jalapeno peppers stemmed, cored, and diced
3 cloves garlic, minced

1 tablespoon of cumin, ground
½ teaspoon of oregano, dried
fresh cilantro, diced for garnish

Directions:
Start by throwing all the Ingredients: into your Crockpot.   Mix well and cover the Crockpot with its lid.   Select the Low settings for 6 hours. Garnish with cilantro, and cheese   Serve warm.
Nutrition Info: Calories 215 Total Fat 21.4 g Saturated Fat 67 g Cholesterol 123 mg Total Carbs 9.4 g Sugar 0.3 g Fiber 2.8 g Sodium 156 mg Potassium 317 mg Protein 3.5 g

836.	Green Bean Leg Of Lamb

Servings: 4   Cooking Time: 6 Hours
Ingredients:

6 cups green beans, trimmed
4 cloves garlic, crushed
2 tablespoons olive oil

¼ cup freshly chopped mint
1 teaspoon freshly ground black pepper
½ teaspoon salt

Directions:
Preheat the Slow Cookerand heat the oil.   Season the lamb with salt and pepper.   Place the lamb into the Slow Cookerand fry until evenly browned. Add the garlic and mint leaves.   Cover and cook for 4 hours.   Transfer the lamb to a plate. Place the green beans in the bottom of the Slow Cookerand place the lamb over them.   Cook for another 2 hours, until the meat is soft and juicy and the beans are crisp and tender.
Nutrition Info: Calories 524 Total Fat 36.4 g Saturated Fat 18.6 g Total Carbs 7 g Dietary Fiber 4.4 g Protein 37.3g

837.	Mushrooms Squash

Servings: 4   Cooking Time: 2 Hours
Ingredients:

3 garlic cloves, minced
1 red bell pepper, diced
2 cups of zucchini squash, peeled and diced
1 ½ cups of cauliflower rice
3 ½ cup of vegetable broth

½ cup of onion, diced
½ cup of dry white wine
8 oz. white mushrooms, sliced
1 teaspoon of salt
1 teaspoon of black pepper
¼ teaspoon of oregano
1 ½ a tablespoon of nutritional yeast

Directions:
Start by throwing all the Ingredients: into your Crockpot.   Cover its lid and cook for 3 hours on Low setting.   Once done, remove its lid and give it a stir.   Garnish as desired.   Serve warm.
Nutrition Info: Calories 295 Total Fat 33.1 g Saturated Fat 2.4 g Cholesterol 69 mg Sodium 58

mg Total Carbs 1.4 g Fiber 0.7 g Sugar 0.3 g Protein 1.4 g

838.	Zucchini And Shrimp

Servings: 4   Cooking Time: 2 Hours
Ingredients:

1 cup zucchini, roughly cubed
1-pound shrimp, peeled and deveined
1/2 cup coconut cream

1 tablespoon butter
1 teaspoon dried oregano
1 teaspoon salt

Directions:
In the slow cooker, mix the zucchini with the shrimp and the other ingredients.   Stir gently and close the slow cooker lid.   Cook the meal for 2 hours on High.   Divide between plates and serve.
Nutrition Info:calories 203, fat 7.7, fiber 1.2, carbs 6.1, protein 12.1

839.	Ginger Broccoli Stew

Servings: 4   Cooking Time: 3 Hours
Ingredients:

A pinch red pepper, crushed
1 small ginger piece, diced
1 garlic clove, minced
1 broccoli head, florets separated

2 teaspoon of coriander seeds
1 tablespoon of olive oil
1 yellow onion, diced
Salt and black pepper- to taste

Directions:
Start by throwing all the Ingredients: into your Crockpot.   Cover its lid and cook for 3 hours on Low setting.   Once done, remove its lid and give it a stir.   Garnish as desired.   Serve warm.
Nutrition Info: Calories 412 Total Fat 16.5 g Saturated Fat 2.4 g Cholesterol 76 mg Sodium 49 mg Total Carbs 5.3 g Fiber 0.5 g Sugar 0.2 g Protein 2.4 g

840.	Beef And Cabbage Roast

Servings: 10.   Cooking Time: 7 Hours On Low + 1 Hour On Low.
Ingredients:

1 red onion, quartered
2 garlic cloves, minced
2-3 stocks celery, diced (approximately 1 cup)
4-6 dry pimento berries
2 bay leaves
5.5 pounds beef brisket (two pieces)

1 teaspoon chilli powder
1 teaspoon ground cumin
2 cups broth, beef + 2 cups hot water
Salt and pepper to taste
1 medium cabbage (approximately 2.2 pounds), cut in half, then quartered

Directions:
Add all ingredients, except cabbage, to crock-pot in order of list.   Cover, cook on low for 7 hours. Uncover, add the cabbage on top of the stew.   Re-cover, cook for 1 additional hour.
Nutrition Info:net C 8g; P 42g; F 40g

841.	**Ham Soup**

Servings: 6   Cooking Time: 4 Hours
Ingredients:
- 4 cups cauliflower florets
- 2 bay leaves
- ¼ teaspoon nutmeg
- 3 cups bone broth

Directions:
Place cauliflower florets in a 6-quarts slow cooker, add remaining ingredients and pour in water until all the ingredients are just submerged.   Plug in the slow cooker, then shut with lid and cook for 4 hours at high heat setting or until cauliflower florets are very tender.   Transfer ham to a bowl, shred with two forms and discard bone and fat pieces.   Puree cauliflower in the slow cooker with a stick blender for 1 to 2 minutes or until smooth, return shredded ham and stir until well combined.   Taste soup to adjust seasoning and serve.
Nutrition Info: Net Carbs: 3g Calories: 349 Total Fat: 23g Saturated Fat: 10g Protein: 34g Carbs: 5g Fiber: 2g Sugar: 2g

842.	**Creamy Coconut Fennel**

Servings: 2   Cooking Time: 3 Hours
Ingredients:
- 2 spring onions, diced
- 2 shallots, minced
- 1 garlic clove, minced
- 1 and ½ cups of coconut cream
- 2 big fennel bulbs, sliced
- ¼ teaspoon of nutmeg, ground
- A pinch of salt and black pepper

Directions:
Start by throwing all the Ingredients: into the Crockpot.   Cover its lid and cook for 3 hours on Low setting.   Once done, remove its lid of the crockpot carefully.   Mix well and garnish as desired.   Serve warm.
Nutrition Info: Calories 279 Total Fat 4.8 g Saturated Fat 1 g Cholesterol 45 mg Sodium 24 mg Total Carbs 5.8 g Sugar 2.3 g Fiber 4.5 g Protein 5 g

843.	**Cinnamon Beef**

Servings: 4   Cooking Time: 10 Hours
Ingredients:
- 1 ½ pound beef sirloin, sliced
- ½ cup keto tomato sauce
- 1 teaspoon cinnamon powder
- 1 teaspoon turmeric
- 1 teaspoon garlic powder
- 1 teaspoon salt
- 1 tablespoon olive oil

Directions:
In the slow cooker, mix the beef with the cinnamon and the other ingredients   Close the lid and cook beef for 10 hours on Low.   When the meat is cooked, remove it from the liquid and slice into the servings.
Nutrition Info:calories 352, fat 14.3, fiber 0.5, carbs 1.3, protein 51.9

844.	**Smoked Fish Dip**

Servings: Makes 1 Large Bowl, About 6 – 8 People As A Starter   Cooking Time: Approximately 1 Hour
Ingredients:
- 1 cup cream cheese
- 2/3 cup smoked fish, (trout or salmon work wonders), flaked
- ½ cup grated cheddar cheese
- 1 cup sour cream
- 2 garlic cloves, crushed
- 1 lemon
- Fresh parsley, finely chopped

Directions:
Place cream cheese, sour cream, fish, garlic, zest and juice of 1 lemon in a medium-sized bowl, mix to combine.   Drizzle some oil into the Crock Pot. Pour the smoked fish dip into the Slow Cookerand spread to evenly cover the bottom of the pot. Sprinkle the cheddar cheese over the dip.   Place the lid onto the pot and set the temperature to LOW. Cook for 1 hour, the cheese on top should melt. Remove the dip and serve in a bowl with a sprinkling of parsley over the top.   Serve warm with an assortment of fresh veggie sticks.

845.	**Lamb Barbacoa**

Servings: 12   Cooking Time: 8 Hours
Ingredients:
- 1 teaspoon chipotle powder
- 2 tablespoons smoked paprika
- 1 tablespoon ground cumin
- 2 tablespoons salt
- 1 tablespoon dried oregano
- ¼ cup dried mustard
- 1 cup water

Directions:
Stir together salt, chipotle powder, paprika, cumin, oregano, and mustard and rub this mixture generously on all over the pork.   Place seasoned pork into a 6-quart slow cooker, plug it in, then shut with lid and cook for 6 hours at high heat setting. When done, shred pork with two forks and stir well until coated well.   Serve straightaway.
Nutrition Info: Net Carbs: 0.7g Calories: 477 Total Fat: 35.8g Saturated Fat: 14.8g Protein: 37.5g Carbs: 1.2g Fiber: 0.5g Sugar: 5g

846.	**Garlic And Chili Brussel's Sprouts With Spicy Mayo Dip**

Servings: 6 As A Starter   Cooking Time: Approximately 2 Hours And 10 Minutes
Ingredients:
- 12 – 16 Brussel's sprouts
- 3 garlic cloves, crushed
- ½ tsp cayenne pepper
- 1 tsp dried chili flakes
- ½ cup egg-based mayonnaise
- ½ lemon

Directions:
Drizzle some olive oil into a skillet and heat.   Once the oil is hot, add the Brussel's sprouts and toss in the hot oil for about 1 minute, until golden on the outside.   Place the sprouts into the Slow Cookerand sprinkle the crushed garlic, chili flakes, salt, and pepper over the top.   Place the lid onto the Slow Cookerand set the temperature to LOW. Leave for 2 hours, turning once after 1 hour.   In a small bowl, mix together the mayonnaise, cayenne pepper, and the juice of half a lemon.   Remove the

sprouts from the Slow Cookerand serve on a platter with the spicy mayonnaise dip.

847.   Tomato Chili

Servings: 4   Cooking Time: 5 Hours

Ingredients:

1 teaspoon chili powder
1-pound tomatoes, roughly cubed
1 jalapeno pepper, chopped
2 spring onions, chopped
1 cup kale, chopped
1 teaspoon oregano, dried
1 teaspoon ground black pepper
1 teaspoon salt
1 green bell pepper, chopped
1/3 cup vegetable stock

Directions:

In the slow cooker, mix the tomatoes with the kale and the other ingredients.   Then close the slow cooker lid and cook on Low for 5 hours.   Divide into bowls and serve.

Nutrition Info:calories 239, fat 8.5, fiber 1.8, carbs 6.8, protein 4.1

848.   Crockpot Pork With Picante Sauce

Servings: 12   Cooking Time: 8 Hours

Ingredients:

3 cloves of garlic, chopped
1 package frozen vegetables
1 jar picante sauce
Salt and pepper to taste

Directions:

Heat skillet over medium flame and add the pork cubes and garlic. Stir until all sides turn slightly brown.   Transfer into the crockpot and add the vegetables and picante sauce.   Season with salt and pepper to taste.   Close the lid and cook on low for 8 hours.

Nutrition Info: Calories: 207 Carbohydrates: 9g Protein: 26 Fat: 10g Sugar: 2g Sodium: 595mg Fiber: 3g

849.   Cream & Cheese Broccoli Soup

Servings: 4   Cooking Time: 3 Hours

Ingredients:

4 cups of vegetable broth
½ cup of heavy cream
⅓ cup of butter
2 cloves garlic, minced
1 onion, diced
cheddar cheese, grated – for garnish
1 head broccoli, cut into florets
salt and black pepper to taste

Directions:

Start by throwing all the Ingredients: into your Crockpot.   Mix well and cover the Crockpot with its lid.   Select the High settings for 3 hours. Serve warm.

Nutrition Info: Calories 287 Total Fat 29.5 g Saturated Fat 3 g Cholesterol 0 mg Total Carbs 5.9 g Sugar 1.4g Fiber 4.3 g Sodium 388 mg Potassium 163 mg Protein 14.2 g

850.   Chicken Chili Soup

Servings: 4   Cooking Time: 6 Hours

Ingredients:

Unsalted butter – 1 tbsp.
Green pepper – ½, chopped
Chicken thighs – 4, boneless
Bacon – 4 slices
Salt and pepper to taste
Minced garlic – ½ tbsp.
Thyme – ½ tbsp.
Coconut flour – ½ tbsp.
Lemon juice – 1 ½ tbsp.
Chicken stock – ½ cup
Tomato paste – 1 ½ tbsp.
Unsweetened coconut milk – 2 tbsp.

Directions:

Add the butter into the Crock-Pot.   Add the sliced onion and peppers.   Then add the chicken on top, and sprinkle with sliced bacon.   Add all the dry ingredients and lastly add the liquids.   Cover and cook on low for 6 hours.   Mix and break apart the chicken.   Serve.

Nutrition Info: Calories: 396 Fat: 21g Carbs: 7g Protein: 41g

851.   Paprika Zucchini

Servings: 3   Cooking Time: 5 Hours

Ingredients:

3 zucchinis, sliced
A pinch of salt and black pepper
1 tablespoon of dill, diced
½ teaspoon of nutmeg (grated)
2 tablespoons of sweet paprika

Directions:

Start by throwing all the Ingredients: into the Crockpot.   Cover its lid and cook for 5 hours on Low setting.   Once done, remove its lid of the crockpot carefully.   Mix well and garnish as desired.   Serve warm.

Nutrition Info: Calories 204 Total Fat 15.7 g Saturated Fat 9.7 g Cholesterol 49 mg Sodium 141 mg Total Carbs 46 g Sugar 3.4 g Fiber 1.5 g

852.   Veggie Shrimps

Servings: 3   Cooking Time: 2-5 Hours

Ingredients:

2 red bell peppers, sliced
2 green bell peppers, sliced
½ onion, sliced
1 small tomato, quartered
1 teaspoon salt
1 teaspoon chili powder
½ teaspoon paprika
½ cup low-sodium broth

Directions:

Pour broth into slow cooker. Add bell peppers, tomato, onion, salt and pepper.   Close the lid and cook on Low for 5 hours or on High for 2 hours. Season shrimps with paprika and chili powder. Put shrimps into slow cooker, coat well with the broth mixture.   Close the lid and cook on High for 30-45 minutes.

Nutrition Info: Calories 111 Fats 21.5g Net carbs 4.8g Protein 16.1g

853. Kale And Chicken Broth Soup

Servings: 4 – 6   Cooking Time: Approximately 4 Hours

Ingredients:

- 6 garlic cloves, finely chopped
- 3 tbsp grated fresh ginger
- 6 cups chicken stock
- 1 large chicken breast, cut into small strips
- 2 cups chopped fresh kale (stalks removed)

Directions:

Drizzle some olive oil into the Crock Pot.   Add the garlic, ginger, stock, chicken breast, kale, salt, and pepper to the pot, stir to combine.   Place the lid onto the pot and set the temperature to HIGH. Cook for 4 hours.   Serve this soup while steaming hot!.

854. Red Pepper Dip With Warming Spices And Avocado Oil

Servings: Makes One Large Bowl Of Dip, About 6 – 8 Servings   Cooking Time: Approximately 2 Hours

Ingredients:

- 6 red peppers (capsicums), seeds and core removed, cut into small chunks
- 3 garlic cloves, crushed
- 1 tsp paprika
- 1 tsp dried chili flakes
- ½ tsp cumin
- ½ tsp dried coriander
- 1 lemon
- ¾ cup sour cream

Directions:

Drizzle some avocado oil into the Crock Pot.   Add the peppers, garlic, all of the spices, salt, pepper, and the finely grated zest of half a lemon to the pot, then add 2 tablespoons of water, stir to combine.   Add the lid to the pot and set the temperature to HIGH. Cook for 3 hours or until the capsicum is very soft. Leave to cool slightly.   With a hand-held stick blender, blend the peppers until a smooth dip forms. Stir the sour cream and juice of half a lemon into the pepper dip.   Serve with a sprinkle of finely chopped fresh parsley and a drizzle of avocado oil.

855. Zucchini Eggplant Spread

Servings: 12   Cooking Time: 5 Hours

Ingredients:

- 3 tablespoon of lemon juice
- 2 zucchinis, diced
- 1 tablespoon of olive oil
- 2 eggplants, diced
- ½ cup of vegetable broth
- 2 tablespoons of dill, diced

Directions:

Start by throwing all the Ingredients: into the Crockpot.   Cover its lid and cook for 5 hours on Low setting.   Once done, remove its lid of the crockpot carefully.   Blend this dip mixture using an immersion blender.   Mix well and garnish as desired.   Serve warm.

Nutrition Info: Calories 132 Total Fat 7.1 g Saturated Fat 1 g Cholesterol 101 mg Sodium 94 mg

Total Carbs 8.2 g Sugar 1.9 g Fiber 0.6 g Protein 13.5 g

856. Hot Beef Stew With Mushrooms(1)

Servings: 2   Cooking Time: 4.5 Hours

Ingredients:

- 2 tablespoons / 28 gr carrot, diced
- 1 clove / 3 gr of garlic, minced
- 1 pinch of onion powder
- 1 pinch of salt and pepper
- 1 tablespoon / 14 gr of Worcester sauce
- 2 tablespoons / 28 gr of olive oil
- 1 tablespoon / 14 gr of coconut oil
- 3 tablespoons / 48 gr mixed mushrooms
- ¼ cup / 100 gr of ripe avocado for garnishing

Directions:

Cut the beef in small pieces   Mince the garlic and carrots, clean and cut the mushrooms   Sauté the onion, carrot and garlic in a frying pan, add the mushrooms after a couple of minutes and sauté the meat for another couple of minutes   Transfer all of the ingredients into the Slow Cooker, add salt, pepper, parsley, Worcester sauce, mix and cook on HIGH for 4 hours and 30 minutes   Sprinkle with a pinch of salt and pepper and with 2 teaspoons of extra virgin olive oil and the coconut oil   Garnish with the fresh avocado slices

Nutrition Info: Calories: 531 Fat: 62.66 g Total carbs: 15.03 Net carbs: 7.85 Protein 39 g

857. Orange Sauce Pork Chops

Servings: 2   Cooking Time: 8 Hours

Ingredients:

- 2 tablespoons / 28 gr of olive oil
- 1 pinch of garlic powder
- 1 pinch of cumin
- 1 pinch of salt
- 1 pinch of black pepper
- 33 cc / 1 fl oz of orange squash
- 1 tablespoon / 14 gr of Mexican sauce

Directions:

Combine the seasonings (except for the orange juice and Mexican sauce) and olive oil in a bowl and mix until you have a homogeneous mixture   Cover the pork chops with the mixture and sauté for 5 minutes per each side on a frying pan (use non-sticking spray for the pan)   Spray your slow cooker pot with non-sticking spray and put the pork inside. Cover with the orange juice and Mexican sauce   Close the pot and cook on LOW for 8 hours

Nutrition Info: Calories: 545 Fat: 46 g Total carbs: 5 Net carbs: 5 Protein 25.5 g

858. Creamy Lemon Chicken Kale Soup

Servings: 8   Cooking Time: 6 Hours

Ingredients:

- 6 cups of bone broth
- 1 bunch of kale, rinsed, drained and sliced into 1/2-inch strips
- 3 lemons
- 2 tablespoons of fresh lemon juice
- 1 cup of onions, diced
- 1/2 cup of olive oil
- salt to taste

Directions:
Start by throwing all the Ingredients: into your Crockpot. Mix well and cover the Crockpot with its lid. Select the Low settings for 6 hours. Serve warm.
Nutrition Info: Calories 392 Total Fat 40.4 g Saturated Fat 6 g Cholesterol 20 mg Total Carbs 7.2 g Sugar 3 g Fiber 4.2 g Sodium 423 mg Potassium 411 mg Protein 22 g

859.   Lemon Pork Stew

Servings: 4   Cooking Time: 10 Hours
Ingredients:

1-pound pork shoulder, boneless and cubed	1 teaspoon salt
	½ cup of water
1 red chili pepper, minced	¼ cup tomatoes, crushed
½ teaspoon garam masala	2 tablespoons lemon zest, grated
½ teaspoon dried rosemary	2 tablespoons lemon juice

Directions:
In the slow cooker, mix the pork with the chili, masala and the other ingredients, toss, close the lid and cook on Low for 10 hours. Divide into bowls and serve.
Nutrition Info:calories 425, fat 18.7, fiber 2.6, carbs 5.4, protein 22.7

860.   Parmesan Tomatoes

Servings: 6   Cooking Time: 4 Hours
Ingredients:

4 garlic cloves, minced	1/4 cup of basil, diced
1/2 teaspoon of oregano, dried	2 lb. cherry tomatoes, halved
1/4 cup of olive oil	Salt and black pepper- to taste
1/2 cup of parmesan, grated	

Directions:
Start by throwing all the Ingredients: into your Crockpot. Cover its lid and cook for 4 hours on Low setting. Once done, remove its lid and give it a stir. Garnish as desired. Serve warm.
Nutrition Info: Calories 231 Total Fat 14.3 g Saturated Fat 3.9 g Cholesterol 349 mg Sodium 45 mg Total Carbs 7.1 g Fiber 3.5 g Sugar 2.1 g Protein 3.6 g

861.   Stockman's Beef Tail

Servings: 3   Cooking Time: 6.5 Hours
Ingredients:

1 pinch of onion powder	1 clove / 3 gr of garlic
2 tablespoons / 28 gr of carrots, diced	2 ounces / 53 gr of lard, diced
2 tablespoons / 28 gr of celery, diced	2 tablespoons / 28 gr tomato pulp
1 tablespoon / 14 gr of coconut oil	1 pinch of salt
33 cc/ 1 fl oz of dry white wine (check that it has less than 2	1 pinch of bitter cocoa
	1 tablespoon / 14 gr of pine nuts
	1 tablespoon / 14 gr of olive oil

gr of cabs per serving)
Directions:
Pour the lard in a frying pan and warm it up, as soon as it starts melting add the onion and garlic with a pinch of salt, then add the tail pieces and sauté all for 2 minutes with the glass of white wine   Turn off and remove the tail from the pan   Lay in your Slow Cooker pot the carrot and celery, then lay the tail pieces, cover it with onion powder and lard, pour the pine nuts, coconut oil, cocoa, sprinkle with salt and pepper, cover with the sauce and finally a dash of extra virgin olive oil   Close the lid and set the Slow Cooker on LOW   After 6 hours remove the lid, stir well and let it cook for another 30 minutes without lid, thus helping the excess liquid to evaporate
Nutrition Info: Calories: 775.5 Fat: 62.5 g Total carbs: 8 Net carbs. 8 Protein 38.5 g

862.   Crockpot Kalua Pig

Servings: 8   Cooking Time: 16 Hours
Ingredients:

5 pounds butt roast, bone removed	1 ½ tablespoon sea salt
5 cloves of garlic, peeled	½ teaspoon black pepper

Directions:
Line the bottom of the slow cooker with the bacon slices. Rub salt all over the meat. Cut some slit on the meat and tuck in the garlic cloves. Place the pork inside the crockpot skin-side up. Close the lid and cook for 16 hours. Once cooked, remove the meat and shred it using two forks.
Nutrition Info: Calories: 621 Carbohydrates: 0.82 g Protein: 80.12g Fat: 30.61g Sugar: 0g Sodium: 1522mg Fiber: 0g

863.   Dill Mixed Fennel Bulbs

Servings: 2   Cooking Time: 3 Hours
Ingredients:

¼ cup of chicken stock	1 tablespoon of dill, diced
A pinch of salt and black pepper	1 tablespoon of parsley, chopped

Directions:
Start by throwing all the Ingredients: into the Crockpot. Cover its lid and cook for 3 hours on Low setting. Once done, remove its lid of the crockpot carefully. Mix well and garnish as desired. Serve warm.
Nutrition Info: Calories 131 Total Fat 10.4 g Saturated Fat 9.5 g Cholesterol 10 mg Sodium 106 mg Total Carbs 9.1 g Sugar 0.5 g Fiber 3.4 g Protein 2.3 g

864.   Kale And Shrimp

Servings: 2   Cooking Time: 2 Hours
Ingredients:

2 cups kale, chopped	1 teaspoon turmeric powder
1 cup of veggie stock	
1-pound shrimp,	1 teaspoon curry

peeled and deveined powder
1 teaspoon dried dill 1 teaspoon salt
Directions:
In the slow cooker, mix the kale with shrimp and the other ingredients, toss and close the lid. Cook meat for 2 hours on High. Divide into bowls and serve.
Nutrition Info:calories 300, fat 7.1, fiber 1.1, carbs 7.6, protein 5.3

865. Chicken In Salsa Verde

Servings: 4. Cooking Time: 6 Hours On Low.
Ingredients:
2.2 pounds chicken breasts

3 bunches parsley, chopped

¾ cup olive oil

¼ cup capers, drained and chopped

3 anchovy fillets

1 lemon, juice and zest

2 garlic cloves, minced

1 teaspoon salt

1 teaspoon fresh ground black pepper

Directions:
Place the chicken breasts in the crock-pot. In a blender, combine rest of ingredients, pour over the chicken. Cover, cook on low for 6 hours. Shred with a fork and serve.
Nutrition Info:net C 5g; P 37g; F 50g

866. Lamb And Rosemary Stew

Servings: 6 Cooking Time: Approximately 8 Hours
Ingredients:
2 lb boneless lamb, cut into cubes

1 onion, roughly chopped

4 garlic cloves, finely chopped

2 tsp dried rosemary

1 lamb stock cube

Directions:
Drizzle some olive oil into the Crock Pot. Brown the lamb in an oiled fry pan or skillet for about 2 minutes. Add the lamb, onion, garlic, rosemary, stock cube, salt, pepper, and 3 cups of water to the pot. Place the lid onto the pot and set the time to LOW. Cook for 8 hours. Remove the lid, stir, and serve while hot.

867. Apricot Salsa Salmon

Servings: 2 Cooking Time: 1 ½ Hours
Ingredients:
3 tablespoon apricot spread, sugar-free

1/4 cup Salsa Verde,

Directions:
Grease a 4-quart slow-cooker with a non-stick cooking spray and place the salmon fillet into it. Stir the remaining ingredients together, and spread this mixture over the salmon. Cover and seal the slow-cooker with its lid, and set the cooking timer for 1 to 1 1/2 hours. Allow to cook at a low heat setting or until salmon is cooked through. When done, flake the salmon fillet with forks and serve. This dish can be eaten hot or cold.
Nutrition Info: Energy: 173.1 Kcal Carbohydrates: 4.6 g Net Carbs: 4.2 g Fats: 6.3 g Protein: 27.1 g

868. Cauliflower Rice Mix

Servings: 2 Cooking Time: 2 Hours
Ingredients:
1 cup cauliflower rice

1 tablespoon coconut butter

¼ teaspoon salt

1 teaspoon cayenne pepper

¾ teaspoon turmeric

1 teaspoon curry powder

2 oz Provolone cheese

1 ½ cups chicken stock

Directions:
In the slow cooker, mix the cauliflower with the butter and the other ingredients except the cheese, close the lid and cook on High for 1 hour. Add the cheese, cook on High for 1 more hour, divide between plates and serve.
Nutrition Info:calories 131, fat 4.5, fiber 2.1, carbs 6.2, protein 4.5

869. Butcher Style Cabbage Rolls – Pork & Beef Version

Servings: 6. Cooking Time: 8.5 Hours On Low.
Ingredients:
1 large head of white cabbage – 3 pounds

1 ¾ cups beef, chopped in small pieces

1 sweet onion, cut into small pieces

1 red bell pepper, cut into small cubes

1 cup mushrooms, chopped small

1 ¾ cups pork, chopped in small pieces

2 Tablespoons olive oil

1 cup beef broth

½ cup cooking cream

Salt and pepper to taste

1 heaping teaspoon ground cumin

Directions:
Cut out the stalk of the cabbage head like a cone shape, place the cabbage in a pot with the hole up, boil some water and pour it over the cabbage. Let it soak in the hot water for 10 minutes. This will soften it considerably and the leaves will separate easily. Chop the meats into small pieces; place them in a mixing bowl. In a pan, heat the olive oil. Sauté the onion, the bell pepper, and the mushrooms for 5 minutes, cool them in the pan and add to the meats. Add the seasoning, mix well with your hands. Separate 8-10 leaves of cabbage, lay each one flat, cut the thick part of the stalk and stuff the leaf with about 2 tablespoons of meat mixture. Roll and put aside until meat mixture used up. Finely cut the remaining cabbage and place in the crock-pot. Place the prepared cabbage rolls seam-side down, pour the broth and the cream evenly over the cabbage rolls. Cover, cook on low for 8.5 hours.
Nutrition Info:net C 17g; P 42g; F 50g

870. Asian Chicken Lettuce Wraps

Servings: 6 Or 12 Wraps Cooking Time: 3 Hours
Ingredients:
3 garlic cloves, minced

1 red bell pepper, cored, finely chopped

½ cup hoisin sauce

1 ½ cups cooked brown rice

½ cup yellow onion, finely chopped
2 tablespoons soy sauce
Salt and pepper to taste
1 (8-ounce) can water chestnuts, sliced

3 green onions, sliced
1 tablespoon rice vinegar
1 ½ teaspoon sesame oil
2 heads iceberg lettuce

Directions:
In a microwave-safe bowl add garlic and ground chicken and cook for 6 minutes or until chicken is no longer pink. Add into Slow Cookeralong with onion, bell pepper, hoisin sauce, soy sauce, salt, pepper, and toss mixture. Cover and cook for 3 hours on LOW heat. Stir in the water chestnuts, cooked rice, green onions, and rice vinegar and sesame oil. Separate iceberg lettuce leaves and serve mixture on top of the leaves.
Nutrition Info: Calories: 359 Total Fat: 8.2 g Saturated Fat: 2 g Sodium: 457 mg Carbs: 39.3 g Fiber: 2.3 g Sugars: 5 g Protein: 30 g Protein: 35 g

871. Radish Soup

Servings: 4   Cooking Time: 2 Hours
Ingredients:

2 cups radishes, halved
½ teaspoon coriander, ground
1 cup coconut cream
1 and ½ cups water

1 tablespoon butter, soft
1 teaspoon black pepper
1 teaspoon salt

Directions:
In the slow cooker, mix the radishes with the coriander and the other ingredients except the cream, close the lid and cook for 2 hours on High. Add the cream, blend the soup and serve.
Nutrition Info:calories 143, fat 7.5, fiber 1.5, carbs 5.4, protein 3.1

872. Garlic Lamb Roast

Servings: 2   Cooking Time: 10 Hours
Ingredients:

1 tsp rosemary
1 leg of lamb
2 tbsp. Worcestershire sauce

Desired veggies: chopped carrots, onions, and butternut squash

Directions:
Put all ingredients in crock-pot. Add seasoning such as garlic, pepper and salt to taste. Cook on low for 6-10 hours or until the lamb is tender.
Nutrition Info: Calories: 435 Fat: 31g Net Carbs: 6g Protein: 44g Cholesterol: 79mg Sodium: 279mg

873. Coconut Okra

Servings: 6   Cooking Time: 3 Hours
Ingredients:

1-pound okra, trimmed
1/3 cup coconut cream
1/3 cup butter
½ teaspoon salt

½ teaspoon turmeric powder
¾ teaspoon ground nutmeg

Directions:

In the slow cooker, mix the okra with cream, butter and the other ingredients. Cook okra for 3 hours on High.
Nutrition Info:calories 203, fat 6.7, fiber 2.5, carbs 6.2, protein 3.3

874. Beef Noodles With Broccoli & Tomato(1)

Servings: 3   Cooking Time: 4 Hours
Ingredients:

2 tablespoons / 28 gr of broccoli, diced
2 teaspoons / 28 gr of olive oil
1 tablespoon / 14 gr of coconut oil

1 pinch of salt
1 pinch of pepper
2 tablespoons / 28 gr of cherry tomatoes, diced

Directions:
Put the beef noodles in the bottom of the Slow Cooker pot Cover with the diced broccoli and tomatoes Sprinkle with a pinch of salt and pepper and with 2 teaspoons of extra virgin olive oil and the coconut oil Set the cooking on LOW temperature, and let it cook for 4 hours Depending on the size of the noodles, the cooking may be a bit longer, so consider whether it is necessary to have an extra hour of cooking (alternatively you can cook on HIGH for about 2 and a half hours)
Nutrition Info: Calories: 590.5 Fat: 48 g Total carbs: 3 g Net carbs: 2 g Protein 38.5 g

875. Capers Eggplant Stew

Servings: 4   Cooking Time: 6 Hours
Ingredients:

1 red onion, diced
1 teaspoon of oregano, dried
2 tablespoons of olive oil
2 tablespoons of capers, diced
2 garlic cloves, diced
1 bunch parsley, a diced

1 handful green olives, pitted and sliced
5 tomatoes, diced
½ cup of vegetable stock
3 tablespoons of herb vinegar
Salt and black pepper- to taste

Directions:
Start by throwing all the Ingredients: except cilantro into your Crockpot. Mix well and cover the Crockpot with its lid. Select the Low settings for 6 hours. Garnish with cilantro. Serve warm.
Nutrition Info: Calories 228 Total Fat 20.2 g Saturated Fat 12.5 g Cholesterol 54 mg Total Carbs 6 g Sugar 2.3 g Fiber 2.4 g Sodium 250 mg Potassium 280 mg Protein 3.7 g

876. Sour Cream Soup

Servings: 6   Cooking Time: 5 Hours
Ingredients:

3 leeks, white part only, sliced
2 bay leaves
2 cloves garlic, minced
½ cup of sour cream
4 cups of vegetable broth

2 tablespoons of butter
2 tablespoons of rosemary
2 tablespoons of fresh chives
salt and black pepper to taste

Directions:
Start by throwing all the Ingredients: into your Crockpot. Mix well and cover the Crockpot with its lid. Select the Low settings for 5 hours. Serve warm.
Nutrition Info: Calories 324 Total Fat 13.4 g Saturated Fat 7 g Cholesterol 20 mg Total Carbs 1.4 g Sugar 2.1 g Fiber 4.8 g Sodium 136 mg Potassium 427 mg Protein 24.2 g

877. Chimichurri Pork Roast

Servings: 12   Cooking Time: 6 Hours
Ingredients:

Salt to taste	3 garlic cloves
4 tbsp. extra-virgin olive oil - divided	1 t. salt
1 sweet onion	1 c. fresh basil/parsley leaves
1 lb. carrots	2 tbsp. lemon juice
1 recipe of the sauce For the Sauce:	¼ t. of each:
½ c. EVOO (olive oil)	Ground black pepper Cayenne pepper

Directions:
Place the roast in the slow cooker. Drizzle with two tablespoons of the olive oil. Season with the salt and pepper. Cover the cooker, and cook on high for six hours or low for 12 hours. After the pork has been in the pot for four hours on high or eight hours on low, add the onions and carrots, arranging them on each the roast. Cook the veggies in the cooker for two more hours on high or four on the low setting. Make the Sauce: Combine all of the ingredients in a blender until the basil is in small bits. Pull the roast apart and place the veggies on a serving platter. Pour the sauce and enjoy.
Nutrition Info: Calories: 167 Net Carbs: 5.0 g Fat: 8.0 g Protein: 17 g

878. Broccoli Yogurt Dip

Servings: 12   Cooking Time: 6 Hours
Ingredients:

8 garlic cloves, minced	1 tablespoon of dill, diced
2 cups of vegetable broth	A pinch of salt and black pepper
6 cups of broccoli florets	½ cup of coconut cream
1 cup of Greek yogurt	

Directions:
Start by throwing all the Ingredients: into the Crockpot. Cover its lid and cook for 6 hours on Low setting. Once done, remove its lid of the crockpot carefully. Blend this dip mixture using an immersion blender. Mix well and garnish as desired. Serve warm.
Nutrition Info: Calories 135 Total Fat 9.9 g Saturated Fat 3.2 g Cholesterol 34 mg Sodium 10 mg Total Carbs 3.1 g Sugar 3.4 g Fiber 1.5 g Protein 8.6 g

879. Swiss Vegetable Soup

Servings: 8   Cooking Time: 6 Hours
Ingredients:

1 bunch swiss chard, a diced	2 cups of water
	2 teaspoons of thyme,
2 zucchinis, diced	diced
1 green bell pepper, diced	1 teaspoon of rosemary, dried
1 lb. sausage, diced	1 tablespoon of fennel, minced
2 garlic cloves, minced	1/2 teaspoon of red pepper flakes
1 cup of cauliflower florets, diced	Grated parmesan for serving
1 cup of green beans, diced	6 carrots, diced
6 cups of chicken stock	4 cups of tomatoes, diced
7 oz. canned tomato paste	Salt and black pepper- to taste

Directions:
Start by throwing all the Ingredients: into your Crockpot. Mix well and cover the Crockpot with its lid. Select the Low settings for 6 hours. Serve warm.
Nutrition Info: Calories 382 Total Fat 36.5 g Saturated Fat 5.5 g Cholesterol 0 mg Total Carbs 9.6 g Sugar 3.4 g Fiber 5.5 g Sodium 73 mg Potassium 539 mg Protein 6.3 g

880. Lamb Shanks

Servings: 2   Cooking Time: 1 Hour And 30 Minutes
Ingredients:

Lamb shanks – 2.5 pounds	Rosemary – 2 tablespoons
Minced garlic – 1 tablespoon	Ground black pepper – 1/2 teaspoon
Medium white onion, peeled and diced – 1	Lamb or chicken broth – 1 cup
Sticks of celery, diced – 2	Diced tomatoes – 14 ounces
Salt – 1 teaspoon	

Directions:
Switch on the instant pot, add half of the oil, press the 'sauté/simmer' button, wait until the oil is hot and lamb shanks in a single layer and cook for 3 to 5 minutes per side or until browned. Transfer lamb shanks to a plate, set aside, then add onion, celery, garlic, and rosemary into the instant pot and cook for 3 minutes. Season with salt and black pepper, pour in the broth, mix well, then add tomatoes, return lamb shanks into the pot and toss until combined. Press the 'keep warm' button, shut the instant pot with its lid in the sealed position, then press the 'manual' button, press '+/-' to set the cooking time to 50 minutes and cook at high-pressure setting; when the pressure builds in the pot, the cooking timer will start. When the instant pot buzzes, press the 'keep warm' button, release pressure naturally for 10 minutes, then do a quick pressure release and open the lid. Transfer lamb shanks to a dish, then press the 'sauté/simmer' button and simmer the sauce for 5 minutes or more until the sauce is reduced by half. Ladle sauce over the lamb shanks and serve.
Nutrition Info: Calories: 410 Fat: 35 g Protein: 51 g Net Carbs: 12 g Fiber: 3 g

881.	**Veggies Dish**

Servings: 4   Cooking Time: 5 Hours
Ingredients:

½ cup of onion, diced
2 zucchinis, cut into
½ inch slices
1 tablespoon of fresh basil, diced
½ tablespoon of olive oil
½ cup of cheddar cheese
½ cup of cream
½ cup of feta cheese
1 garlic clove, minced
Salt and black pepper, to taste
½ (7 oz.) can sugar-free crushed tomatoes with juice

Directions:
Start by throwing all the Ingredients: into your Crockpot.   Cover its lid and cook for 5 hours on Low setting.   Once done, remove its lid and give it a stir.   Garnish as desired.   Serve warm.
Nutrition Info: Calories 381 Total Fat 18.1 g Saturated Fat 2.4 g Cholesterol 139 mg Sodium 78 mg Total Carbs 4.4 g Fiber 0.5 g Sugar 3.3 g Protein 5.4 g

882.	**Capers Zucchini Dip**

Servings: 10   Cooking Time: 5 Hours
Ingredients:

1 and ½ lbs. zucchinis, diced
1 tablespoon of olive oil
-1 tablespoon of capers, drained and diced
2 garlic cloves, minced
A pinch of salt and black pepper
¼ cup of vegetable broth
1 bunch basil, diced

Directions:
Start by throwing all the Ingredients: into the Crockpot.   Cover its lid and cook for 5 hours on Low setting.   Once done, remove its lid of the crockpot carefully.   Blend this dip mixture using an immersion blender.   Mix well and garnish as desired.   Serve warm.
Nutrition Info: Calories 194 Total Fat 21.7 g Saturated Fat 9.4 g Cholesterol 105 mg Sodium 384 mg Total Carbs 8.3 g Sugar 1.6 g Fiber 1.3 g Protein 3.2 g

883.	**Mushrooms Balsamic Mix**

Servings: 2   Cooking Time: 3 Hours
Ingredients:

2 spring onions, diced
1 garlic clove, minced
2 endives, trimmed and halved
1 tablespoon of balsamic vinegar
1 tablespoon of chives, diced
1 cup of chicken stock

Directions:
Start by throwing all the Ingredients: into the Crockpot.   Cover its lid and cook for 3 hours on Low setting.   Once done, remove its lid of the crockpot carefully.   Mix well and garnish as desired.   Serve warm.
Nutrition Info: Calories 204 Total Fat 15.7 g Saturated Fat 9.7 g Cholesterol 49 mg Sodium 141 mg Total Carbs 46 g Sugar 3.4 g Fiber 1.5 g Protein 6.3 g

884.	**Creamy Portobello Mix**

Servings: 4   Cooking Time: 7 Hours
Ingredients:

4 Portobello mushrooms
½ cup Monterey Jack cheese, grated
1 teaspoon curry powder
½ cup heavy cream
1 teaspoon basil, dried
½ teaspoon salt
1 teaspoon olive oil

Directions:
In the slow cooker, mix the mushrooms with the cheese and the other ingredients.   Close the lid and cook the meal for 7 hours on Low.
Nutrition Info:calories 126, fat 5.1, fiber 1.6, carbs 5.9, protein 4.4

885.	**Chilli Con Steak**

Servings: 6.   Cooking Time: 6 Hours On High.
Ingredients:

3 pounds beef steak, cubed
½ teaspoon chilli powder
1 teaspoon dried oregano
½ teaspoon ground cumin
1 Tablespoon paprika
Salt and pepper to taste
4 Tablespoons butter
½ cup sliced leeks
2 cups Italian diced tomatoes
1 cup broth, beef

Directions:
Place all the ingredients in the crock-pot by order on list.   Stir together.   Cover, cook on high for 6 hours.
Nutrition Info:net C 9g; P 62g; F 26g

886.	**Bacon, Paprika, And Cauliflower Soup**

Servings: 6   Cooking Time: Approximately 4 Hours
Ingredients:

1 large head of cauliflower, cut into chunks
4 garlic cloves, crushed
5 slices streaky bacon, cut into small pieces
1 onion, finely chopped
2 cups chicken stock
1 tsp smoked paprika
1 tsp chili powder (optional)
1 cup heavy cream

Directions:
Drizzle some olive oil into the pot.   Add the cauliflower, garlic, onion, bacon, stock, paprika, chili, salt, and pepper to the pot, stir to combine.   Place the lid onto the pot and set the temperature to HIGH.   Cook for 4 hours.   With a hand-held stick blender, blend until smooth.   Mix the cream into the soup.   Serve while hot, with a sprinkling of paprika on top!

887.	**Mexican Chicken Low Carb Soup**

Servings: 4   Cooking Time: 4 Hours
Ingredients:

15.5 oz. chunky salsa
15 oz. chicken broth
8 oz. Monterey, shredded

Directions:

Start by throwing all the Ingredients: into your Crockpot. Mix well and cover the Crockpot with its lid. Select the High settings for 4 hours. Serve warm.
Nutrition Info: Calories 474 Total Fat 40.8 g Saturated Fat 25.5 g Cholesterol 105 mg Total Carbs 3.9 g Sugar 1.8 g Fiber 0.8 g Sodium 345 mg Potassium 228 mg Protein 24.5 g

888.   Lamb & Feta Meatballs

Servings: 3   Cooking Time: 4.5 Hours
Ingredients:

1 small egg	1 pinch of chopped parsley (plus a small amount to garnish)
3 tablespoons / 42 gr of parmesan cheese, grated	¼ lemon (only the peel)
2 tablespoons / 28 gr of smoked feta cheese	1 pinch of salt and pepper
1 clove / 3 gr of garlic, finely chopped	A dash of white wine
1 pinch of onion powder	1 tablespoon / 14 gr of olive oil
	1 pinch of oregano

Directions:
To prepare the meatballs, put all the ingredients in a bowl. Mix well and form small meatballs with your hands   Heat a frying pan with the olive oil, onion powder, the garlic clove and oregano. Pour a dash of white wine and make it evaporate   Pour the content of the frying pan in your Slow Cooker with a spoon   Clean the frying pan with clean kitchen paper. Add a little oil and drizzle the meatballs on all sides   After a few minutes lay the meatballs on the bottom of the Slow Cooker. Cover and cook on LOW for 4.5 hours
Nutrition Info: Calories: 813.7 Fat: 70.28 Total carbs: 4.84 Net carbs: 4.84 Protein 41.8 g

889.   Mini Lamb And Eggplant Skewers With Yogurt Dip

Servings: 4 As A Starter   Cooking Time: Approximately 4 Hours
Ingredients:

1 lb minced lamb	1 lemon
2 garlic cloves, crushed	¾ cup full-fat Greek yoghurt
1 egg, lightly beaten	2 tbsp fresh mint leaves, finely chopped
1 large eggplant, cut into 12 even chunks	

Directions:
In a medium-sized bowl, mix together the minced lamb, garlic cloves, egg, salt, pepper, and zest of one lemon.   Roll the lamb mixture into 12 balls. Place the eggplant chunks on a damp tea towel and sprinkle them with salt and leave while you prepare the yoghurt dip in advance.   Mix together the yoghurt, fresh mint, and juice of the lemon in a small bowl, cover and store in the fridge until needed. Rub the eggplant chunks with olive oil.   Take 4 skewers and "fill" them with alternating lamb mince balls and eggplant chunks, so that each skewer has 3 lamb mince balls and 3 eggplant chunks.   Drizzle some olive oil into the Crock Pot.   Lay the skewers into the Slow Cookerand set the temperature at

LOW.   Cook for 4 hours, turning once, after the 2-hour mark.   Remove the skewers from the pot and serve on a platter with the yoghurt dip.

890.   Creamy Parmesan Green Beans

Servings: 4   Cooking Time: 2 Hours
Ingredients:

1/2 cup of heavy cream	2 teaspoon of lemon zest, grated
1 cup of mozzarella, shredded	Salt and black pepper- to taste
2/3 cup of parmesan, grated	A pinch red pepper flake

Directions:
Start by throwing all the Ingredients: into your Crockpot.   Cover its lid and cook for 2 hours on Low setting.   Once done, remove its lid and give it a stir.   Garnish as desired.   Serve warm.
Nutrition Info: Calories 331 Total Fat 16.2 g Saturated Fat 8.4 g Cholesterol 47 mg Sodium 63 mg Total Carbs 6.4 g Fiber 0.7 g Sugar 0.3 g Protein 3.4 g

891.   Simple Chicken Chilli

Servings: 8.   Cooking Time: 6 Hours On Low.
Ingredients:

1 Tablespoon butter	1 teaspoon chilli powder
1 red onion, sliced	Salt and pepper to taste
1 bell pepper, sliced	1 cup chicken broth
2 garlic cloves, minced	¼ cup coconut milk
3 pounds boneless chicken thighs	3 Tablespoons tomato paste
8 slices bacon, chopped	

Directions:
Add all ingredients to the crock-pot, starting with the butter.   Cover, cook on low for 6 hours. Shred the chicken with a fork in the crock-pot. Serve.
Nutrition Info:net C 7g; P 41g; F 21g

892.   Sausage Stew

Servings: 4   Cooking Time: 3.5 Hours
Ingredients:

7 oz sausages, sliced	1 cup of water
3 spring onions, chopped	1 cup keto tomato sauce
1 tomato, chopped	1 teaspoon minced garlic
1 tablespoon Cajun seasonings	1 teaspoon olive oil

Directions:
In the slow cooker, combine the sausages with the spring onions and the other ingredients and toss. Close the lid and cook gumbo for 3 hours and 30 minutes.
Nutrition Info:calories 329, fat 24, fiber 1.5, carbs 3.4, protein 17.5

893.   Balsamic Collard Greens

Servings: 2   Cooking Time: 2 Hours
Ingredients:

2 tablespoon of olive oil	2 tablespoon of tomato puree

1 teaspoon of swerve
1 yellow onion, diced
3 garlic cloves, minced

1 tablespoon of balsamic vinegar
Salt and black pepper- to taste

Directions:
Start by throwing all the Ingredients: into your Crockpot.   Cover its lid and cook for 2 hours on Low setting.   Once done, remove its lid and give it a stir.   Garnish as desired.   Serve warm.
Nutrition Info: Calories 371 Total Fat 14.5 g Saturated Fat 3.4 g Cholesterol 361 mg Sodium 66 mg Total Carbs 4.8 g Fiber 0.7 g Sugar 0.3 g Protein 5.1 g

894.   Slightly Addictive Pork Curry

Servings: 6.   Cooking Time: 8 Hours On Low.
Ingredients:
2.2 pounds pork shoulder, cubed
1 Tablespoon coconut oil
1 yellow onion, diced
2 garlic cloves, minced
2 Tablespoons tomato paste
1 small can coconut milk – 12 fl ounces

1 cup water
½ cup white wine
1 teaspoon turmeric
1 teaspoon ginger powder
1 teaspoon curry powder
½ teaspoon paprika
Salt and pepper to taste

Directions:
In a pan, heat 1 tablespoon olive oil. Sauté the onion and garlic for 2-3 minutes.   Add the pork and brown it. Finish with tomato paste.   In the crock-pot, mix all remaining ingredients, submerge the meat in the liquid.   Cover, cook on low for 8 hours.
Nutrition Info:net C 7g; P 30g; F 34g

895.   Crispy Zucchini Wedges

Servings: 2   Cooking Time: 2 Hours
Ingredients:
1 yellow onion, diced
1 small carrot, roughly chopped
1 ½ tablespoon of almond flour
1/2 cup of chicken stock

1 bay leaf
2 tablespoons of Greek yogurt
2 tablespoons of butter, melted
Salt and black pepper- to taste

Directions:
Start by throwing all the Ingredients: into your Crockpot and mix well.   Cover its lid and cook for 5 hours on Low setting.   Once done, remove its lid and give it a stir.   Garnish as desired.   Serve warm.
Nutrition Info: Calories 355 Total Fat 4.2 g Saturated Fat 21.4 g Cholesterol 53 mg Sodium 67 mg Total Carbs 4.4 g Fiber 0.8 g Sugar 0.5 g Protein 6.1 g

896.   Butter Green Peas

Servings: 4   Cooking Time: 3 Hours
Ingredients:
1 cup green peas
1 teaspoon minced garlic
1 tablespoon butter,

1 tablespoon olive oil
¾ teaspoon salt
1 teaspoon paprika
1 teaspoon garam

softened
½ teaspoon cayenne pepper

masala
½ cup chicken stock

Directions:
In the slow cooker, mix the peas with butter, garlic and the other ingredients,   Close the lid and cook for 3 hours on High.
Nutrition Info:calories 121, fat 6.5, fiber 3, carbs 3.4, protein 0.6

897.   Greek Style Lamb Shanks

Servings: 8.   Cooking Time: 6 Hours On Medium High.
Ingredients:
3 Tablespoons butter
4 lamb shanks, approximately 1 pound each
2 Tablespoons olive oil
8-10 pearl onions
5 garlic cloves, minced
2 beef tomatoes, cubed
¼ cup green olives

4 bay leaves
1 sprig fresh rosemary
1 teaspoon dry thyme
1 teaspoon ground cumin
1 cup fresh spinach
¾ cup hot water
½ cup red wine, Merlot or Cabernet
Salt and pepper to taste

Directions:
In a pan, melt the butter, brown the shanks on each side.   Remove from pan, add oil, onions, garlic. Cook for 3-4 minutes. Add tomatoes, olives, spices. Stir well. Add liquids and return the meat. Bring to boil for 1 minute.   Transfer everything to the crock-pot.   Cover, cook on medium-high for 6 hours.
Nutrition Info:net C 3g; P 71g; F 53g

898.   Brussel Sprouts Saute

Servings: 5   Cooking Time: 3 Hours
Ingredients:
11 oz Brussels sprouts, trimmed and halved
½ teaspoon coriander, ground
½ teaspoon turmeric powder
½ teaspoon salt

¾ teaspoon cayenne pepper
¾ teaspoon sage
¼ teaspoon caraway seeds
1 teaspoon almond butter
1 cup chicken stock

Directions:
Put Brussels sprouts in the slow cooker.   Add the rest of the ingredients and toss.   Close the lid and cook vegetables for 3 hours on High.   Divide between plates and serve.
Nutrition Info:calories 130, fat 2.3, fiber 3.4, carbs 4.9, protein 3.3

899.   Pork Carnitas

Servings: 10   Cooking Time: 12 Hours
Ingredients:
½ cup lime juice, freshly squeezed
½ cup lemon juice, freshly squeezed

½ tablespoon salt
1 teaspoon ground coriander

| 1 tablespoon ground cumin | 1 teaspoon black pepper |
| 1 tablespoon garlic powder | 1 teaspoon cayenne pepper |

Directions:
Place all ingredients in the Slow Cookerand stir. Close the lid and cook on low for 12 hours.   Once cooked, shred the meat using two forks and mix into the sauce.   Serve warm.

Nutrition Info: Calories: 469 Carbohydrates: 2.7g Protein: 30.9g Fat: 37.2g Sugar: 0.7g Sodium: 473mg Fiber: 0.4g

---

900. Beef Noodles With Broccoli & Tomato(2)

Servings: 2   Cooking Time: 4 Hours

Ingredients:

2 tablespoons / 28 gr of broccoli, diced	1 pinch of salt
2 teaspoons / 28 gr of olive oil	1 pinch of pepper
1 tablespoon / 14 gr of coconut oil	2 tablespoons / 28 gr of cherry tomatoes, diced

Directions:
Put the beef noodles in the bottom of the Slow Cooker pot   Cover with the diced broccoli and tomatoes   Sprinkle with a pinch of salt and pepper and with 2 teaspoons of extra virgin olive oil and the coconut oil   Set the cooking on LOW temperature, and let it cook for 4 hours   Depending on the size of the noodles, the cooking may be a bit longer, so consider whether it is necessary to have an extra hour of cooking (alternatively you can cook on HIGH for about 2 and a half hours)

Nutrition Info: Calories: 590.5 Fat: 48 g Total carbs: 3 Net carbs: 2 Protein 38.5 g

---

901. Butternut Pumpkin Soup

Servings: 4   Cooking Time: 6 Hours

Ingredients:

1 onion, diced	1 tablespoon of olive oil
2 chipotle peppers, seeded and minced	¼ teaspoon of nutmeg, grated
1 pinch cinnamon, ground	¼ teaspoon of cloves, ground
1 cup of half and half cream	1 teaspoon of black pepper
4 cups of vegetable broth	1 teaspoon of salt

Directions:
Start by throwing all the Ingredients: except half and half cream into your Crockpot.   Mix well and cover the Crockpot with its lid.   Select the Low settings for 6 hours.   Stir in half, and half cream then blend using a hand blender until smooth. Serve warm.

Nutrition Info: Calories 334 Total Fat 11.4 g Saturated Fat 1.2 g Cholesterol 0 mg Total Carbs 9.1 g Sugar 2.7 g Fiber 5.2 g Sodium 10 mg Potassium 557 mg Protein 21.3 g

---

902. Slow CookerCreole Seafood

Servings: 4   Cooking Time: 2 Hours

Ingredients:

2 cloves of garlic, minced	1 teaspoon thyme
2 stalks of celery, chopped	5oz. catfish fillets, cut into strips, deboned
1 ½ cups tomatoes, crushed	½ pound shrimps, shelled and deveined
1 bay leaf	Salt and pepper to taste
A dash of Tabasco sauce	

Directions:
Place all ingredients in the Slow Cookerand stir. Close the lid and cook on high for 2 hours. Discard the bay leaf and garnish with chopped green onions if desired.

Nutrition Info: Calories: 229 Carbohydrates: 8.9g Protein: 21g Fat: 12.2g Sugar: 5.5g Sodium: 349mg Fiber: 3.5g

---

903. Mexican Flavor Chicken Soup

Servings: 8.   Cooking Time: 8 Hours On Low.

Ingredients:

2.2 pounds chicken thighs, cut in half	1 teaspoon chilli powder
2 cups chicken broth	1 teaspoon dry oregano
1 ½ cups salsa:	1 teaspoon dry thyme
1 regular can diced Italian tomatoes	1 cup shredded cheese, your choice
1 red onion, diced	Salt and pepper to taste
2 garlic cloves, minced	

Directions:
Add all ingredients to the crock-pot, starting with chicken pieces.   Cover, cook on low for 8 hours. Remove the bones, shred the chicken with a fork. Serve.

Nutrition Info:net C 8g; P 60g; F 55g

---

904. Cabbage Stew

Servings: 4   Cooking Time: 7 Hours

Ingredients:

1-pound white cabbage, shredded	1 teaspoon salt
1 cup cherry tomatoes, halved	1 teaspoon chili flakes
1 ½ cup ground pork	¾ tablespoon keto tomatoes sauce
1 teaspoon ground black pepper	1/3 cup water
1/2 cup spring onions, chopped	1 tablespoon dill, chopped

Directions:
In the slow cooker, mix the cabbage with the tomatoes and the other ingredients.   Close the lid and cook the stew for 7 hours on Low.   Divide into bowls and serve.

Nutrition Info:calories 305, fat 14.7, fiber 1.7, carbs 4.1, protein 8.3

---

905. Lamb Shanks With Tomatoes

Servings: 2   Cooking Time: 8 Hours

Ingredients:

| 1 x 400g tin diced tomatoes | 1/3 tbsp. sundried tomato pesto |
| 1/3 cup beef stock | 2 lb. lamb shanks |

Directions:
Heat oil in a saucepan and cook onions until translucent. Add garlic and cook for 3 minutes. Add tomato paste and cook for another 2 minutes, stirring.   Add diced tomatoes, sundried tomato pesto and beef stock. Bring to a boil.   Put the lamb into the crock-pot and pour tomato sauce over. Cook for 8 hours on low.
Nutrition Info: Calories: 397 Fat: 34g Net Carbs: 5g Protein: 29g Cholesterol: 110mg Sodium: 654mg

906.   Beef And Mushrooms

Servings: 4   Cooking Time: 8 Hours
Ingredients:

1 shallot, chopped	1 cup ground beef
2 spring onions, chopped	1 teaspoon butter
1/3 cup white mushrooms, chopped	1 teaspoon dried basil
½ cup tomatoes, crushed	1 teaspoon salt
	½ teaspoon ground black pepper

Directions:
In the slow cooker, mix the beef with the shallot and the other ingredients and toss.   Close the slow cooker lid and cook pizza casserole for 8 hours on Low.
Nutrition Info:calories 326, fat 16.8, fiber 5.1, carbs 6.3, protein 22.9

907.   Chicken Cacciatore With Zoodles

Servings: 6   Cooking Time: 7 Hours
Ingredients:

1 cup chicken stock	½ cup onions, sliced
1 cup tomatoes, chopped	1 teaspoon dried parsley
2 tablespoons olive oil	1 teaspoon salt
3 cloves garlic, minced	Parmesan cheese (optional)
1 teaspoon dried oregano	For zoodles:
1 teaspoon dried thyme	1 zucchini
	2 teaspoons coconut oil

Directions:
Zoodles: Wash the zucchini and trim the ends off. Using a spiralizer, create zucchini noodles (zoodles). Heat coconut oil in a non-stick pan.   Place the zoodles into the pan.   Cook briefly for 3–5 minutes, depending on how tender you prefer the zoodles.   Chicken: Heat the oil in the Slow Cookeron high   Add the onions and cook until golden brown.   Add the chicken mince and garlic and cook for another 3 minutes.   Mix the remaining ingredients in a large mixing bowl and add them to the chicken.   Cook on low for about 6–7 hours.   Serve hot over zoodles, with some grated Parmesan cheese if desired.
Nutrition Info: Calories 347 Total Fat 17 g Saturated Fat 13.6 g Total Carbs 6 g Dietary Fiber 1 g Protein 28 g

908.   Ground Beef Soup

Servings: 4   Cooking Time: 3.5 Hour

Ingredients:

1 cup ground beef	2 spring onions, chopped
1 teaspoon garam masala	1 red bell pepper, chopped
1 cup tomatoes, crushed	3 and ½ cups of water
½ teaspoon chili flakes	1 teaspoon olive oil
1 teaspoon salt	1 teaspoon fresh dill, chopped

Directions:
Grease the slow cooker with the oil and combine all the ingredients inside.   Close the lid and cook the soup on High for 3 hours and 30 minutes.   Divide the soup into bowls and serve.
Nutrition Info:calories 325, fat 16.7, fiber 2.5, carbs 5.8, protein 10.5

909.   Shredded Pork Tacos

Servings: 12   Cooking Time: 10 Hours
Ingredients:

½ cup sugar-free bottled salsa	1 cup chicken broth
2 tablespoon green chilies, chopped	Salt and pepper to taste

Directions:
Place the pork inside the crockpot.   Add the chicken broth and salsa. Stir in the green chilies and season with salt and pepper.   Close the lid and cook on low for 10 hours.   Using two forks, shred the meat.   Serve with shredded lettuce, avocado, sour cream, olives, or tomatoes.
Nutrition Info: Calories: 616 Carbohydrates: 12g Protein: 61g Fat: 31g Sugar: 2g Sodium: 846mg Fiber: 3g

910.   Green Beans, Leeks And Artichokes

Servings: 5   Cooking Time: 5 Hours
Ingredients:

1-pound green beans, trimmed and halved	½ cup of coconut milk
2 artichokes, trimmed and halved	1 teaspoon salt
2 leeks, sliced	1 teaspoon curry powder
1 cup Cheddar cheese, shredded	1 teaspoon butter, softened

Directions:
In the slow cooker, mix the green beans with the artichokes and the other ingredients, toss and close the slow cooker lid.   Cook the mix for 5 hours on Low.
Nutrition Info:calories 162, fat 5.5, fiber 2.2, carbs 7.6, protein 7.1

911. Rustic Crockpot Ham

Servings: 12   Cooking Time: 5 Hours
Ingredients:

1 teaspoon ground mustard	1 cooked boneless ham
1 teaspoon horseradish	A dash of black pepper

Directions:

Place all ingredients in the crockpot.   Give a good stir to incorporate all ingredients.   Close the lid and cook on low for 5 hours.
Nutrition Info: Calories: 120 Carbohydrates: 6.4g Protein: 12.9 g Fat: 12.09g Sugar: 3.2g Sodium: 978mg Fiber: 0.1g

912. Cauliflower Rice And Tomatoes

Servings: 4   Cooking Time: 2 Hours
Ingredients:
- 2 cups cauliflower, riced
- 1 cup cherry tomatoes, halved
- 1/2 cup veggie stock
- 1 teaspoon turmeric
- 1 teaspoon smoked paprika
- 1 teaspoon salt
- 1 teaspoon butter
- ½ cup of coconut milk

Directions:
In the slow cooker, mix the cauliflower with tomatoes and the other ingredients.   After this, close the lid of the slow cooker and cook the meal for 2 hours on high.   When the time is over, open the slow cooker lid, stir, divide into bowls and serve.
Nutrition Info:calories 207, fat 11.5, fiber 2.5, carbs 5.5, protein 7.1

913. Lemongrass Short Ribs

Servings: 6   Cooking Time: 6 Hours
Ingredients:
- 16 oz beef short ribs, boneless
- 2 tablespoons lemon juice
- 2 tablespoons lemon zest, grated
- 1 tablespoon lemongrass, crushed
- 1 cup of water
- ½ cup fresh cilantro, chopped
- 1 tablespoon Keto tomato sauce
- 1 teaspoon minced garlic
- 1 teaspoon butter
- 1 teaspoon salt

Directions:
Place the short ribs in the slow cooker.   Add the rest of the ingredients and toss.   Close the lid and cook the meat for 6 hours on High.   Divide between plates and serve.
Nutrition Info:calories 358, fat 30.7, fiber 1., carbs 8.7, protein 24.9

914. Spicy Salmon With Spinach

Servings: 4   Cooking Time: 2 Hours
Ingredients:
- 4 cups fresh spinach
- 1-inch ginger knob, peeled and sliced thinly
- 2 lemons, sliced, seeds removed
- 1 teaspoon dried dill
- ½ cup dry white wine or chicken stock
- 3 tbsp. olive oil
- Salt and pepper, to taste

Directions:
Place the spinach in the bottom of your crock pot. Top with salmon and sliced ginger.   Add the olive oil over the top of the salmon and season to taste with salt and pepper.   Add the dill and lemon slices.   Finally, pour in the stock or dry white wine. Cover and cook on low for 2 hours.   The fish is done when it flakes easily with a fork.   Serve warm.

Nutrition Info: Calories: 284 Carbohydrates: 6.5g Protein: 23.8g Fat: 18.1g Sugar: 1.7g Sodium: 116mg Fiber: 1.9g

915. Eggplant Mushroom Soup

Servings: 6   Cooking Time: 6 Hours
Ingredients:
- 2 eggplant, peeled and diced
- 1 cup of creme fraiche
- 4 cups of vegetable stock
- 1 cup of spinach, chopped
- 2 tablespoons of white wine
- 1 red onion, diced
- 1 tablespoon of olive oil
- 1 tablespoon of dry porcini mushrooms, soaked and drained
- ½ teaspoon of salt
- ½ teaspoon of black pepper

Directions:
Start by throwing all the Ingredients: except crème Fraiche and slice mushrooms into your Crockpot. Mix well and cover the Crockpot with its lid. Select the Low settings for 6 hours.   Stir in crème Fraiche and puree the soup until smooth. Garnish with sliced mushrooms.   Serve warm.
Nutrition Info: Calories 266 Total Fat 26.9 g Saturated Fat 15.8 g Cholesterol 184 mg Total Carbs 2.5 g Sugar 0.4 g Fiber 0 g Sodium 218 mg Potassium 53 mg Protein 4.5 g

916. Broccoli Soup

Servings: 4   Cooking Time: 2.5 Hours
Ingredients:
- 8 oz broccoli, shredded
- 4 cups water
- 1 teaspoon sweet paprika
- 1 teaspoon oregano, dried
- 2 spring onions, chopped
- 1/3 cup organic almond milk
- 1 tablespoon chives, chopped
- 1 teaspoon salt

Directions:
In the crock pot, mix the broccoli with the water and the other ingredients, toss and close the slow cooker lid.   Cook casserole for 5 hours on High.
Nutrition Info:calories 223, fat 13.2, fiber 3.8, carbs 11.2, protein 10.2

917. Bacon And Zucchinis

Servings: 4   Cooking Time: 5 Hours
Ingredients:
- 1-pound zucchinis, roughly cubed
- 5 oz bacon, chopped
- 1 teaspoon sweet paprika
- 1 teaspoon minced garlic
- 1 teaspoon salt
- 1 teaspoon ground black pepper
- 1/2 cup Cheddar cheese, shredded
- ¼ cup heavy cream
- 1 teaspoon butter

Directions:
Grease the slow cooker with the butter and arrange all the ingredients except the cheese.   Sprinkle the cheese on top.   Close the lid and cook it for 5 hours on Low.
Nutrition Info:calories 312, fat 13.2, fiber 0.7, carbs 3.6, protein 14.6

| **918.** | **Pesto Salmon With Vegetables** |

Servings: 2   Cooking Time: 3 Hours
Ingredients:

8 oz fresh green beans, trimmed	10 cherry tomatoes, quartered
4 teaspoons basil pesto	3 lemons, juiced

Directions:
Grease a 4-quart slow-cooker with a non-stick cooking spray and place the cherry tomatoes and green beans inside.   Rub the salmon fillets with salt and black pepper, and place on top of the vegetables.   Mix together the pesto and the lemon juice, then drizzle over the salmon fillets and vegetables.   Cover and seal slow-cooker with its lid, and set the cooking timer for 2 to 3 hours. Allow to cook at a low heat setting or until fillets are cooked through.   Serve fish fillet and vegetables with cooked cauliflower rice.
Nutrition Info: Energy: 435 Kcal Carbohydrates: 9 g Net Carbs: 5 g Fats: 26 g Protein: 33 g

| **919.** | **Turkey Squash Stew** |

Servings: 4   Cooking Time: 8 Hours
Ingredients:

2 cups of zucchini squash, diced	1 teaspoon of coriander, ground
1 cup of chicken stock	2 teaspoons of cumin, ground
Salt and black pepper- to taste	
1 teaspoon of garlic, minced	¼ cup of tomato, diced
½ cup of sugar-free Salsa Verde	1 tablespoon of parsley, chopped

Directions:
Start by throwing all the Ingredients: except cilantro into your Crockpot.   Mix well and cover the Crockpot with its lid.   Select the Low settings for 8 hours.   Garnish with cilantro.   Serve warm.
Nutrition Info: Calories 260 Total Fat 22.9 g Saturated Fat 7.3 g Cholesterol 0 mg Total Carbs 2.7 g Sugar 1.8 g Fiber 1.4 g Sodium 9 mg Potassium 209 mg Protein 35.6 g

| **920.** | **Red Wine Beef Stew** |

Servings: 3   Cooking Time: 9 Hours
Ingredients:

2 tablespoons / 28 gr of carrot, diced	2 tablespoons / 28 gr of olive oil
2 tablespoons / 28 gr of celery	1 tablespoon / 14 gr of coconut oil
2 tablespoons / 28 gr of white onion	1 pinch of salt
1 clove / 3 gr of garlic	33 cc / 1 fl oz of red wine (verify the type you choose has max 2 gr of carbs per fl oz)
1 tablespoon / 14 gr of Sukrin coconut flour	

Directions:
Chop the carrots, onion and garlic   Roll the meat pieces in the coconut flour and coconut oil   In a pan, sauté the onion, carrot, celery and garlic with the olive oil   Add the meat and sauté for a minute stirring   Pour everything into the Slow Cooker pot and add Guinness beer and salt   Set the Slow Cooker on LOW and let it cook for 8 hours   After 8 hours, the stew is ready yet there will be an excess of liquids, which we will have to reduce to get a delicious cream. To do this remove the lid and cook another one hour on HIGH
Nutrition Info: Calories: 585.56 Fat: 48 g Total carbs: 9.5 Net carbs: 8.5 Protein 27.66 g

| **921.** | **Chinese Pulled Pork** |

Servings: 6   Cooking Time: 7 Hours And 30 Minutes
Ingredients:

2 tablespoons garlic paste	4 tablespoons soy sauce
2 teaspoons ginger paste	1 tablespoon tomato paste
1 teaspoon smoked paprika	4 tablespoons tomato sauce, sugar-free
5 drops Erythritol sweetener	1 cup chicken broth

Directions:
Place pork in a 6-quart slow cooker.   Whisk together remaining ingredients until smooth and then pour over the pork.   Plug in the slow cooker, then shut with lid and cook for 7 hours at low heat setting or until pork is tender.   Then shred pork with two forks and stir well until evenly coated with sauce.   Continue cooking pork for 30 minutes or more at low heating setting until sauce is thicken to desired consistency.   Serve straightaway.
Nutrition Info: Net Carbs: 2g Calories: 447 Total Fat: 35g Saturated Fat: 13g Protein: 30g Carbs: 3g Fiber: 1g Sugar: 2g

| **922.** | **Coconut Halibut** |

Servings: 4   Cooking Time: 7 Hours
Ingredients:

14 oz halibut fillet, cut into serving steaks	½ cup coconut cream
1 teaspoon turmeric powder	1 garlic clove, peeled, crushed
1 teaspoon sweet paprika	½ teaspoon ground black pepper
	1 teaspoon butter

Directions:
In the slow cooker, mix the halibut with the cream and the other ingredients.   Close the slow cooker lid and cook the fish for 7 hours on Low.
Nutrition Info:calories 226, fat 11.2, fiber 1, carbs 2.8, protein 17.9

| **923.** | **Rabbit & Mushroom Stew** |

Servings: 6.   Cooking Time: 6 Hours On High.
Ingredients:

1 rabbit, in portion size pieces	1 red onion, sliced
2 cups spicy Spanish sausage, cut in chunks	1 teaspoon cayenne pepper
2 Tablespoons butter, divided	1 teaspoon sweet paprika
1 cup button	1 teaspoon salt
	1 teaspoon fresh ground black pepper

mushrooms, washed and dried | 1 cup chicken broth+1 cup hot water

Directions:
Butter the crock-pot.   In a large pan, melt the butter, add the pieces of rabbit, brown on all sides. Transfer to crock-pot.   In the same pan, sauté the onions, sausage chunks, and spices for 2-3 minutes. Pour in chicken broth to deglaze the pan, heat on high for 1 minute then pour the mixture over the rabbit.   Add the mushrooms. Adjust the seasoning, if needed.   Add the water. Cover, cook on high for 6 hours. Serve.

Nutrition Info:net C 12g; P 54g; F 38g

---

924.   Scallops In Lemon Butter

Servings: 4   Cooking Time: 3 Hours

Ingredients:

Salt and pepper to taste	3 tablespoons lemon juice, freshly squeezed
2 tablespoons olive oil	¼ cup cilantro, chopped
4 tablespoons butter	

Directions:
Place all the ingredients in the Slow Cookerand stir together briefly.   Close the lid and cook on low for 3 hours.   Garnish with fresh parsley and serve.

Nutrition Info: Calories: 265 Carbohydrates: 3.5g Protein: 19.2g Fat: 19.4g Sugar: 0.3g Sodium: 267mg Fiber: 0.1g

---

925.   Salmon Stew

Servings: 4   Cooking Time: 3 Hours

Ingredients:

¼ teaspoon minced ginger	¾ teaspoon ground cinnamon
1 teaspoon turmeric powder	2 tablespoons butter
1 teaspoon cumin, ground	8 oz celery stalk, roughly chopped
1 cup heavy cream	14 oz salmon fillet, roughly chopped

Directions:
In the slow cooker, mix the salmon with the celery and the other ingredients and toss.   Close the slow cooker lid and cook the stew for 3 hours on High.

Nutrition Info:calories 315, fat 13.2, fiber 3.1, carbs 7.1, protein 12.6

---

926.   Mushroom Soup

Servings: 4   Cooking Time: 7 Hours

Ingredients:

1 cup cremini mushrooms, chopped	1 garlic clove, diced
2 spring onions, chopped	1 teaspoon olive oil
1 tablespoon oregano, chopped	¾ teaspoon ground black pepper
	2 cups of water
	1 cup of coconut milk

Directions:
In your slow cooker, mix the mushrooms with spring onions and the other ingredients and close the lid. Cook the soup for 7 hours on Low.   When the soup is cooked, blend with an immersion blender and serve.

Nutrition Info:calories 214, fat 12..5, fiber 2.2, carbs 6.7, protein 2.3

---

927.   Hot Sweet Ribs

Servings: 4   Cooking Time: 6 Hours

Ingredients:

2 tablespoons of olive oil	1 clove / 3 gr of garlic
2 tablespoons of liquid Stevia (plus another teaspoon for baking in the oven)	1 pinch of pepper
	1 pinch of thyme
	1 pinch of rosemary
	1 pinch of oregano
1 teaspoon of apple cider vinegar	½ / 100 gr of ripe avocado for garnishing, sliced
1 pinch of salt	

Directions:
Chop the aromas (adding more to your liking) Crush the garlic clove   Mix all the ingredients except the meat and create a mixture   Cover the ribs with the mixture   Put the ribs in the Slow Cooker possibly vertically from the bottom   Cook for 6 hours on HIGH (or 10 on LOW)   Put the meat over an oven plate, and brush over the Stevia Bake on grill mode for 10 minutes, then garnish with the avocado slices

Nutrition Info: Calories: 671g Fat: 59.66 Total carbs: 9.53 Net carbs: 2.83 Protein 28 g

---

928.   Paprika Bok Choy

Servings: 6   Cooking Time: 2.5 Hours

Ingredients:

1-pound bok choy, torn	1 teaspoon ground paprika
½ cup of coconut milk	1 teaspoon turmeric
1 tablespoon almond butter, softened	½ teaspoon cayenne pepper

Directions:
In the slow cooker, mix the bok choy with the coconut milk and the other ingredients, toss and close the lid.   Cook the meal for 5 hours on High.

Nutrition Info:calories 128, fat 3.2, fiber 3.9, carbs 4.9, protein 4.1

---

929.   Coriander Broccoli

Servings: 3   Cooking Time: 1 Hour

Ingredients:

2 cups broccoli florets	¾ cup organic almond milk
1 tablespoon butter	
1 teaspoon turmeric powder	1 teaspoon coriander, ground

Directions:
In the slow cooker, combine the broccoli with the butter and the other ingredients and close the lid. Cook broccoli mix for 1 hour on High.   Divide between plates and serve.

Nutrition Info:calories 132, fat 7.1, fiber 3.5, carbs 2.9, protein 3.4

---

930.   Spinach Leeks Dip

Servings: 6   Cooking Time: 6 Hours

Ingredients:

2 tablespoons of
avocado oil
2 leeks, diced
-2 garlic cloves,
minced
4 cups of spinach,
torn

¼ cup of vegetable
broth
¼ cup of lime juice
1 bunch basil, diced
A pinch of salt and
black pepper

Directions:
Start by throwing all the Ingredients: into the Crockpot.   Cover its lid and cook for 6 hours on Low setting.   Once done, remove its lid of the crockpot carefully.   Blend this dip mixture using an immersion blender.   Mix well and garnish as desired.   Serve warm.
Nutrition Info: Calories 136 Total Fat 18.3 g Saturated Fat 2.6 g Cholesterol 75 mg Sodium 104 mg Total Carbs 0.6 g Sugar 6.2 g Fiber 2.9 g Protein 5.9 g

931. Butter Green Beans

Servings: 6   Cooking Time: 4.5 Hours
Ingredients:

2 cups green beans,
trimmed and halved

½ cup butter
1 teaspoon salt

Directions:
Mix up together snap peas with salt and transfer them in the slow cooker.   Add butter and close the lid.   Cook the vegetables on Low for 4.5 hours.
Nutrition Info:calories 175, fat 15.5, fiber 2.5, carbs 7, protein 2.8

932. Pot Roast Beef Brisket

Servings: 10.   Cooking Time: 12 Hours On Low.
Ingredients:

6.6 pounds beef
brisket, whole
2 Tablespoons olive
oil
2 Tablespoons apple
cider vinegar
1 teaspoon dry
oregano
1 teaspoon dry thyme

1 teaspoon dried
rosemary
2 Tablespoons
paprika
1 teaspoon Cayenne
pepper
1 tablespoon salt
1 teaspoon fresh
ground black pepper

Directions:
In a bowl, mix dry seasoning, add olive oil, apple cider vinegar.   Place the meat in the crock-pot, generously coat with seasoning mix.   Cover, cook on low for 12 hours.   Remove the brisket from the liquid, place on a pan. Sear it under the broiler for 2-4 minutes, watch it carefully so the meat doesn't burn.   Cover the meat with foil, let it rest for 1 hour. Slice and serve.
Nutrition Info:net C 1g; P 70g; F 54g

933. Cauliflower Bowls

Servings: 2   Cooking Time: 3 Hours
Ingredients:

1 and ½ cups
cauliflower, shredded
1/2 cup Mozzarella,
shredded
1 teaspoon chili flakes

½ cup tomatoes,
cubed
1 teaspoon dried
oregano
3 eggs, beaten
1 teaspoon olive oil

Directions:
Place the oil in the bottom of the slow cooker. Combine the cauliflower with the Mozzarella and the other ingredients and toss.   Close the slow cooker lid.   Cook the hash for 3 hours on High.
Nutrition Info:calories 228, fat 11.2, fiber 0.9, carbs 2.5, protein 13.8

934. Beef Stew

Servings: 5   Cooking Time: 5 Hours
Ingredients:

Coconut oil – 3 tbsp.
Beef broth – 3 cups
Medium onion – 1,
chopped
Apple cider vinegar –
2 tbsp.
Fresh thyme - 1 tbsp.
Ground cinnamon –
2 tsp.

Erythritol – 2 tsp.
Minced garlic – 1 ½
tbsp.
Bay leaves – 2
Black pepper – 1 ½
tsp.
Sage, rosemary, salt,
fish sauce, soy sauce
– 1 tsp. each

Directions:
Cut up the beef into 1-inch cubes, dice the veggies. Season the meat with salt and pepper.   Add oil in a hot skillet and brown the meat in batches. Once done, add the veggies and cook for a couple of minutes.   Add everything (except for thyme, rosemary, and sage) in the Crock-Pot.   Cover and cook on high for 3 hours. Add the thyme, rosemary, and sage and cook 1 to 2 hours on the same setting. Serve.
Nutrition Info: Calories: 337.6 Fat: 13.8g Carbs: 5.5g Protein: 42.1g

935. Coconut Pulled Pork

Servings: 2   Cooking Time: 8 Hours
Ingredients:

2 tablespoons / 28 gr
of olive oil
2 tablespoons / 28 gr
of coconut milk
1 tablespoon / 14 gr
of ginger, shredded
1 pinch of onion
powder

2 tablespoons / 28 gr
of apple cider vinegar
Pinch of garlic
powder
1 pinch of salt and
pepper

Directions:
Make a zig zag cut on the fat part of the shoulder Lay the ginger on the bottom of your Slow Cooker pot   In a small bowl combine the olive oil and seasonings until you obtain a homogeneous mixture Pour the mixture over the pork and lay in the Slow Cooker pot   Cover the Slow cooker and leave the meat to marinate for a night   The day after, add the coconut milk and cook on LOW for 8 hours Once cooked, the pork meat shreds naturally
Nutrition Info: Calories: 604.4 Fat: 51.74 g Total carbs: 4.18 Net carbs: 3.56 Protein 26.6 g

936. Zucchini Dip

Servings: 6   Cooking Time: 2 Hours
Ingredients:

1-pound zucchinis,
chopped

1 teaspoon cumin,
ground

1 tablespoon butter
¼ cup cream cheese
1 teaspoon minced garlic
½ cup of coconut milk
1 teaspoon turmeric powder

1 tablespoon fresh parsley, chopped
¼ teaspoon ground coriander
¾ teaspoon sweet paprika

Directions:
In the slow cooker, mix the zucchinis with the butter and the other ingredients.   Close the lid and cook it on Low for 2 hours.   Blend using an immersion blender, divide into bowls and serve.
Nutrition Info:calories 209, fat 4.5, fiber 1.3, carbs 6.4, protein 4.3

937. Cauliflower Bolognese On Zucchini Noodles

Servings: 2   Cooking Time: 4 Hours
Ingredients:

1 tsp dried basil flakes
1/2 cup vegetable broth

28 oz. diced tomatoes
5 zucchinis, spiral cut

Directions:
Place ingredients in the crockpot except for the zucchini. Season with 2 garlic cloves, 3.4 diced onions, salt and pepper to taste and desired spices. Cover and cook for 4 hours.   Smash florets of the cauliflower with a fork to form "Bolognese." Transfer the dish on top of the zucchini noodles.
Nutrition Info: Calories: 164 Fat: 5 g Net carbs: 6 g Protein: 12 g

938. Bacon Beef Bolognese

Servings: 4   Cooking Time: 4 Hours
Ingredients:

4 oz. bacon, diced
2 (28 oz.) cans crushed tomatoes
3 bay leaves
1 large onion, minced
2 celery stalks, minced
2 large carrots, minced
½ cup of yogurt

1/4 cup of diced fresh basil
1 tablespoon of butter, melted
3 tablespoons of dry white wine
1 teaspoon of salt
½ teaspoon of black pepper

Directions:
Start by throwing all the Ingredients: into your Crockpot.   Mix well and cover the Crockpot with its lid.   Select the Low settings for 4 hours. Serve warm.
Nutrition Info: Calories 191 Total Fat 8.4 g Saturated Fat 0.7 g Cholesterol 0 mg Total Carbs 7.1 g Sugar 0.1 g Fiber 1.4 g Sodium 226 mg Potassium 323 mg Protein 26.3 g

939. Lamb With Mint And Green Beans

Servings: 2   Cooking Time: 6 Hours
Ingredients:

1 tbsp. ghee, tallow or lard

3 cups green beans, trimmed

1/8 cup freshly chopped mint leaves

Directions:
Pat the lamb dry with paper towels and season it with salt and pepper.   Grease the crock-pot with ghee, tallow or lard, then put the lamb inside. Sprinkle with garlic and mint all over. If it makes you more comfortable, add up to half a cup of water. Cover and cook for 4 hours on high.   Transfer the lamb to a plate, then place the green beans on the bottom of the crock-pot. Add the lamb again inside. Cover and cook for another two hours on high.
Nutrition Info: Calories: 525 Fat: 36.4g Net Carbs: 7.6g Protein: 37.3g

940. Fish Stock

Servings: 6   Cooking Time: 4-8 Hours
Ingredients:

1 tablespoon olive oil
1 onion, sliced
1 carrot, sliced
2 bay leaves
1/3 cup parsley stems
2 tablespoons dry white wine

1/3 cup dill stems
½ teaspoon rosemary
½ teaspoon dried thyme
Salt, pepper, to taste
11 cups water

Directions:
Heat oil in a slow cooker on High. Add onion, cook until translucent stirring constantly.   Add carrot, parsley and dill stems, stir for 1 minute. Pour wine into the pan and sauté for 2 minutes.   Transfer the vegetables and wine mixture into a slow cooker, add fish. Add salt, pepper, rosemary and dried thyme. Pour water to cover the fish by 1 inch.   Close the lid and cook on Low for 6-8 hours or on High for 3-4 hours.
Nutrition Info: Calories 40 Fats 11g Net carbs 0g Protein 5.27g

941. Nutritious Bean Bowl

Servings: 2   Cooking Time: 9 Hours
Ingredients:

½ onion, diced
½ tablespoon of fresh ginger, minced
½ tablespoon of garlic, minced
½ teaspoons of curry powder
½ teaspoon of cumin, ground
½ teaspoon of ground coriander

1 medium tomato, diced
½ cup of edamame beans
½ cup of water
Pinch of salt
Black pepper, to taste
1 tablespoon of fresh parsley, chopped

Directions:
Start by throwing all the Ingredients: into your Crockpot.   Cover its lid and cook for 3 hours on Low setting.   Once done, remove its lid and give it a stir.   Garnish as desired.   Serve warm.
Nutrition Info: Calories 265 Total Fat 15.5 g Saturated Fat 12.4 g Cholesterol 154 mg Sodium 57 mg Total Carbs 7.4 g Fiber 0.9 g Sugar 1.6 g Protein 5.4 g

| **942.** | **Chicken And Spinach Stew** |

Servings: 6 – 8   Cooking Time: Approximately 8 Hours

Ingredients:

2 lb chicken thighs and legs, bone in, skin on	6 garlic cloves, crushed
2 cups spinach, roughly chopped	1 tsp dried tarragon
1 onion, finely chopped	2 cups chicken stock
	½ cup dry white wine
	½ cup heavy cream

Directions:

Drizzle some olive oil into the Crock Pot.   Add the chicken, spinach, onion, 4 cloves of garlic, stock, tarragon, salt, and pepper to the pot, stir to combine. Add the lid to the pot and set the temperature to LOW.   Cook for 8 hours.   Drizzle some olive oil into a small pot and add the remaining 2 cloves of garlic.   Pour the wine into the pot and simmer until reduced.   Add the cream to the pot with the wine and stir to combine.   Remove the lid from the Slow Cookerand stir the wine and cream mixture into the stew.   Serve while hot!

| **943.** | **Creamy Coconut Cauliflower** |

Servings: 2   Cooking Time: 3 Hours

Ingredients:

1 cup of red onion, diced	2 tablespoons of balsamic vinegar
¼ cup of chicken stock	1 cup of coconut cream
A pinch of salt and black pepper	

Directions:

Start by throwing all the Ingredients: into the Crockpot.   Cover its lid and cook for 3 hours on Low setting.   Once done, remove its lid of the crockpot carefully.   Mix well and garnish as desired.   Serve warm.

Nutrition Info: Calories 173 Total Fat 16.2 g Saturated Fat 9.8 g Cholesterol 100 mg Sodium 42 mg Total Carbs 9.4 g Sugar 0.2 g Fiber1 g Protein 3.3 g

| **944.** | **Dill Leeks** |

Servings: 3   Cooking Time: 3 Hours

Ingredients:

2 cups leeks, sliced	1 teaspoon sweet paprika
1 cup chicken stock	
2 tablespoons fresh dill, chopped	1 tablespoon coconut cream
½ teaspoon turmeric powder	1 teaspoon butter

Directions:

In the slow cooker, mix the beets with the stock, dill and the other ingredients.   Cook on Low for 3 hours and serve.

Nutrition Info:calories 123, fat 2.9, fiber 2.2, carbs 7.5, protein 4.3.

| **945.** | **Rich Creamy Endives** |

Servings: 4   Cooking Time: 3 Hours

Ingredients:

4 endives, trimmed and halved	1 tablespoon of dill, diced
½ cup of chicken stock	1 tablespoon of smoked paprika

Directions:

Start by throwing all the Ingredients: into the Crockpot.   Cover its lid and cook for 3 hours on Low setting.   Once done, remove its lid of the crockpot carefully.   Mix well and garnish as desired.   Serve warm.

Nutrition Info: Calories 191 Total Fat 8.4 g Saturated Fat 0.7 g Cholesterol 743 mg Total Carbs 7.1 g Sugar 0.1 g Fiber 1.4 g Sodium 226 mg Protein 6.3 g

| **946.** | **Cider Dipped Greens With Bacon** |

Servings: 2   Cooking Time: 2 Hours

Ingredients:

2 tablespoon of chicken stock	1 tablespoon of apple cider vinegar
3 bacon strips, diced	Salt and black pepper- to taste
1/4 cup of cherry tomatoes, halved	

Directions:

Start by throwing all the Ingredients: into your Crockpot.   Cover its lid and cook for 2 hours on Low setting.   Once done, remove its lid and give it a stir.   Garnish as desired.   Serve warm.

Nutrition Info: Calories 421 Total Fat 19.5 g Saturated Fat 2.4 g Cholesterol 69 mg Sodium 58 mg Total Carbs 5.3 g Fiber 0.7 g Sugar 0.3 g Protein 1.4 g

| **947.** | **Korean Barbecue Beef** |

Servings: 4   Cooking Time: 25 Minutes

Ingredients:

Beef broth – ½ cup	Apple cider vinegar – 1 tablespoon
Erythritol sweetener – 1/3 cup	
Liquid aminos – ¼ cup	Grated ginger – 1 tablespoon
Minced garlic – 2 tablespoons	Sriracha sauce – 1 ½ teaspoon
Avocado oil – 2 tablespoons	Ground black pepper – ½ teaspoon

Directions:

Switch on the instant pot, add all the ingredients, and stir until mixed.   Shut the instant pot with its lid in the sealed position, then press the 'manual' button, press '+/-' to set the cooking time to 25 minutes and cook at high-pressure setting; when the pressure builds in the pot, the cooking timer will start.   When the instant pot buzzes, press the 'keep warm' button, release pressure naturally for 10 minutes, then do a quick pressure release and open the lid.   Garnish beef with cilantro and serve.

Nutrition Info: Calories: 635.7 Fat: 31.7 g Protein: 69.3 g Net Carbs: 10.5 g Fiber: 17.3 g

| **948.** | **Spinach Stuffed Portobello** |

Servings: 8   Cooking Time: 3 Hours

Ingredients:

3 tablespoons olive oil
½ onion, chopped
2 cups fresh spinach, rinsed and chopped
3 garlic cloves, minced
1 cup chicken broth
3 tablespoons parmesan cheese, grated
1/3 teaspoon dried thyme
salt, pepper, to taste

Directions:
Heat oil in a medium pan over high heat. Add onion, cook until translucent stirring steadily. Add spinach and thyme, cook for 1-2 minutes until spinach is wilted.   Brush each mushroom with olive oil. Put 1 tablespoon of onion and spinach stuffing into each mushroom.   Pour chicken broth into slow cooker. Put stuffed mushrooms on the bottom. Close the lid and cook on High for 3 hours.   Once cooked, sprinkle mushrooms with parmesan cheese and serve.
Nutrition Info: Calories 310g Fats 21g Net carbs 3g Protein 12g

949.   Cheesy Tuna Casserole

Servings: 4   Cooking Time: 6 Hours
Ingredients:
1-inch ginger, peeled and grated
1 tablespoon lemon juice
2 tablespoons soy sauce
Zest of ½ lemon
¼ cup butter, melted
4 cloves of garlic, peeled, minced
1 cup heavy cream
9 ounces fresh spinach, rinsed and drained
4 large eggs, beaten
Salt and pepper to taste
1 cup whole-milk mozzarella cheese, shredded

Directions:
In a mixing bowl, combine the tuna, ginger, lemon juice, soy sauce, and lemon zest.   Place the bowl in the fridge and marinate for at least 2 hours.   After 2 hours, discard liquid from the tuna. Transfer marinated tuna into the crock pot.   Stir in the butter, garlic, heavy cream, and spinach.   Add the eggs and season with salt and pepper to taste. Sprinkle the mozzarella cheese on top.   Close the lid and cook on high for 4 hours or on low for 6 hours.
Nutrition Info: Calories: 484 Carbohydrates: 6.3g Protein: 31.9g Fat: 36.8g Sugar: 0.6g Sodium: 828mg Fiber: 1.6g

950.   Bacon And Cauliflower Soup

Servings: 4   Cooking Time: 4 Hours
Ingredients:
Garlic – 3 cloves, crushed
Onion – ¾, finely chopped
Bacon – 4 slices, cut into small pieces
Chicken stock – 2 cups
Smoked paprika – ½ tsp.
Chili powder – ½ tsp.
Heavy cream – ¾ cup
Olive oil – 2 tbsp.
Salt and pepper to taste
Paprika to taste

Directions:

Add olive oil into the Crock-Pot.   Add the garlic, cauliflower, onion, bacon, stock, paprika, chili, salt, and pepper to the pot. Stir to mix.   Cover with the lid and cook on high for 4 hours.   Open the lid and blend with a hand mixer.   Add the cream and mix. Serve sprinkled with paprika.
Nutrition Info: Calories: 265 Fat: 22.3g Carbs: 6.1g Protein: 10.4g

951.   Ground Lamb Casserole

Servings: 2   Cooking Time: 8 Hours
Ingredients:
1/2 lb. ground lamb
1/8 cup diced green bell pepper
2 cups thinly sliced cabbage
1 cup tomato sauce

Directions:
Add the ground lamb, bacon, pepper, onion, and garlic to taste into the crock-pot.   Cover and cook for 6 hours in low.   Add the cabbage and tomato sauce to the pot, stir, then cook for another 2 hours.
Nutrition Info: Calories: 295 Fat: 19g Net Carbs: 6g Protein: 22g Cholesterol: 67mg Sodium: 360mg

952.   Lazy Man's Pork Ribs

Servings: 6   Cooking Time: 10 Hours
Ingredients:
2 teaspoon Cajun seasoning
1 cup water
¼ cup yacon syrup
Salt and pepper to taste

Directions:
Place all ingredients in the crockpot.   Give a stir to incorporate all ingredients.   Close the lid and cook on low for 10 hours.
Nutrition Info: Calories: 464 Carbohydrates: 12g Protein: 37.4g Fat: 30g Sugar: 4.7g Sodium: 190mg Fiber: 0.2g

953.   Broccoli Sauté

Servings: 4   Cooking Time: 5 Hours
Ingredients:
2 cups broccoli florets
1 teaspoon salt
1 teaspoon ground nutmeg
1 teaspoon coriander, ground
1 tablespoon olive oil
1 teaspoon cumin, ground
½ cup chicken stock
1 oz Cheddar cheese, shredded

Directions:
In the slow cooker, mix the broccoli with the coriander, salt and the other ingredients.   Close the lid and cook on Low for 5 hours.
Nutrition Info:calories 143, fat 4.1, fiber 2.3, carbs 5.2, protein 5.2

954.   Cube Steak

Servings: 8   Cooking Time: 8 Hours
Ingredients:
1 ¾ t. adobo seasoning/garlic salt
1 can (8 oz.) tomato sauce
1 c. water
Black pepper to taste
½ med. onion
1 small red pepper
1/3 c. green pitted olives (+) 2 tbsp. brine

Directions:

Slice the peppers and onions into ¼-inch strips. Sprinkle the steaks with the pepper and garlic salt as needed and place in the cooker. Fold in the peppers and onion along with the water, sauce, and olives (with the liquid/brine from the jar). Close the lid. Prepare using the low-temperature setting for eight hours.

Nutrition Info: Calories: 154 Net Carbs: 4 g Protein: 23.5 g Fat: 5.5 g

955. Vegetable Salad

Servings: 2   Cooking Time: 1 Hour

Ingredients:
- ½ carrot, peeled and shredded
- 1 cup of water
- ¼ teaspoon of salt
- ½ cup of cabbage, sliced
- ½ cup of green onions, diced
- ½ cup of red onions, sliced
- 1 tablespoon of brown swerve
- 2 tablespoons, balsamic vinegar
- 1 tablespoon of vegetable oil
- 1 tablespoon of ginger, grated
- 1 tablespoon of sunflower seeds
- 1 garlic clove, minced
- Black pepper, to taste

Directions:
Start by adding throwing all the Ingredients: into your Crockpot.   Cover its lid and cook for 1 hour on Low setting.   Once done, remove its lid and give it a stir.   Garnish as desired.   Serve fresh.

Nutrition Info: Calories 254 Total Fat 23.5 g Saturate Fat 2.4 g Cholesterol 69 mg Sodium 58 mg Total Carbs 2.49 g Fiber 0.7 g Sugar 0.3 g Protein 7.9 g

956. Trout & Broccoli Chowder

Servings: 6   Cooking Time: 2 Hours

Ingredients:
- 1 onion, chopped
- 1 tablespoon butter, unsalted
- 1 cup soy milk, unsweetened
- 1 cup water
- 1 package (10 oz) frozen broccoli, thawed
- ¼ teaspoon garlic powder
- Salt, pepper, to taste
- 1 cup cheddar cheese, shredded
- 1 tablespoon parsley, chopped

Directions:
Melt butter in a pan over high heat, add onions. Sauté for 2-3 minutes until onion softens. Transfer onion to a slow cooker. Add milk, broccoli, cheese, fish, garlic powder and salt.   Close the lid and cook on High for 2 hours. Check if the fish is soft. Serve topped with parsley.

Nutrition Info: Calories 403 Fats 20.9g Net carbs 6.7g Protein 15.2g

957. Chicken And Egg Soup

Servings: 6   Cooking Time: Approximately 4 Hours

Ingredients:
- 4 chicken thighs, boneless, skinless, cut into medium-sized pieces
- 4 garlic cloves, finely chopped
- 1 red chili, finely chopped
- 1 tbsp finely grated fresh ginger
- 1 lemon
- 4 cups chicken stock
- 6 eggs (1 egg per person)
- Fresh coriander

Directions:
Drizzle some olive oil into the Crock Pot.   Add the chicken, garlic, chili, ginger, juice of one lemon, stock, salt, and pepper to the pot, stir to combine. Place the lid onto the pot and set the temperature to HIGH.   Cook for 4 hours.   Remove the lid and stir the soup.   At this stage, you can either crack the eggs straight into the hot soup to lightly poach, or you can simply poach them in water in a separate pot and place them into each serving bowl of soup. Sprinkle each bowl of soup with fresh coriander!

958. French Onion Soup

Servings: 3   Cooking Time: 4 Hours

Ingredients:
- 3 spring onions, chopped
- ½ cup coconut milk
- ½ teaspoon minced garlic
- 1 teaspoon turmeric powder
- ½ cup coconut cream
- ½ teaspoon ground black pepper
- 7 oz Parmesan, grated
- 2 tablespoon butter
- 1 cup of water

Directions:
Melt butter and pour it in the slow cooker.   Add the onions and the other ingredients except the cheese.   Close the lid and cook soup for 2 hours on High.   After this, add grated cheese and stir well. Cook the soup for 2 hours more on Low.

Nutrition Info:calories 371, fat 22.2, fiber 5.8, carbs 10, protein 23.9

959. Beef Stroganoff

Servings: 8   Cooking Time: 6 Hours

Ingredients:
- 2 teaspoons salt
- ½ teaspoon white ground pepper
- 4 cloves of garlic, minced
- 2 teaspoons paprika
- 1 onion, chopped finely
- 1 teaspoon thyme
- 1 cup fresh Portobello mushrooms, sliced
- 1/3 cup heavy cream
- ½ cup olive oil
- 2 teaspoon wine vinegar

Directions:
Place all ingredients in the crock pot. Close the lid and cook on high for 6 hours.   Open the lid and stir gently halfway through.   Serve warm over egg noodles.

Nutrition Info: Calories: 381 Carbohydrates: 2.4g Protein: 25.9g Fat: 29.7g Sugar: 0.7g Sodium: 640mg Fiber: 0.6g

960. Kale And Celery Stock

Servings: 8   Cooking Time: 5 Hours

Ingredients:
- 2 carrots, diced
- 4 garlic cloves
- 10 peppercorns
- 2 bay leaves
- 2 cups of celery, diced
- 1 cup of kale

8 cups of cold water, filtered
1 cup of bell pepper, diced
a handful rosemary
a handful parsley
salt to taste

Directions:
Start by throwing all the Ingredients: into your Crockpot. Mix well and cover the Crockpot with its lid. Select the Low settings for 5 hours. Strain the cooked soup and add it to a jar. Serve warm.
Nutrition Info: Calories 143 Total Fat 16.7 g Saturated Fat 9.7 g Cholesterol 32 mg Total Carbs 8.6 g Sugar 2.4 g Fiber 5.7 g Sodium 141 mg Potassium 478 mg Protein 3.4 g

961. Nutty Green Beans With Avocado

Servings: 4   Cooking Time: 2 Hours
Ingredients:
½ cup of chicken stock
½ cup of walnuts, diced
1 avocado (peeled, pitted and cubed)
¼ teaspoon of sweet paprika
A pinch of salt and black pepper
2 teaspoons of balsamic vinegar

Directions:
Start by throwing all the Ingredients: into the Crockpot. Cover its lid and cook for 2 hours on Low setting. Once done, remove its lid of the crockpot carefully. Mix well and garnish as desired. Serve warm.
Nutrition Info: Calories 134 Total Fat 21.4 g Saturated Fat 1.2 g Cholesterol 244 mg Sodium 10 mg Total Carbs 10.1 g Sugar 2.7 g Fiber 5.2 g Protein 2.3 g

962. Zucchini Balls

Servings: 4   Cooking Time: 30 Minutes
Ingredients:
1 cup zucchini, grated
½ cup almond flour
¼ cup Parmesan, grated
1 egg, whisked
1 tablespoon avocado oil
¾ cup of coconut milk
½ teaspoon salt

Directions:
In the mixing bowl zucchinis with flour and the other ingredients except the coconut milk and the oil and shape medium balls. Preheat avocado oil in the skillet and add zucchini balls. Roast them for 2 minutes from each side. After this, transfer the zucchini balls in the slow cooker. Add coconut milk and close the lid. Cook the meal for 30 minutes on High.
Nutrition Info:calories 207, fat 5.5, fiber 1.8, carbs 4.5, protein 3.6

963. Steak And Tomato Salad

Servings: 2   Cooking Time: 5 Hours
Ingredients:
1-pound beef steaks, cut into strips
1 cup cherry
1 cup baby spinach
2 bell peppers, roughly chopped
tomatoes, halved
1 tablespoon olive oil
1/3 cup vegetable stock
1 tablespoon fresh cilantro, chopped
½ cup spring onions, chopped
1 tablespoon lime juice
1 teaspoon chili flakes

Directions:
In the slow cooker, mix the beef with the tomatoes and the other ingredients. Close the lid and cook meal for 5 hours on High. Divide into bowls and serve.
Nutrition Info:calories 347, fat 11.4, fiber 1.7, carbs 9, protein 27.2

964. Buttermilk Curry

Servings: 6   Cooking Time: 8 Hours
Ingredients:
4 spring onions, diced into lengths
4 cups of chicken stock
½ cup of buttermilk
1½ teaspoon of cumin, ground
¼ teaspoon of cayenne pepper
1½ teaspoon of ground turmeric
2 tablespoon of curry powder
2 bay leaves
1 bunch cilantro leaves, diced
salt and black pepper to taste

Directions:
Start by throwing all the Ingredients: except cilantro into your Crockpot. Mix well and cover the Crockpot with its lid. Select the Low settings for 8 hours. First, discard the bay leaves then puree the soup. Pass this soup through a fine sieve. Garnish with cilantro. Serve warm.
Nutrition Info: Calories 149 Total Fat 14.5 g Saturated Fat 8.1 g Cholesterol 56 mg Total Carbs 11.6 g Sugar 0.3 g Fiber 0 g Sodium 56 mg Potassium 39 mg Protein 2.6 g

965. Spinach And Tomato Soup

Servings: 2   Cooking Time: 3 Hours
Ingredients:
3 cups of water
1/3 cup tomatillos, chopped
1 teaspoon sweet paprika
½ teaspoon ground black pepper
2 cups baby spinach
1 teaspoon salt
1 tablespoon dried dill
1 tablespoon butter, melted

Directions:
In the slow cooker, mix the water with spinach and the other ingredients, toss and close the lid. Cook soup for 3 hours on Low.
Nutrition Info:calories 322, fat 5.3, fiber 2.9, carbs 4.8, protein 4.5

966. Sugar Snap Peas Soup

Servings: 4   Cooking Time: 3 Hours
Ingredients:
2 cups sugar snap peas
½ cup celery stalk, chopped
1 teaspoon garlic,
1 teaspoon chili powder
1 teaspoon salt
1 tablespoon chives, chopped

diced
3 cups of water

½ teaspoon thyme
1 teaspoon olive oil

Directions:
Grease the slow cooker with the oil and combine all the ingredients inside.   Close the lid and cook soup for 3 hours on High.
Nutrition Info:calories 226, fat 5.8, fiber 1.8, carbs 6.3, protein 6.3

967.   Creamy Eggplant Soup

Servings: 4   Cooking Time: 8 Hours
Ingredients:

4 tomatoes
1 teaspoon of garlic, minced
1/4 yellow onion, diced
2 tablespoons of basil, diced
4 tablespoons of parmesan, grated

1 tablespoon of olive oil
2 cups of chicken stock
1 bay leaf
1/2 cup of heavy cream
salt and black pepper - to taste

Directions:
Start by throwing all the Ingredients: except cilantro into your Crockpot.   Mix well and cover the Crockpot with its lid.   Select the Low settings for 8 hours.   Garnish with cilantro.   Serve warm.
Nutrition Info: Calories 304 Total Fat 15.7 g Saturated Fat 9.7 g Cholesterol 49 mg Total Carbs 2.6 g Sugar 3.4 g Fiber 1.5 g Sodium 141 mg Potassium 178 mg Protein 6.3 g

968.   Pork And Chive Meatballs

Servings: 6 As A Starter   Cooking Time: Approximately 4 Hours
Ingredients:

1 lb minced pork
1 egg
2 garlic cloves, crushed

¼ cup ground almonds
2 tbsp finely chopped chives

Directions:
In a large bowl, mix together the pork, egg, garlic, ground almonds, chives, salt, and pepper until combined.   Roll the mixture into about 18 balls. Drizzle the Slow Cookerwith olive oil.   Lay the meatballs into the Slow Cookerand drizzle with olive oil.   Place the lid onto the pot and set the timer to LOW.   Cook for 4 hours.   Once the meatballs are cooked, take them out of the pot and serve on a serving platter with a small bowl of toothpicks.

969.   Chipotle Barbacoa

Servings: 9   Cooking Time: 4 Hours
Ingredients:

2 med. chilis in adobo (with the sauce, it's about 4 teaspoons)
3 lb. chuck roast/beef brisket
5 minced garlic cloves
2 tbsp. of each:
Lime juice

Apple cider vinegar
2 t. of each:
Sea salt
Cumin
1 tbsp. dried oregano
1 t. black pepper
2 whole bay leaves

Optional: ½ t. ground cloves

Directions:

Mix the chilis in the sauce, and add the broth, garlic, ground cloves, pepper, cumin, salt, vinegar, and lime juice in a blender, mixing until smooth. Chop the beef into two-inch chunks, and toss it in the slow cooker. Empty the puree on top. Toss in the two bay leaves.   Cook four to six hrs. on the high setting or eight to ten using the low setting. Dispose of the bay leaves when the meat is done. Shred and stir into the juices to simmer for five to ten minutes.
Nutrition Info: Calories: 242 Net Carbs: 2 g Fat: 11 g Protein: 32 g

970.   Beet And Goat Cheese

Servings: 4   Cooking Time: 3 Hours
Ingredients:

2 tablespoon of olive oil
4-ounce goat cheese, crumbled
1 tablespoon of balsamic vinegar
1 red onion, sliced

2 tablespoons of swerves
1-pint mixed cherry tomatoes, halved
2-ounce pecans
Salt and black pepper- to taste

Directions:
Start by throwing all the Ingredients: into your Crockpot except cheese.   Cover its lid and cook for 3 hours on Low setting.   Once done, remove its lid and give it a stir.   Garnish with goat cheese. Serve warm.
Nutrition Info: Calories 355 Total Fat 26.2 g Saturated Fat 7.4 g Cholesterol 98 mg Sodium 75 mg Total Carbs 5.7 g Fiber 0.7 g Sugar 0.9 g Protein 5.4 g

971.Pork Chops

Servings: 8   Cooking Time: 6 Hours
Ingredients:

1 tablespoon dried thyme
1 tablespoon dried rosemary
1 tablespoon ground cumin
1 tablespoon dried curry powder

1 teaspoon salt
1 tablespoon chopped fresh chives
1 tablespoon fennel seeds
4 tablespoons avocado oil

Directions:
Place 2 tablespoons oil in a small bowl, add remaining ingredients except for pork and stir until well mixed.   Rub this mixture on all sides of pork chips until evenly coated.   Grease a 6-quart slow cooker with remaining oil, add seasoned pork chops and shut with lid.   Plug in the slow cooker and cook pork for 6 hours at low heat setting or 4 hours at high heat setting.   Serve straightaway.
Nutrition Info: Net Carbs: 1g Calories: 235 Total Fat: 15g Saturated Fat: 3g Protein: 24g Carbs: 1g Fiber: 0g Sugar: 0g

972.   Coco-loco Shrimp

Servings: 8   Cooking Time: 2 Hours
Ingredients:

1 tablespoon garlic, minced
1 tablespoon ginger,

1 teaspoon garam masala
½ teaspoon cayenne

grated
½ teaspoon turmeric powder
½ cup shredded toasted coconut, unsweetened

pepper
½ can coconut milk, unsweetened
Salt and pepper to taste

Directions:
Place all the ingredients except the shredded coconut, in the Slow Cookerand stir well. Close the lid and cook on low for 2 hours. Serve warm, sprinkled with coconut.
Nutrition Info: Calories: 301 Carbohydrates: 8.7g Protein: 13g Fat: 23.8g Sugar: 2.9g Sodium: 170mg Fiber: 2.2g

973.	**Tuna-zucchini Spaghetti**

Servings: 4   Cooking Time: 1 Hour
Ingredients:

1/3 cup chicken broth
1 cup whole milk
2 tablespoons parsley flakes
½ pound ground tuna, boiled

2 zucchinis, spiralized or peeled into long strips
1 tablespoons butter
Salt and pepper to taste

Directions:
Place all ingredients in the Slow Cookerand stir well. Close the lid and cook on high for 1 hour. Serve warm.
Nutrition Info: Calories: 208 Carbohydrates: 12.1g Protein: 18.9g Fat: 9.3g Sugar: 9.8g Sodium: 172mg Fiber: 1.5g

974.	**Winter Keto Stew**

Servings: 3   Cooking Time: 5 Hours
Ingredients:

2 tablespoons / 28 gr red onion, diced
2 tablespoons / 28 gr of ghee
A dash of red wine
¼ cup / 50 gr of plain firm tofu, crumbled

2 tablespoons / 28 gr of olive oil
1 pinch of salt
1 pinch of oregano
1 pinch of parsley
1 pinch of sweet paprika

Directions:
With a frying pan, sauté the meat and onion with olive oil   Pour the other ingredients and the meat in your Slow-Cooker, and cook on LOW for 7 hours
Nutrition Info: Calories: 631 Fat: 55 g Total carbs: 5 Net carbs: 5 Protein 30 g

975.	**Mayo Artichokes Hearts**

Servings: 4   Cooking Time: 4 Hours
Ingredients:

8-ounce cream cheese
16-ounce parmesan cheese, grated
10-ounce spinach
1/2 cup of chicken stock
1/2 cup of mayonnaise

8-ounce mozzarella, shredded
1/2 cup of sour cream
3 garlic cloves, minced
1 teaspoon of onion powder

Directions:

Start by throwing all the Ingredients: into your Crockpot.   Cover its lid and cook for 4 hours on Low setting.   Once done, remove its lid and give it a stir.   Garnish as desired.   Serve warm.
Nutrition Info: Calories 412 Total Fat 16.5 g Saturated Fat 2.4 g Cholesterol 76 mg Sodium 49 mg Total Carbs 5.3 g Fiber 0.5 g Sugar 0.2 g Protein 2.4 g

976.	**Smoky Barbecue Pulled Pork**

Servings: 4   Cooking Time: 12 Hours And 20 Minutes
Ingredients:

1 bottle sugar-free barbecue sauce
Salt and pepper to taste

1 can yacon syrup
2 tablespoons smoked paprika

Directions:
Place all ingredients in the crockpot and make sure to rub the meat with the sauce mixture.   Close the lid and cook on low for 12 hours or until the pork is very tender.   Take out the pork and place in a baking sheet.   Use two forks to shred the meat. Place the shredded meat back in the crockpot and stir to coat the sauce.   Cook on high for 20 minutes to infuse the meat with the sauce.
Nutrition Info: Calories per Servings: 283 Carbohydrates: 2.9g Protein: 47.6g Fat: 10.6g Sugar: 1.4g Sodium: 132mg Fiber: 0 g

977.	**Zesty Garlic Pulled Pork**

Servings: 6   Cooking Time: 8 Hours
Ingredients:

5 cloves of garlic, peeled and sliced
1 tablespoon of salt
1/2 teaspoon ground black pepper

1 teaspoon oregano
1/2 teaspoon cumin
1 lime, zested and juiced

Directions:
Make cut into the meat of pork and stuff with garlic slices.   Stir together garlic, salt, black pepper, oregano, cumin, lime zest, and juice until smooth paste comes together and then brush this paste all over the pork.   Place pork into a large resealable bag, seal it and let marinate in the refrigerator for overnight.   When ready to cook, transfer pork to a 6-quart slow cooker and shut with lid.   Plug in the slow cooker and cook for 8 hours at low heat setting or until pork is very tender.   When done, shred pork with two forks and serve as a lettuce wrap.
Nutrition Info: Net Carbs: 1.2g Calories: 616 Total Fat: 43g Saturated Fat: 11.5g Protein: 55.4g Carbs: 1.5g Fiber: 0.3g Sugar: 0g

978.	**Lamb And Coconut Stew**

Servings: 4   Cooking Time: 5.10 Hours
Ingredients:

2-pound lamb fillet, cubed
1 teaspoon cumin, ground
3 spring onions, chopped

1 cup of water
½ cup of coconut milk
1 teaspoon salt
1 teaspoon turmeric
¼ cup spinach,

| 1 tablespoon coconut cream | chopped |
| | 1/2 teaspoon black pepper |

Directions:
In the slow cooker, mix the lamb with cumin, spring onions and the other ingredients except the spinach, stir and close the lid.   Cook stew for 5 hours on High.   Then add spinach and stir the stew well. Cook it on High for 10 minutes more.
Nutrition Info:calories 257, fat 13.9, fiber 1.1, carbs 2.7, protein 24.7

979.   Creamy Broccoli

Servings: 4   Cooking Time: 1 Hour
Ingredients:

2 cups broccoli florets	½ cup coconut cream
1 teaspoon mint, dried	1 teaspoon salt
1 teaspoon garam masala	1 tablespoon almonds flakes
	½ teaspoon turmeric

Directions:
In the slow cooker, mix the broccoli with the mint and the other ingredients.   Close the lid and cook vegetables for 1 hour on High.   Divide between plates and serve.
Nutrition Info:calories 102, fat 9, fiber 1.9, carbs 4.3, protein 2.5

980.   Hot Eggplant Mix

Servings: 4   Cooking Time: 2 Hours
Ingredients:

1 teaspoon coconut oil, melted	1 teaspoon keto tomato sauce
3 eggplants, sliced	1 tablespoon butter
1 teaspoon minced garlic	1 teaspoon hot paprika
1 red chili pepper, minced	1 teaspoon chives, chopped

Directions:
In the slow cooker, mix the eggplants with the coconut oil and the other ingredients and close the lid.   Cook the eggplant mix for 2 hours on Low.
Nutrition Info:calories 202, fat 5.2, fiber 6.5, carbs 4.5, protein 5.1

981.   Swiss Cheese Onion Soup

Servings: 8   Cooking Time: 3 Hours 4 Minutes
Ingredients:

½ cup of dry white wine	2 tablespoons of butter, melted
4 cups of beef stock	2 teaspoons of swerves
1 cup of swiss cheese, shredded	1 teaspoon of salt
½ cup of water	½ teaspoon of black pepper
2 sprigs fresh thyme	
2 bay leaves	

Directions:
Start by throwing all the Ingredients: except cheese into your Crockpot.   Mix well and cover the Crockpot with its lid.   Select the Low settings for 3 hours.   Divide the cooked soups into servings bowl.   Top each bowl with ¼ of the cheese.

Place these bowls in the baking sheet.   Broil the soup for 4 minutes in the oven at 350 degrees F. Serve warm.
Nutrition Info: Calories 345 Total Fat 23.1 g Saturated Fat 9.1 g Cholesterol 96 mg Total Carbs 24 g Sugar 1.2 g Fiber 1.5 g Sodium 35 mg Potassium 37 mg Protein 13.5 g

982.   Okra Sauté

Servings: 5   Cooking Time: 4 Hours
Ingredients:

1 chili pepper, minced	1-pound okra, chopped
1 teaspoon coriander, ground	1 tablespoon curry paste
1 teaspoon turmeric powder	2 tablespoons sour cream
	½ cup heavy cream

Directions:
In the slow cooker, mix the okra with the chili pepper and the other ingredients.   Close the lid and cook for 4 hours on Low.
Nutrition Info:calories 133, fat 4.4, fiber 3.3, carbs 4.9, protein 2.5

983.   Slow CookerHungarian Goulash

Servings: 8   Cooking Time: 4 Hours
Ingredients:

2 tablespoons Hungarian paprika	2 cups daikon radishes, cubed
1 cup onion, chopped	1 yellow or green pepper, chopped
2 garlic cloves, minced	2 stalks celery, sliced
2 lbs. beef stew meat, cubed	1 (15-ounce) can diced tomatoes
1 teaspoon sea salt	1 ½ cups chicken or beef broth
½ teaspoon black pepper	1 bay leaf
½ teaspoon caraway seeds	

Directions:
Heat bacon grease over medium heat. Add in onions, garlic, paprika and stir for about 1 minute.   Add cubed beef and brown beef all over. Stir in salt and pepper, as well as caraway seeds.   Add mixture to Crock Pot.   Add radish, celery, pepper, tomatoes, broth and bay leaf. Mix well.   Cook on HIGH for 4 hours.
Nutrition Info: Calories: 345 Total Fat: 23.88 g Cholesterol: 3 mg Carbohydrate: 8.33 g Dietary Fiber: 2.81 g Protein: 23.84 g

984.   Tuna Steaks

Servings: 4   Cooking Time: 3 Hours
Ingredients:

Garlic – 3 cloves, crushed	White wine – ½ cup
Lemon – 1, sliced into 8 slices	Olive oil – 2 tbsp.
	Salt and pepper to taste

Directions:
Reduce the white wine in a pan by simmering until the strong alcohol smell is cooked off.   Rub the

tuna steaks with olive oil, and season with salt and pepper.   Place the tuna steaks into the Crock-Pot. Sprinkle the crushed garlic on top of the tuna steaks. Place 2 lemon slices on top of each tuna steak. Pour the reduced wine into the pot.   Cover with the lid and cook on high for 3 hours.   Transfer fish on serving plates. Drizzle with pot liquid and serve.
Nutrition Info: Calories: 269 Fat: 8.6g Carbs: 2.9g Protein: 40.4g

985.   Lamb And Eggplant Stew

Servings: 4   Cooking Time: 8 Hours 30 Minutes
Ingredients:

- Onion – 1, finely chopped
- Garlic – 3 cloves, crushed
- Large eggplant – ½, cut into small cubes
- Tomatoes – 1, chopped
- Lamb stock cube – 1
- Dried rosemary – 1 tsp.
- Grated mozzarella – ¾ cup
- Olive oil – 2 tbsp.
- Water – 2 cups
- Salt and pepper to taste

Directions:
Add olive oil into the Crock-Pot.   Add water, lamb, onion, garlic, eggplant, stock cube, tomatoes, rosemary, salt, and pepper to the pot. Stir to mix. Cover with the lid and cook on high for 8 hours. Remove the lid and stir the stew.   Sprinkle the mozzarella on top, cover with the lid, and cook 30 minutes more.   Serve.
Nutrition Info: Calories: 432 Fat: 21g Carbs: 8.8g Protein: 50.9g

986.   Red Cabbage And Walnuts

Servings: 4   Cooking Time: 6 Hours
Ingredients:

- 2 cups red cabbage, shredded
- 3 spring onions, chopped
- ½ cup chicken stock
- 1 tablespoon olive oil
- 1 teaspoon cumin, ground
- 1 teaspoon salt
- 1 teaspoon hot paprika
- 1 tablespoon keto tomato sauce
- 1 oz walnuts
- 1/3 cup fresh parsley, chopped

Directions:
In the slow cooker, mix the cabbage with the spring onions and the other ingredients.   Close the lid and cook cabbage for 6 hours on Low.   Divide into bowls and serve.
Nutrition Info:calories 112, fat 5.1, fiber 2, carbs 5.8, protein 3.5

987.   Shrimp And Tomatoes

Servings: 7   Cooking Time: 2 Hours
Ingredients:

- 1-pound shrimp, peeled and deveined
- 1 avocado, peeled, pitted
- 1 teaspoon chili flakes
- 1 teaspoon salt
- 1 teaspoon chili powder
- 1 cup cherry tomatoes, halved
- 1 cup fresh cilantro, chopped

Directions:

In the slow cooker, mix the shrimp with the avocado and the other ingredients, put the lid on and cook on High for 2 hours.   Divide into bowls and serve.
Nutrition Info:calories 280, fat 5.7, fiber 3.6, carbs 6.5, protein 7.7

988.   German-style Pork Stew

Servings: 5   Cooking Time: 8 Hours
Ingredients:

- 1 cauliflower head, cut into florets
- 2 jars of mushroom gravy
- 2 teaspoon caraway seeds
- Salt and pepper to taste

Directions:
Coat a skillet with cooking spray and heat over medium flame. Add the pork and cook until the surface turns slightly brown.   In the crockpot, mix all ingredients together and add the pork.   Close the lid and cook on low for 8 hours.
Nutrition Info: Calories: 607 Carbohydrates: 6.65g Protein: 55.51g Fat: 38g Sugar: 1.6 g Sodium: 580mg Fiber: 1.8g

989.   Chili-lime Chicken Wings

Servings: 10   Cooking Time: 6 Hours And 15 Minutes
Ingredients:

- ¼ cup fresh lime juice
- 4 garlic cloves, minced
- 1 tablespoon ginger, chopped
- 1 tablespoon chili sauce
- 1 tablespoon fish sauce
- ¼ cup coconut aminos
- ¼ cup coconut oil
- 1 teaspoon dried oregano
- 1 teaspoon black pepper
- 1 teaspoon salt
- Lemon, sliced, for serving

Directions:
Preheat the Slow Cookeron high.   In a large bowl, mix all the ingredients until well combined. Transfer into the crock pot.   Cover and cook on high for 4–6 hours.   Preheat the oven to 350°F. Transfer the wings onto a parchment-lined baking tray.   Bake for 15 minutes until nice golden brown. Serve hot with some lemon slices.
Nutrition Info: Calories 176 Total Fat 9 g Saturated Fat 5 g Total Carbs 4 g Dietary Fiber 1 g Protein 30 g

990.   Lime Green Beans

Servings: 5   Cooking Time: 2.5 Hours
Ingredients:

- 1-pound green beans, trimmed and halved
- 2 spring onions, chopped
- 2 tablespoons lime juice
- ¾ teaspoon salt
- ½ teaspoon lime zest, grated
- 2 tablespoons olive oil
- ¼ teaspoon ground black pepper
- ¾ cup of water

Directions:

In the slow cooker, mix the green beans with the spring onions and the other ingredients and close the lid. Cook for 5 hours on High.
Nutrition Info:calories 67, fat 5.6, fiber 2, carbs 4, protein 2.1

991.	Tomato Cheese Soup

Servings: 2   Cooking Time: 6 Hours
Ingredients:

1 carrot, peeled and diced	1 onion, diced
1 garlic clove, minced	1 cup of heavy cream
1 cup of vegetable stock	2 tablespoon of olive oil
4 tablespoons of butter, at room temperature	2 tablespoons of parsley, a diced
	salt and black pepper to taste

Directions:
Start by throwing all the Ingredients: into your Crockpot. Mix well and cover the Crockpot with its lid. Select the Low settings for 6 hours. Serve warm.
Nutrition Info: Calories 244 Total Fat 24.8 g Saturated Fat 15.6 g Cholesterol 32 mg Total Carbs 11.1 g Sugar 0.4 g Fiber 0.1 g Sodium 204 mg Potassium 81 mg Protein 14 g

992.	Sausage Soup

Servings: 5   Cooking Time: 4.15 Hour
Ingredients:

9 oz Italian sausages, chopped	1 cup broccoli, chopped
1 teaspoon sweet paprika	3 cups of water
1 teaspoon salt	1 cup spinach
½ teaspoon ground black pepper	1/3 cup heavy cream
	1 tablespoon cream cheese

Directions:
In the slow cooker, mix the sausage with the paprika and the other ingredients except the cream and cream cheese. Close the slow cooker lid and cook soup for 4 hours on High. Then open the lid and add the remaining ingredients. Cook the meal for 15 minutes more on High.
Nutrition Info:calories 362, fat 22.2, fiber 0.9, carbs 6.5, protein 12.1

993.	Chicken Cordon Bleu Soup

Servings: 8   Cooking Time: 6 Hours
Ingredients:

12 oz. diced ham	4 oz. onion, diced
5 oz. mushrooms, diced	4 cloves garlic, minced
2 teaspoons of dried tarragon	3 tablespoons of salted butter
1 teaspoon of salt, more to taste	1 1/2 cups of heavy cream
1 teaspoon of black pepper	1/2 cup of sour cream
1 lb. chicken breast, cubed	1/2 cup of grated Parmesan cheese
	4 oz. Swiss cheese

Directions:
Start by throwing all the Ingredients: into your Crockpot. Mix well and cover the Crockpot with its lid. Select the Low settings for 6 hours. Serve warm.
Nutrition Info: Calories 266 Total Fat 26.4 g Saturated Fat 4 g Cholesterol 13 mg Total Carbs 11.4 g Sugar 2 g Fiber 1.6 g Sodium 455 mg Potassium 94 mg Protein 20.6 g

994.	Cheddar Artichoke

Servings: 6   Cooking Time: 3 Hours
Ingredients:

1 teaspoon garlic, diced	3 oz Cheddar cheese, shredded
1 tablespoon olive oil	1 teaspoon curry powder
1-pound artichoke hearts, chopped	1 teaspoon butter
1 cup chicken stock	1 teaspoon garam masala

Directions:
In the slow cooker, mix the artichokes with garlic, oil and the other ingredients. Cook the artichoke hearts for 3 hours on High. Divide between plates and serve.
Nutrition Info:calories 135, fat 3.9, fiber 4.3, carbs 4.9, protein 4.3

995.	Keto Slow Cooker Chili

Servings: 3   Cooking Time: 8 Hours
Ingredients:

2 tablespoons1 / 28 gr of tomato sauce	1 pinch of hot pepper
2 tablespoons / 28 gr of red beans	1 pinch of cumin
2 tablespoons / 28 gr of olive oil	1 pinch of ground coriander
1 tablespoon / 14 gr of coconut oil	1 tablespoon of Stevia powder
1 pinch of onion powder	1 pinch of sweet paprika
1 clove / 3 gr of garlic	1 pinch of ground pepper
	1 pinch of salt
	1 dash of tabasco

Directions:
First place 2/3rds of the seasonings and Stevia and oil on the bottom of the Slow Cooker   Add the beef, trying to distribute it homogeneously   Cover with the beans   Add salt and the rest of the spices   We cover it all with the sauce   Close the lid and turn on the Slow Cooker on "LOW" temperature for 8 hours   After 8 hours, open the lid, stir well and ensure that the meat is distributed evenly   At this point add a dash of tabasco
Nutrition Info: Calories: 503.5 Fat: 50 g Total carbs: 8 Net carbs: 8 Protein 39.5 g

996.	Squash And Zucchinis

Servings: 6   Cooking Time: 4 Hours
Ingredients:

4 cups spaghetti squash, cubed	½ cup coconut milk
2 zucchinis, cubed	¾ teaspoon ground ginger
½ teaspoon ground cinnamon	3 tablespoons oregano
	1 teaspoon butter

Directions:

In the slow cooker, mix the squash with the zucchinis, milk and the other ingredients.   Close the lid and cook the vegetables on Low for 4 hours.
Nutrition Info:calories 40, fat 2.2, fiber 1.8, carbs 4.3, protein 1.1

997.   Fish With Tomatoes

Servings: 2   Cooking Time: 1 ½ Hours
Ingredients:
- 1 white onion, peeled and sliced
- 1 can diced tomatoes
- 1 1/2 teaspoon minced garlic
- 1/4 cup chicken broth

Directions:
Season the cod with a pinch of salt and pepper and red chili flakes.   Mix the remaining ingredients together, and place into a 4-quart slow-cooker. Gently place the seasoned cod on top, then cover and seal the slow-cooker with its lid, setting the cooking timer for 1 to 1 1/2 hours.   Allow to cook at a high heat setting or until fish is cooked through.   Serve warm.
Nutrition Info: Energy: 220 Kcal Carbohydrates: 3.64 g Net Carbs: 2.5 g Fats: 6.7 g Protein: 34.8 g

998.   Saucy Ranch Pork

Servings: 6   Cooking Time: 8 Hours
Ingredients:
- 2 cans cream of chicken soup
- 1 envelope ranch salad dressing
- 1 cup milk
- A sprig of parsley, chopped

Directions:
Place the pork loin chops in the crockpot and add the chicken soup, milk and ranch salad dressing. Close the lid and cook on low for 8 hours.   Garnish with a sprig of parsley.
Nutrition Info: Calories: 448 Carbohydrates: 9.4g Protein: 44.3g Fat: 24g Sugar: 2g Sodium: 790mg Fiber: 0.2g

999.   Cauliflower With Eggplants

Servings: 4   Cooking Time: 5 Hours
Ingredients:
- 1/2 cup of cauliflower, diced
- 1 teaspoon of oregano, diced
- 1/2 cup of parsley, chopped
- Salt and black
- 10 tablespoons of olive oil
- 1 green bell pepper, diced
- 1 yellow onion, diced
- 1 tablespoon of garlic, minced

pepper- to taste
2 ½ lb. tomatoes, cut into halves and grated

3-ounce feta cheese, crumbled
½ cup of vegetable stock

Directions:
Start by throwing all the Ingredients: into your Crockpot except cheese.   Cover its lid and cook for 5 hours on Low setting.   Once done, remove its lid and give it a stir.   Garnish with feta cheese. Serve warm.
Nutrition Info: Calories 288 Total Fat 25.5 g Saturated Fat 7.4 g Cholesterol 66 mg Sodium 73 mg Total Carbs 4.4 g Fiber 0.6 g Sugar 0.1 g Protein 3.4 g

1000.   Cheese Asparagus

Servings: 4   Cooking Time: 3 Hours
Ingredients:
- 10 oz asparagus, trimmed
- 4 oz Cheddar cheese, sliced
- 1/3 cup butter, soft
- 1 teaspoon turmeric powder
- ½ teaspoon salt
- ¼ teaspoon white pepper

Directions:
In the slow cooker, mix the asparagus with butter and the other ingredients, put the lid on and cook for 3 hours on High.
Nutrition Info:calories 214, fat 6.2, fiber 1.7, carbs 3.6, protein 4.2

1001.   Cod And Vegetables

Servings: 4   Cooking Time: 1-3 Hours
Ingredients:
- 1 bell pepper, sliced or chopped
- 1 onion, sliced
- ½ fresh lemon, sliced
- 1 zucchini, sliced
- 3 garlic cloves, minced
- ¼ cup low-sodium broth
- 1 teaspoon rosemary
- ¼ teaspoon red pepper flakes
- Salt, pepper, to taste

Directions:
Season cod fillets with salt and pepper.   Pour broth into slow cooker, add garlic, rosemary, bell pepper, onion and zucchini into slow cooker.   Put fish into your crockpot, add lemon slices on top. Close the lid and cook on Low for 2-3 hours or on High for 1 hour.
Nutrition Info: Calories 150 Fats 11.6g Net carbs 6.2g Protein 26.9g

www.ingramcontent.com/pod-product-compliance
Lightning Source LLC
Chambersburg PA
CBHW081951260726
48657CB00009BA/2546